I0644704

50 Landmark Papers *every* Neurosurgeon Should Know

This indispensable resource provides a comprehensive guide to the most impactful studies that have shaped the field of neurosurgery. It distils the key findings and clinical relevance of 50 landmark papers across the full spectrum of neurosurgical subspecialties.

Designed with the needs of neurosurgery residents, fellows, and junior faculty in mind, this book provides a concise, high-yield format that is ideal for preparing for the ABNS oral board exam, and the FRCS and FRCSC certifications. Each chapter is authored by leading experts in the field, offering unique insights into the rationale, methodologies, and clinical impact of these pivotal studies. Key points are highlighted in a clear and concise manner, supported by tables, line diagrams, and practical commentaries to ensure rapid comprehension and retention.

The challenge of navigating the ever-increasing neurosurgical literature can be daunting and this one-stop resource for evidence-based practice helps readers access the core literature. Whether you are preparing for certification exams or seeking to deepen your understanding of the field, *50 Landmark Papers every Neurosurgeon Should Know* is your definitive guide to the foundational studies that continue to shape neurosurgical practice worldwide, making it an essential tool for neurosurgery trainees, practicing neurosurgeons, and educators seeking to enhance their knowledge and improve outcomes in patient care.

Jignesh K Tailor is currently Assistant Professor of Neurological Surgery at Indiana University School of Medicine and a Pediatric Neurosurgeon at Riley Hospital for Children. He received his medical degree from the University of Oxford Medical School and holds a PhD in Stem Cell Biology from the University of Cambridge. During neurosurgery training in London, Tailor received a highly competitive Wellcome Trust Post-Doctoral Research Award, which allowed him to complete neurosurgery training at the Hospital for Sick Children in Toronto, Ontario while doing an enfolded Postdoctoral Research Fellowship at the University of Toronto. He completed fellowship training in Pediatric Neurosurgery at Johns Hopkins University Hospital in Baltimore in July 2021.

50 Landmark Papers Series

50 Landmark Papers every Spine Surgeon Should Know
Alexander R Vaccaro, Charles G Fisher, Jefferson R Wilson

50 Landmark Papers every Trauma Surgeon Should Know
Stephen M Cohn and Ara J Feinstein

50 Landmark Papers every Acute Care Surgeon Should Know
Stephen M Cohn and Peter Rhee

50 Landmark Papers every Vascular and Endovascular Surgeon Should Know
Juan Carlos Jimenez and Samuel Eric Wilson

50 Landmark Papers every Oral and Maxillofacial Surgeon Should Know
Niall MH McLeod and Peter A Brennan

50 Landmark Papers every Intensivist Should Know
Stephen M Cohn, Alan Lisbon, Stephen Heard

50 Landmark Papers every Thyroid and Parathyroid Surgeon Should Know
Sam Wiseman and Sebastian Aspinall

50 Landmark Papers every Pediatric Surgeon Should Know
Mark Davenport, Bashar Aldeiri and Joseph Davidson

50 Landmark Papers every Breast Surgeon Should Know
Lynda Wyld, Ramsey Cutress and Jenna Morgan

50 Landmark Papers every Colorectal Surgeon Should Know
John RT Monson, Lawrence Lee, Fergal J Fleming

50 Landmark Papers every Plastic Surgeon Should Know
Tor Wo Chiu

50 Landmark Papers every Neurosurgeon Should Know
Jignesh K Tailor

For more information about this series, please visit
www.routledge.com/50-Landmark-Papers/book-series/50LP

50 Landmark Papers *every* Neurosurgeon Should Know

EDITED BY

Jignesh K Tailor

Pediatric Neurosurgeon
Assistant Professor of Neurological Surgery
Division of Pediatric Neurosurgery
Indiana University School of Medicine
Riley Hospital for Children at IU Health
Indianapolis, IN, USA

CRC Press
Taylor & Francis Group
Boca Raton London New York

CRC Press is an imprint of the
Taylor & Francis Group, an **informa** business

First edition published 2027
by CRC Press
2385 NW Executive Center Drive, Suite 320, Boca Raton FL 33431

and by CRC Press
4 Park Square, Milton Park, Abingdon, Oxon, OX14 4RN

CRC Press is an imprint of Taylor & Francis Group, LLC

© 2027 selection and editorial matter, Jignesh K. Tailor; individual chapters, the contributors

This book contains information obtained from authentic and highly regarded sources. While all reasonable efforts have been made to publish reliable data and information, neither the author[s] nor the publisher can accept any legal responsibility or liability for any errors or omissions that may be made. The publishers wish to make clear that any views or opinions expressed in this book by individual editors, authors or contributors are personal to them and do not necessarily reflect the views/opinions of the publishers. The information or guidance contained in this book is intended for use by medical, scientific or health-care professionals and is provided strictly as a supplement to the medical or other professional's own judgement, their knowledge of the patient's medical history, relevant manufacturer's instructions and the appropriate best practice guidelines. Because of the rapid advances in medical science, any information or advice on dosages, procedures or diagnoses should be independently verified. The reader is strongly urged to consult the relevant national drug formulary and the drug companies' and device or material manufacturers' printed instructions, and their websites, before administering or utilizing any of the drugs, devices or materials mentioned in this book. This book does not indicate whether a particular treatment is appropriate or suitable for a particular individual. Ultimately it is the sole responsibility of the medical professional to make his or her own professional judgements, so as to advise and treat patients appropriately. The authors and publishers have also attempted to trace the copyright holders of all material reproduced in this publication and apologize to copyright holders if permission to publish in this form has not been obtained. If any copyright material has not been acknowledged please write and let us know so we may rectify in any future reprint.

Except as permitted under U.S. Copyright Law, no part of this book may be reprinted, reproduced, transmitted, or utilized in any form by any electronic, mechanical, or other means, now known or hereafter invented, including photocopying, microfilming, and recording, or in any information storage or retrieval system, without written permission from the publishers.

For permission to photocopy or use material electronically from this work, access www.copyright.com or contact the Copyright Clearance Center, Inc. (CCC), 222 Rosewood Drive, Danvers, MA 01923, 978-750-8400. For works that are not available on CCC please contact mpkbookspermissions@tandf.co.uk

For Product Safety Concerns and Information please contact our EU representative GPSR@taylorandfrancis.com. Taylor & Francis Verlag GmbH, Kaufingerstraße 24, 80331 München, Germany.

Trademark notice: Product or corporate names may be trademarks or registered trademarks and are used only for identification and explanation without intent to infringe.

ISBN: 9781032542935 (hbk)
ISBN: 9781032535777 (pbk)
ISBN: 9781003416197 (ebk)

DOI: 10.1201/9781003416197

Typeset in Times
by KnowledgeWorks Global Ltd.

To my family –
to my wife, Priti,
and to our children, Ronav and Sanya –
for your love, patience, and unwavering support.
Everything I accomplish is grounded in you.

Contents

Section Two Vascular

Section Four Functional Epilepsy

Section Seven Spine

Contributors

Laurie L Ackerman
Indiana University School of Medicine
Indianapolis, IN, USA

Joao Paulo Almeida
Indiana University School of Medicine
Indianapolis, IN, USA

Miracle Anokwute
Indiana University School of Medicine
Indianapolis, IN, USA

Kholoud Arab
Indiana University School of Medicine
Indianapolis, IN, USA

Keyoumars Ashkan
King's College Hospital NHS Foundation Trust
London, UK

Mark Bain
Cleveland Clinic
Cleveland, OH, USA

Chetan Bettegowda
Johns Hopkins University School of Medicine
Baltimore, MD, USA

Rob Blake
Indiana University School of Medicine
Indianapolis, IN, USA

Brad Bohnstedt
Indiana University School of Medicine
Indianapolis, IN, USA

Jamie Bradbury
Indiana University School of Medicine
Indianapolis, IN, USA

Paul Brennan
The University of Edinburgh
Edinburgh, UK

Shu Kiat Chan
National Neuroscience Institute
Singapore

Anoop Chinthala
Indiana University School of Medicine
Indianapolis, IN, USA

Eisha Christian
The Hospital for Children
Toronto, Canada

Jason Chu
Indiana University School of Medicine
Indianapolis, IN, USA

Felicia Hui Zhuang Chua
National Neuroscience Institute
Singapore

Alan R Cohen
The Johns Hopkins University School of Medicine
Baltimore, MD, USA

Benjamin M Davies
University of Cambridge
Cambridge, UK

Günther Deuschl
Christian-Albrechts-University Kiel
Kiel, Germany

Michael G Fehlings
University of Toronto
Toronto, Canada

Chiara A Flores
Indiana University School of Medicine
Indianapolis, IN, USA

Ryan Gensler
Johns Hopkins University School of Medicine
Baltimore, MD, USA

Allie Heineman
University of Cincinnati College of Medicine
Cincinnati, OH, USA

Melanie Alfonzo Horowitz
Johns Hopkins University School of Medicine
Baltimore, MD, USA

Judy Huang
Johns Hopkins University School of Medicine
Baltimore, MD, USA

Meng Huang
Houston Methodist Hospital
Houston, TX, USA

Alice L Hung
Johns Hopkins University School of Medicine
Baltimore, MD, USA

Peter J Hutchinson
University of Cambridge
Cambridge, UK

George Ibrahim
The Hospital for Sick Children
Toronto, Canada

Abdurrahman I Islim
The University of Manchester
Manchester, UK

Michael D Jenkinson
University of Liverpool
Liverpool, UK

Fezaan A Kazi
Indiana University School of Medicine
Indianapolis, IN, USA

Richard Kerr
Oxford University Hospitals NHS Foundation Trust
Oxford, UK

Ramez Wadie Kirollos
National Neuroscience Institute
Singapore

Angelos G Kolias
University of Cambridge
Cambridge, UK

Aditya Kondajji
Cleveland Clinic
Cleveland, OH, USA

Abdulbaki Kozan
Indiana University School of Medicine
Indianapolis, IN, USA

Abhaya V Kulkarni
The Hospital for Sick Children
Toronto, Canada

Jae Hyun Kwon
Indiana University School of Medicine
Indianapolis, IN, USA

Brandon Lane
Indiana University School of Medicine
Indianapolis, IN, USA

Tom Larrew
Indiana University School of Medicine
Indianapolis, IN, USA

Jose Lavrador
King's College Hospital NHS Foundation Trust
London, UK

Adriel Z Leong
National Neuroscience Institute
Singapore

Jia Xu Lim
National Neuroscience Institute
Singapore

Trenton A Line
Indiana University School of Medicine
Indianapolis, IN, USA

Armaan K Malhotra
University of Toronto
Toronto, Canada

Conor L Mallucci
Alder Hey Children's NHS Foundation Trust
Liverpool, UK

Gordan Mao
Indiana University School of Medicine
Indianapolis, IN, USA

Kyle Mcgrath
University of Cincinnati College of Medicine
Cincinnati, OH, USA

Sydney McQueen
University of Toronto
Toronto, Canada

Derryl Miller
Indiana University Indianapolis School of Medicine
Indianapolis, IN, USA

Hiba J Mustafa
Indiana University School of Medicine
Indianapolis, IN, USA

Laura B Ngwenya
University of Cincinnati College of Medicine
Cincinnati, OH, USA

Thomas Noh
Houston Methodist Hospital
Houston, TX, USA

Barnabas Obeng-Gyasi
Indiana University School of Medicine
Indianapolis, IN, USA

Josue Ordaz
Indiana University School of Medicine
Indianapolis, IN, USA

Lu-Ann Papile
University of New Mexico
Albuquerque, NM, USA

Omar N Pathmanaban
The University of Manchester
Manchester, UK

Karlo M Pedro
University of Toronto
Toronto, Canada

Bruce E Pollock
Mayo Clinic
Rochester, MN, USA

Dilon Putzler
Houston Methodist Hospital
Houston, TX, USA

Rabia Qaiser
Indiana University School of Medicine
Indianapolis, IN, USA

Angela M Richardson
Indiana University School of Medicine
Indianapolis, IN, USA

Thomas Santarius
University of Cambridge
Cambridge, UK

Mitesh Shah
Indiana University School of Medicine
Indianapolis, IN, USA

Edward R Smith
Harvard Medical School
Cambridge, MA, USA

Robert F Spetzler
Barrow Neurological Institute
Phoenix, AZ, USA

David Stockwell
Indiana University School of Medicine
Indianapolis, IN, USA

Walter Stummer
Neurochirurgische Klinik
Universitätsklinikum Münster
Münster, Germany

Jignesh Tailor
Indiana University School of Medicine
Indianapolis, IN, USA

Shelly D Timmons
Medical College of Wisconsin
Milwaukee, WI, USA

Matthew Tobin
Indiana University School of Medicine
Indianapolis, IN, USA

Alexander Vaccaro
Thomas Jefferson University Hospital
Philadelphia, PA, USA

Francesco Vergani
King's College Hospital NHS Foundation Trust
London, UK

Ken Virgin
Indiana University School of Medicine
Indianapolis, IN, USA

Piiamaria S Virtanen
Indiana University School of Medicine
Indianapolis, IN, USA

Daniel C Walsh
King's College Hospital NHS Foundation Trust
London, UK

Mark Wilson
Imperial College London
London, UK

CHAPTER 1

Radiotherapy Plus Concomitant and Adjuvant Temozolomide for Glioblastoma

Stupp R, Mason WP, van den Bent MJ, Weller M, Fisher B, Taphoorn MJB, Belanger K, Brandes AA, Marosi C, Bogdahn U, Curschmann J, Janzer RC, Ludwin SK, Gorlia T, Allgeier A, Lacombe D, Cairncross JG, Eisenhauer E, Mirimanoff RO, N Engl J Med. 2005 Mar 10;352(10):987–996

Reviewed by Ryan Gensler, Melanie Alfonzo Horowitz, and Chetan Bettegowda

Research Question/Objective Does the addition of temozolomide in combination with radiotherapy and as an adjuvant therapy improve overall survival in patients with newly diagnosed glioblastoma (GBM), compared to radiotherapy alone?

Study Design Randomized, multicenter, phase III clinical trial.

Sample Size A total of 573 patients were enrolled from 85 centers.

Follow-Up Median follow-up of 28 months.

Inclusion/Exclusion Criteria

- Inclusion Criteria
  - Patients with newly diagnosed and histologically confirmed GBM/WHO grade IV astrocytoma and a WHO performance status of 2 or less were included.
  - Patients were required to have adequate hematologic, renal, and hepatic function (absolute neutrophil count $\geq 1500/mm^3$, platelet count $\geq 100{,}000/mm^3$, serum creatinine ≤ 1.5 times the upper limit of normal, total serum bilirubin ≤ 1.5 times the upper limit of normal, and liver function values <3 times the upper limit of normal).
  - Patients were required to have a stable or decreasing corticosteroid dose for at least 14 days before randomization.

- Exclusion Criteria
  - N/A

DOI: 10.1201/9781003416197-1

Intervention or Treatment Received

- **Radiotherapy group**: Standard focal radiotherapy (2 Gy per fraction, 5 days/week for 6 weeks, total 60 Gy).
- **Radiotherapy plus temozolomide group**: Standard focal radiotherapy with daily temozolomide (75 mg/m^2/day) during radiotherapy (concomitant phase), followed by six 28-day cycles of adjuvant temozolomide (150–200 mg/m^2/day for 5 days per cycle).

Results This phase III clinical trial conducted by Stupp et al. demonstrated that patients with a newly diagnosed GBM who underwent combined radiotherapy-temozolomide vs radiotherapy only had a significantly improved median overall survival (OS) (14.6 vs 12.1 months), median progression-free survival (PFS) (6.9 months vs 5.0 months), and 2-year survival rate (26.5% vs 10.4%). The unadjusted hazard ratio for death in the radiotherapy-temozolomide group was 0.63 (95% confidence interval (CI), 0.52–0.75; $p < 0.001$), and for progression or death, the hazard ratio was 0.54 (95% CI, 0.45–0.64; $p < 0.001$).

During the concomitant radiation-temozolomide phase, 7% of patients experienced grade III–IV hematologic toxicity (4% neutropenia, 3% thrombocytopenia), increasing to 14% during the adjuvant temozolomide phase, with 11% developing thrombocytopenia. The most common adverse nonhematologic complication in the concomitant phase was moderate-to-severe fatigue (33%). Other complications during the concomitant phase included 3% of patients having severe infections, increasing to 5% during the adjuvant temozolomide phase.

In the combined therapy cohort, 85% of patients were compliant in completing both radiotherapy and concomitant temozolomide as planned, but this dropped to 47% of patients completing all six cycles of temozolomide during the adjuvant period. The reasons for discontinuation in either phase included progression of their GBM (39%), temozolomide toxicity (8%), patient decision (4%), and other reasons (3%).

Conclusion The combination of temozolomide with radiotherapy for a newly diagnosed GBM resulted in a statistically and clinically significant improvement in OS and PFS compared to radiotherapy alone. The survival rate at 2 years more than doubled in the combined therapy cohort, with toxicity being minimal and manageable. The findings from this landmark study established radiotherapy plus temozolomide as the new standard of care for GBM, as this combination offered improved outcomes with acceptable safety.

Reviewer Commentary The landmark Stupp et al. study built upon the initial temozolomide work done in 1993 by O'Reilly et al. and marked a major advancement in the management of GBM.[1] By adding temozolomide to standard radiotherapy, patients had a significant improvement in OS, PFS, and a 2-year survival rate compared to radiotherapy alone. The results of this trial have established radiotherapy plus temozolomide as one of the major treatment options for the initial treatment of GBM. Compared to previous studies that utilized chemotherapeutics, such as Walker et al., with 1,3-bis(2-chloroethyl)-1-nitrosourea (BCNU), temozolomide offers several advantages, including its ease of oral administration and lower toxicity, a major obstacle of previous chemotherapy protocols like radiation with BCNU. Owing to its relatively low toxicity and oral administration, temozolomide can be taken by patients at home and used as both concomitant and adjuvant therapy for GBM, thereby enabling an extended treatment period.

The study demonstrated a significant survival difference in temozolomide-treated GBM patients based on O^6-methylguanine-DNA methyltransferase (MGMT) promoter methylation status, establishing MGMT as a predictive marker of response to combined therapy. In doing so, Stupp et al. helped lay the groundwork for personalized medicine by incorporating molecular profiling into treatment selection.

The findings of this study remain a cornerstone of neuro-oncology and continue to guide treatment today.

Study Limitations The study was not designed to differentiate the effects of concomitant versus adjuvant temozolomide therapy, which limited its ability to assess the contribution of the concomitant phase versus the adjuvant phase of treatment. This study did not compare the efficacy of temozolomide to already established chemotherapeutic protocols, including BCNU. Additionally, long-term toxicity outcomes, such as potential cognitive effects or secondary malignancies, were not evaluated in this trial, but were followed up in a future study by Stupp and colleagues at 5 years. As with any study, the inclusion and exclusion criteria, such as patients requiring adequate liver and kidney function, limit the findings of this study. For patients who do not fit the inclusion criteria, the findings may not be similar, and the effects of temozolomide may be more toxic and less beneficial.

Relevant Studies The 1970s–1980s Brain Tumor Cooperative Group phase III trials (7201 and 7501) were among the first to show that chemotherapeutics, specifically BCNU, could provide a modest clinical yet statistically significant survival benefit when added to radiotherapy compared to radiotherapy alone.[2] Additionally, the joint Radiation Therapy Oncology Group and the Eastern Cooperative Oncology Group study during the 1980s further showed the survival benefits from BCNU, but that the effects were mainly isolated to patients between the ages of 40 and 60.[3] Building on earlier studies of BCNU delivery, Brem et al. demonstrated the feasibility and safety of using biodegradable polymer implants for localized interstitial chemotherapy in recurrent gliomas, which showed promise in prolonging survival with minimal systemic toxicity. However, BCNU still had limitations due to its toxicity.[4]

O'Reilly et al.'s study in 1993 marked a turning point, being the first to show the efficacy of temozolomide for the treatment of gliomas.[1] This early phase I trial demonstrated significant clinical and radiographic responses in patients with recurrent gliomas following radiotherapy, which laid the foundation for future studies, including Stupp's landmark trial.

Following Stupp's trial in 2005, Jalali et al. made the study more generalizable as they found the same efficacy in a predominantly Indian cohort, reporting a median survival of 16.4 months.[5] Muni et al. demonstrated the protocol's utility in achieving survival benefits in the poor-prognosis/high-risk population by combining temozolomide with short-course radiotherapy.[6]

Later, Erpolat et al. worked to standardize Stupp's protocol by demonstrating that patients should complete at least four cycles of adjuvant temozolomide to maximize survival, with a median survival of 20 months.[7] Chinot et al. then attempted to modify the Stupp protocol with the addition of bevacizumab and found a significant improvement in the PFS but no effect on OS, highlighting the difficulty of enhancing an already robust treatment.[8]

To address a major limitation of the original Stupp trial, the same team conducted a 5-year follow-up, which showed the combined treatment group's 5-year survival rate being significantly higher at 9.8% compared to 1.9% with radiotherapy alone, solidifying the efficacy of temozolomide in GBM management.[9]

These studies collectively demonstrate the foundational research that preceded Stupp et al.'s trial and the subsequent investigations that expanded upon it. In doing so, they underscore how the work of Stupp et al. has fundamentally shaped glioblastoma treatment, guiding future research and informing refinements in therapeutic strategies to improve patient outcomes.

REFERENCES

1. O'Reilly SM, Newlands ES, Glaser MG, et al. Temozolomide: a new oral cytotoxic chemotherapeutic agent with promising activity against primary brain tumours. Eur J Cancer. 1993;29A(7):940–942. doi:10.1016/s0959-8049(05)80198-4
2. Shapiro WR. Combined Modality Treatment of Malignant Glioma. In: Clifford Rose F, Fields WS, eds. Progress in Tumor Research. Vol 29. S. Karger AG; 1985:219–224. doi:10.1159/000411643
3. Chang CH, Horton J, Schoenfeld D, et al. Comparison of postoperative radiotherapy and combined postoperative radiotherapy and chemotherapy in the multidisciplinary management of malignant gliomas. A joint Radiation Therapy Oncology Group and Eastern Cooperative Oncology Group Study. Cancer. 1983;52(6):997–1007. doi:10.1002/1097-0142(19830915)52:6<997::aid-cncr2820520612>3.0.co;2-2
4. Brem H, Mahaley MS, Vick NA, et al. Interstitial chemotherapy with drug polymer implants for the treatment of recurrent gliomas. J Neurosurg. 1991;74(3):441–446. doi:10.3171/jns.1991.74.3.0441
5. Jalali R, Basu A, Gupta T, et al. Encouraging experience of concomitant temozolomide with radiotherapy followed by adjuvant temozolomide in newly diagnosed glioblastoma multiforme: single institution experience. Br J Neurosurg. 2007;21(6):583–587. doi:10.1080/02688690701604574

6. Muni R, Minniti G, Lanzetta G, et al. Short-term radiotherapy followed by adjuvant chemotherapy in poor-prognosis patients with glioblastoma. Tumori. 2010;96(1):60–64. doi:10.1177/030089161009600110
7. Erpolat OP, Akmansu M, Goksel F, Bora H, Yaman E, Büyükberber S. Outcome of newly diagnosed glioblastoma patients treated by radiotherapy plus concomitant and adjuvant temozolomide: a long-term analysis. Tumori. 2009;95(2):191–197. doi:10.1177/030089160909500210
8. Chinot OL, Wick W, Mason W, et al. Bevacizumab plus radiotherapy-temozolomide for newly diagnosed glioblastoma. N Engl J Med. 2014;370(8):709–722. doi:10.1056/NEJMoa1308345
9. Stupp R, Hegi ME, Mason WP, et al. Effects of radiotherapy with concomitant and adjuvant temozolomide versus radiotherapy alone on survival in glioblastoma in a randomised phase III study: 5-year analysis of the EORTC-NCIC trial. Lancet Oncol. 2009;10(5):459–466. doi:10.1016/S1470-2045(09)70025-7

Chapter 2

MGMT Gene Silencing and Benefit from Temozolomide in Glioblastoma

Hegi ME, Diserens AC, Gorlia T, Hamou MF, de Tribolet N, Weller M, Kros JM, Hainfellner JA, Mason W, Mariani L, Bromberg JEC, Hau P, Mirimanoff RO, Cairncross JG, Janzer RC, Stupp R, N Engl J Med. 2005 Mar 10;352(10):997–1003

Reviewed by Melanie Alfonzo Horowitz, Ryan Gensler, and Chetan Bettegowda

Research Question/Objective This study was conducted to investigate if O^6-methylguanine-DNA methyltransferase (MGMT) promoter methylation in glioblastoma patients is associated with an improved response to temozolomide treatment.

Study Design Randomized clinical trial.

Sample Size 573 patients were enrolled. MGMT methylation status could only be determined in 206 of the patient glioblastoma samples.

Inclusion/Exclusion Criteria

- Inclusion Criteria
  - Patients between 18 and 70 years of age with a newly diagnosed and histologically confirmed glioblastoma (a World Health Organization (WHO) grade IV astrocytoma) were included in this study.
  - To be eligible, patients also needed a WHO performance status of 2 or less and to meet the following laboratory test parameters: hematologic absolute neutrophil count, ≥1500 per cubic millimeter; platelet count ≥100,000 per cubic millimeter; renal ≤1.5 times the upper limit of normal in the laboratory where it was measured; total serum bilirubin level ≤1.5 times the upper limit of normal; and hepatic (liver function tests <3 times the upper limit of normal). All patients provided written informed consent.
- Exclusion Criteria
  - N/A

DOI: 10.1201/9781003416197-2

Intervention or Treatment Received

- Patients were randomly assigned to receive either standard focal radiotherapy alone or radiotherapy plus concomitant daily temozolomide, followed by adjuvant temozolomide, within 6 weeks of a histological confirmation of glioblastoma diagnosis.
- Treatment began within a week of randomization.

Results Among the 206 patients in whom MGMT promoter methylation status of the tumors could be assessed, overall survival differed significantly between those with and without MGMT promoter methylation ($p < 0.001$), independent of temozolomide treatment. In this cohort, patients without MGMT promoter methylation had a median overall survival of 12.2 months (95% confidence interval (CI), 11.4–13.5), whereas patients with MGMT promoter methylation had a median overall survival of 18.2 months (95% CI, 15.5–22.0). Consistent with these findings, MGMT promoter methylation was associated with a hazard ratio for death of 0.45 (95% CI, 0.32–0.61), corresponding to a 55% reduction in mortality risk.

Among patients with MGMT promoter-methylated tumors, those treated with radiotherapy plus temozolomide experienced significantly improved survival compared with patients who received radiotherapy alone (46.0% vs 22.7%, $p = 0.007$). In contrast, among patients with unmethylated MGMT promoter status, there was no statistically significant difference in median survival between treatment groups ($p = 0.06$).

With respect to progression-free survival, patients with MGMT promoter methylated tumors who received radiotherapy plus temozolomide had a significantly longer median progression-free survival compared with those treated with radiotherapy alone (10.3 vs 5.9 months, $p = 0.001$). A similar, though less pronounced, benefit was observed among patients with unmethylated MGMT promoter status: those treated with radiotherapy plus temozolomide had a median progression-free survival of 5.3 months, compared with 4.4 months in patients who received radiotherapy alone ($p = 0.02$).

The majority of patients in both treatment groups received salvage chemotherapy, including 70% of patients in the radiotherapy alone group, of whom 57.8% were treated with temozolomide. This likely accounts for the longer overall survival relative to progression-free survival observed in patients with MGMT promoter methylated tumors, underscoring the effectiveness of salvage therapy in this glioblastoma subgroup.

Paper Significance and Impact The significance of this study lies in its demonstration that MGMT promoter methylation status is a strong predictor of glioblastoma response to temozolomide, which remains the standard first-line chemotherapeutic agent for this disease. The findings provide a framework for identifying patients who are most likely to derive a survival benefit from combined radiotherapy and temozolomide. Conversely, because tumors lacking MGMT promoter methylation derive minimal benefit from the addition of temozolomide to radiotherapy, the study underscores the need for alternative therapeutic strategies to improve outcomes in this patient population.

By identifying a molecular biomarker capable of guiding treatment selection, this work has contributed to the personalization of glioblastoma therapy and has helped advance the broader development of biomarker-driven approaches to cancer treatment.

Study Limitations The most significant limitation of this study is that not all 573 glioblastoma patients were included in the analysis. This was due to inadequate paraffin-embedded tumor tissue and a variable success rate of methylation-specific polymerase chain reaction on glioblastoma tumor samples. This study was not properly powered to test the interactions between the magnitude of the treatment effect and MGMT promoter methylation status with respect to overall survival. Providing salvage therapy in the radiotherapy only group could serve as a potential confounder.

Relevant Studies In 2005, Stupp et al. conducted a landmark clinical trial evaluating whether the addition of temozolomide to radiotherapy could improve survival in patients with glioblastoma.[1] Prior to this study, the standard of care for these highly aggressive tumors consisted of a maximal safe surgical resection followed by adjuvant radiotherapy. The trial demonstrated that temozolomide, an oral alkylating chemotherapeutic agent administered in combination with radiotherapy, was associated with a significantly reduced risk of death compared with radiotherapy alone following surgical resection. As a result, the standard of care evolved to include maximal surgical resection followed by combined adjuvant radiotherapy and temozolomide. Despite this advancement, the therapeutic landscape for glioblastoma has changed little over the past two decades.[2]

Temozolomide induces DNA damage that is repaired by O^6-methylguanine-DNA methyltransferase (MGMT). Silencing of MGMT through promoter methylation impairs this repair mechanism, thereby enhancing the cytotoxic effect of temozolomide. As a result, MGMT promoter- methylation status has emerged as an important prognostic indicator in glioblastoma. A systematic review by Zhao et al. of 66 studies involving 7,886 patients confirmed that MGMT promoter methylation is predictive of prognosis in newly diagnosed, elderly, and recurrent glioblastoma patients.[3] The authors additionally reported that, in elderly patients, temozolomide monotherapy may confer greater benefit than radiotherapy alone.[3] MGMT promoter-methylation frequency increases with age, and multiple studies have demonstrated a survival benefit associated with temozolomide treatment in elderly glioblastoma patients.[4–6] In contrast, Egaña et al. reported no association between MGMT promoter-methylation status and survival in a single-institution cohort of 334 patients.[7]

Given these findings, it has been argued that patients with unmethylated MGMT promoters should have temozolomide omitted from their therapy course. A meta-analysis by Alnahhas et al. found that the median overall survival in glioblastoma patients with unmethylated MGMT promoters who received combination temozolomide and radiotherapy treatment was 14.11 months, compared to 24.59 months in methylated patients receiving the same treatments.[8] The authors concluded that further investigation is warranted to determine if temozolomide therapy should be withheld in MGMT unmethylated patients.

It is worth noting that there have also been inconsistencies between methylation status, protein/gene expression, and patient outcome.[9] Additional challenges include variability among methylation detection assays and the absence of standardized cutoff values across diagnostic platforms.[9] Furthermore, MGMT expression may be upregulated in response to temozolomide exposure, contributing to treatment resistance and the emergence of resistant tumor subclones.[10]

Overall, these studies underscore the clinical significance of Hegi et al.'s work in identifying the survival benefit associated with MGMT promoter methylation in glioblastoma patients treated with temozolomide.

Conclusion Patients with MGMT promoter methylated tumors demonstrate significantly improved survival when treated with temozolomide compared with patients whose tumors lack MGMT promoter methylation. Accordingly, assessment of MGMT promoter methylation status can help identify patients most likely to benefit from temozolomide therapy and can inform more effective, individualized treatment strategies for glioblastoma.

REFERENCES

1. Stupp R, Mason WP, van den Bent MJ, et al. Radiotherapy plus concomitant and adjuvant temozolomide for glioblastoma. N Engl J Med. 2005;352(10):987–996. doi:10.1056/NEJMoa043330
2. Jia JL, Alshamsan B, Ng TL. Temozolomide chronotherapy in glioma: a systematic review. Curr Oncol. 2023;30(2):1893–1902. doi:10.3390/curroncol30020147
3. Zhao YH, Wang ZF, Cao CJ, et al. The clinical significance of O^6-methylguanine-DNA methyltransferase promoter methylation status in adult patients with glioblastoma: a meta-analysis. Front Neurol. 2018;9:127. doi:10.3389/fneur.2018.00127
4. Reifenberger G, Hentschel B, Felsberg J, et al. Predictive impact of MGMT promoter methylation in glioblastoma of the elderly. Int J Cancer. 2012;131(6):1342–1350. doi:10.1002/ijc.27385
5. Perry JR, Laperriere N, O'Callaghan CJ, et al. Short-course radiation plus temozolomide in elderly patients with glioblastoma. N Engl J Med. 2017;376(11):1027–1037. doi:10.1056/NEJMoa1611977
6. Malmström A, Grønberg BH, Marosi C, et al. Temozolomide versus standard 6-week radiotherapy versus hypofractionated radiotherapy in patients older than 60 years with glioblastoma: the Nordic randomised, phase 3 trial. Lancet Oncol. 2012;13(9):916–926. doi:10.1016/S1470-2045(12)70265-6

7. Egaña L, Auzmendi-Iriarte J, Andermatten J, et al. Methylation of MGMT promoter does not predict response to temozolomide in patients with glioblastoma in Donostia Hospital. Sci Rep. 2020;10:18445. doi:10.1038/s41598-020-75477-9
8. Alnahhas I, Alsawas M, Rayi A, Palmer JD, Raval R, Ong S, Giglio P, Murad MH, Puduvalli V. Characterizing benefit from temozolomide in MGMT promoter unmethylated and methylated glioblastoma: a systematic review and meta-analysis. Neurooncol Adv. 2020 Oct 30;2(1):vdaa082. doi: 10.1093/noajnl/vdaa082. Erratum in: Neurooncol Adv. 2021 Jul 10;3(1):vdab095. doi: 10.1093/noajnl/vdab095. PMID: 33150334; PMCID: PMC7596890.
9. Butler M, Pongor L, Su YT, et al. MGMT status as a clinical biomarker in glioblastoma. Trends Cancer. 2020;6(5):380–391. doi:10.1016/j.trecan.2020.02.010
10. Kitange GJ, Carlson BL, Schroeder MA, et al. Induction of MGMT expression is associated with temozolomide resistance in glioblastoma xenografts. Neuro Oncol. 2009;11(3):281–291. doi:10.1215/15228517-2008-090

CHAPTER 3

Fluorescence-Guided Surgery with 5-Aminolevulinic Acid for the Resection of Malignant Gliomas: A Randomized Controlled Multicentre Phase III Trial

Stummer W, Pichlmeier U, Meinel T, Wiestler OD, Zanella F, Reulen HJ, for the ALA-Glioma Study Group, Lancet Oncol. 2006;7(5):392–401

Reviewed by Walter Stummer

Research Question/Objective 5-Aminolevulinic acid is a nonfluorescent prodrug that results in the intracellular accumulation of fluorescent porphyrins within malignant gliomas. This study aimed to evaluate the impact of 5-aminolevulinic acid–guided fluorescence resection on the extent of resection, progression-free survival, overall survival, and surgical morbidity.

Study Design This was a phase III interventional, randomized controlled trial.

Sample Size and Methods 322 patients aged 23–73 years with a suspected malignant glioma amenable to the complete resection of a contrast-enhancing tumour were randomly assigned to 20 mg/kg body weight 5-aminolevulinic acid for fluorescence-guided resection ($n = 161$) or to conventional microsurgery with white light ($n = 161$). The primary endpoints were the number of patients without a contrast-enhancing tumour on an early magnetic resonance imaging (MRI) scan (i.e. obtained within 72 hours after surgery) and 6-month progression-free survival as assessed by an MRI. Secondary endpoints were the volume of the residual tumour on a postoperative MRI, overall survival, neurological deficit, and toxic effects.

Follow-Up Median follow-up of 35.4 months (95% confidence interval (CI), 1.0–56.7).

Inclusion/Exclusion Criteria

- Inclusion Criteria
  - Radiological suspicion of a unilocular malignant glioma with distinct ring- or garland-shaped contrast agent accumulating tumour structures and a core of reduced intensity in the MRI (central necroses) with no significant non-staining tumour tissue (exclusion of a secondary malignant glioma).

DOI: 10.1201/9781003416197-3

- Indication for surgical tumour resection. If radical resection is planned, the location of the contrast agent accumulating tumour should allow complete resection.
- First operation of the tumour; no other tumour-specific pretreatment.
- Karnofsky Performance Status at least 70%.
- Patient's written informed consent.
- Age 18–72 years.

- Exclusion Criteria
  - Tumour location in the midline, basal ganglia, cerebellum, or brainstem.
  - More than one contrast agent accumulating lesion unrelated to the primary tumour or extracerebral metastases.
  - Porphyria, hypersensitivity to porphyrins.
  - Renal insufficiency: Creatinine >2.0 mg/dL.
  - Hepatic insufficiency: Bilirubin >3.0 mg/dL.
  - Quick test <60%.
  - Gamma-glutamyl transferase >70 U/I.
  - Malignancies other than basaliomas.
  - Existing or planned pregnancy or lactation, or inadequate contraception.
  - Simultaneous participation in another clinical trial or participation in another clinical trial in the 30 days preceding randomization.

Intervention or Treatment Received 20 mg/kg body weight 5-aminolevulinic acid for fluorescence-guided resection surgery.

Analysis An interim analysis was conducted in a full-analysis population of 270 patients (139 assigned to 5-aminolevulinic acid and 131 to white-light surgery). Patients with ineligible histological or radiological findings, as determined by centrally masked reviewers, were excluded. The interim analysis met the prespecified protocol criteria for study termination. All primary and secondary endpoints were analyzed according to the intention-to-treat principle within the full analysis population.

Results The contrast-enhancing tumour was resected completely in 90 (65%) of 139 patients assigned 5-aminolevulinic acid compared with 47 (36%) of 131 assigned white light (difference between groups 29% [95% CI, 17–40], $p < 0.0001$). Patients allocated 5-aminolevulinic acid had a higher 6-month progression-free survival than did those allocated white light (41% [32.8–49.2] vs 21.1% [14.0–28.2]; difference between groups 19.9% [9.1–30.7], $p = 0.0003$, Z test). Groups did not differ in the frequency of severe adverse events or adverse events in any organ system class reported within 7 days after surgery.

Conclusion Tumour fluorescence derived from 5-aminolevulinic acid enables more complete resections of a contrast-enhancing tumour, leading to improved progression-free survival in patients with a malignant glioma.

Reviewer Commentary In the 1900s, neurosurgeons were not uniformly convinced that resections for malignant gliomas were relevant for outcome. In retrospect, this was due to two reasons: one being the difficulty in discerning a marginal contrast-enhancing tumour from a normal brain during surgery, the second being the lack of routine postoperative imaging providing objective data on the degree of resection, leaving neurosurgeons unaware of how much tumour had been left behind.

Publications during the early 1990s provided evidence that neurosurgeons were systematically overestimating resection rates based on their intraoperative impressions only, and that patients with complete resections of enhancing tumours would have the best prognosis.[1] The problem remained as to how to best identify a residual-enhancing tumour as the greatest hurdle for achieving optimal resections. Neuronavigation was becoming available at the time, but the issue of brain shift could not completely resolve the problem of correct tissue identification.

In the early 1990s, I worked with a group studying photodynamic therapy of malignant tumours. I was specifically investigating various drugs for the photosensitization of malignant gliomas. One molecule known for its photosensitizing properties was 5-aminolevulinic acid (5-ALA). This molecule differs from other compounds as it is the body's metabolite in the heme biosynthesis pathway and thus is virtually non-toxic. Its photosensitizing properties are based on an intracellular conversion of 5-ALA into protoporphyrin IX (PPIX), another metabolite in the heme biosynthesis pathway, and a moiety further characterized by its brilliant fluorescence when illuminated with blue light. In the presence of excess, externally administered 5-ALA, PPIX cannot be cleared by a tumour and accumulates intracellularly.[2]

I first used this fluorescence for quantifying PPIX accumulation, and I found PPIX accumulation to be highly specific for malignant gliomas.[2] Observing this selective and crisp fluorescence under the microscope led me to change gears and to contemplate using 5-ALA-induced tissue fluorescence for detecting tumours intraoperatively. I was able to convince my former programme director about the potential and with the help of Medac, a medium-sized company in Hamburg (Germany) specializing in innovative pharmaceuticals for rare diseases, we collaborated in a development programme that culminated in the pivotal approval study presented here.[3]

In the forefront of the pivotal study, however, we were involved in intense discussions with the European Medicines Agency (EMA) on study design as the concept of fluorescence-guided resections with the aim of improving resections for improving outcome was novel. The EMA decided to treat 5-ALA as an anti-cancer drug rather than as an intraoperative diagnostic agent. Hence, the EMA required a randomized study with an outcome endpoint as one of two co-primary endpoints, apart from resection rates. Ultimately, the EMA agreed with progression-free survival as being sufficient if the safety profile of 5-ALA and surgery with 5-ALA was acceptable.

The study met its primary endpoints, i.e. significantly greater rates of resection rates when surgeons used 5-ALA, and a doubling of progression-free survival at 6 months. No major safety concerns of extended resections were identified, so that ultimately, 5-ALA received marketing authorization in the European Union in 2007 and consequently, by the Food and Drug Administration (FDA) in 2017.[4]

Paper Significance and Impact The paper presented here marks the first large, randomized study of fluorescence-guided resections, not only for malignant gliomas, but also for any other surgery discipline in general, leading to the first approval in the field. The study also represents the largest randomized study on a neurosurgical technique so far. It took until 2021 for a second fluorochrome, pafolacianine, an infrared dye for identifying ovarian cancer during abdominal surgery, to be approved by the FDA.[5] Furthermore, our paper has been widely regarded as a strong indicator for the benefit of surgery in malignant gliomas.

Relevant Studies While progression-free survival was significantly improved when surgeons used 5-ALA for improving resection rates, the study only showed a marginal improvement of overall survival when resection rates were doubled. Retrospectively, outcome data apart from the safety and extent of resection must be considered inappropriate for establishing the efficacy of an intraoperative tissue imaging method using a drug for identifying tissue. The reason is simply that it is not the drug driving oncological benefit but rather, it is the degree of resection in the hands of the surgeon. Thus, while the frequency of complete resections of enhancing tumours was higher in patients in the fluorescence group of the study (65%), there was still a portion of patients (35%) who also had complete resections of enhancing tumours, thus diluting any effects on progression-free and overall survival. We later restratified survival results from our study based on degrees of resection and accounted for possible biases from restratification, again corroborating the strong influence of resection on survival in glioblastoma patients.[6]

Conversely, one decade later, approval with the FDA relied on safety, as well as the observation from our study and other studies[7] that 5-ALA helps to selectively identify additional tissue not primarily identified by conventional means, in a disease where the community agrees that the greater the degree of safe resection, the more benefit there is for the patient.

This study was conducted by neurosurgeons at a time when intraoperative mapping and monitoring were rarely used in the context of malignant gliomas, possibly impacting safety in the study overall. However, no significant differences were noted regarding major neurological deficits in the 5-ALA arm compared to the control arm. Furthermore, surgeons who engaged in surgery, which was conducted in 17 German neurosurgical centres, had little experience with 5-ALA, and the results of the study mark the beginner's experience with fluorescence-guided resections. The study may thus have underestimated the true potential of the technology.

On the other hand, this study was conducted during a period in which the intraoperative MRI was not widely used, and none of the study centres had access to an intraoperative MRI. The study design further precluded using any other methods for tissue identification, such as neuronavigation or ultrasound. This decision has been criticized and it was argued that the use of neuronavigation would have allowed surgeons to improve resection rates in the control arm.

Considering a more widespread use of the intraoperative MRI (ioMRI) several years later, the question was again brought forward on whether intraoperative MRI was superior for improving resections in malignant gliomas compared to fluorescence guidance using 5-ALA. In fact, a second, albeit single-centre, prospective study randomizing between conventional surgery (without fluorescence) and the ioMRI was published in 2011 by Senft and coauthors.[8] In that study, rates of complete resection of enhancing tumours were achieved in >90% of patients using ioMRI, suggesting that ioMRI is far superior to 5-ALA for resections of malignant gliomas.

To address the question regarding which method was superior, a German consortium consisting of seven centres operating only with ioMRI and 11 centres operating only using 5-ALA designed a prospective, controlled study employing a strategy of pseudo-randomization, with the two groups of centres basically competing against each other. The pseudo-randomization strategy was chosen because of an anticipated lack of equipoise and fear of bias in individual centres, in which both technologies were available. In contrast to our older study, no restrictions were imposed regarding any other technologies for tissue localization, e.g. neuronavigation or intraoperative ultrasound.

The recruitment strategy succeeded in creating cohorts that were highly comparable regarding nonsurgical prognostic factors. Importantly, resection rates of enhancing tumours in both study groups were very similar, with 80% in either cohort. However, surgery took approximately 100 minutes longer in patients operated on using ioMRI.[9] Progression-free and overall survival were statistically equivalent in both cohorts, as was safety regarding neurological deficits from surgery. Interestingly, in the MRI cohort, surgeons found that they had only achieved resections in 41% of patients as observed in the first intraoperative scan. This value was slightly better than that achieved in the white-light arm in our randomized study from 20 years before, indicating that surgery for malignant gliomas requires tools allowing better identification of residual-enhancing tumours. Ultimately, a combination of both technologies would be optimal.

It is noteworthy that overall survival in this study in patients with complete resections of enhancing tumours was comparable to the best cohort from the Response Assessment in Neuro-Oncology (RANO) resect group, with supramarginal resections (28 vs 29 months). The RANO resect study was published in 2023.[10]

REFERENCES

1. Albert FK, Forsting M, Sartor K, Adams HP, Kunze S. Early postoperative magnetic resonance imaging after resection of malignant glioma: objective evaluation of residual tumour and its influence on regrowth and prognosis. Neurosurgery. 1994;34(1):45–60; discussion 60-1. doi:10.1097/00006123-199401000-00008
2. Stepp H, Stummer W. 5-ALA in the management of malignant glioma. Lasers Surg Med. 2018;50(5):399–419. doi:10.1002/lsm.22933
3. Stummer W, Pichlmeier U, Meinel T, et al. Fluorescence-guided surgery with 5-aminolevulinic acid for resection of malignant glioma: a randomised controlled multicentre phase III trial. Lancet Oncol. 2006;7(5):392–401. doi:10.1016/S1470-2045(06)70665-9
4. Hadjipanayis CG, Stummer W. 5-ALA and FDA approval for glioma surgery. J Neurooncol. 2019;141(3):479–486. doi:10.1007/s11060-019-03098-y
5. Tanyi JL, Randall LM, Chambers SK, et al. A Phase III study of pafolacianine injection (OTL38) for intraoperative imaging of folate receptor-positive ovarian cancer (study 006). J Clin Oncol. 2023;41(2):276–284. doi:10.1200/JCO.22.00291
6. Stummer W, Reulen HJ, Meinel T, et al. Extent of resection and survival in glioblastoma multiforme: identification of and adjustment for bias. Neurosurgery. 2008;62(3):564–576; discussion 564-76. doi:10.1227/01.neu.0000317304.31579.17
7. Stummer W, Tonn JC, Goetz C, et al. 5-Aminolevulinic acid-derived tumour fluorescence: the diagnostic accuracy of visible fluorescence qualities as corroborated by spectrometry and histology and postoperative imaging. Neurosurgery. 2014;74(3):310–319; discussion 319–20. doi:10.1227/NEU.0000000000000267
8. Senft C, Bink A, Franz K, Vatter H, Gasser T, Seifert V. Intraoperative MRI guidance and extent of resection in glioma surgery: a randomised, controlled trial. Lancet Oncol. 2011;12(11):997–1003. doi:10.1016/S1470-2045(11)70196-6
9. Roder C, Stummer W, Coburger J, et al. Intraoperative MRI-guided resection is not superior to 5-aminolevulinic acid guidance in newly diagnosed glioblastoma: a prospective controlled multicentre clinical trial. J Clin Oncol. 2023;41(36):5512–5523. doi:10.1200/JCO.22.01862
10. Karschnia P, Young JS, Dono A, et al. Prognostic validation of a new classification system for extent of resection in glioblastoma: a report of the RANO resect group. Neuro Oncol. 2023;25(5):940–954. doi:10.1093/neuonc/noac193

CHAPTER 4

A Randomized Trial of Surgery in the Treatment of Single Metastases to the Brain

Patchell RA, Tibbs PA, Walsh JW, Dempsey RJ, Maruyama Y, Kryscio RJ, Markesbery WR, Macdonald JS, Young B,
N Engl J Med. 1990 Feb 22;322(8):494–500

Reviewed by Jose Lavrador, Francesco Vergani, and Keyoumars Ashkan

Objective/Research Question To assess if surgical resection followed by whole brain radiotherapy offers a clinical benefit over whole brain radiotherapy alone in patients with a single brain metastasis from an extracranial systemic cancer.

Study Design Single-centre randomized clinical trial (RCT) with two treatment groups: surgical resection followed by whole brain radiotherapy (Sx + WBRT) vs WBRT alone. Patients were stratified according to location (supra vs infratentorial), extent (brain metastasis alone vs brain metastasis) and cancer in the primary site vs brain metastasis, cancer in the primary site and at least one other site), and type of disease (primary tumour).

Sample Size 56 patients were screened from 1985 to 1988; two patients declined study enrolment, and six patients were excluded after neuropathology confirmed the non-metastatic origin of the lesions. Therefore, 48 patients were included in the study, with 25 in the Sx + WBRT group and 23 in the WBRT alone group.

Inclusion/Exclusion Criteria

- Inclusion Criteria
  - Patients with a radiological suggestion of a single brain metastasis.
  - Age >18 years old.
  - Karnofsky Performance Status (KPS) >70%.
  - Histological evidence of extracranial systemic cancer within 5 years of treatment for the query brain metastasis.

DOI: 10.1201/9781003416197-4

- Exclusion Criteria
    - Non-resectable metastases.
    - Previous cranial radiotherapy.
    - Leptomeningeal disease.
    - Impending neurological deterioration requiring acute intervention.
    - Radiosensitive primary tumours (small-cell lung cancer, germ-cell tumours, leukaemia, lymphoma, and multiple myeloma).

Intervention or Treatment Received

- **Sx + WBRT** Craniotomy for a tumour resection within 72 hours of study enrolment, followed by WBRT (36 Gy in 12 sessions during weekdays, 3 Gy per session) within 14 days after surgery.
- **WBRT alone** Stereotaxic biopsy for supratentorial lesions within 72 hours, followed by WBRT as per above within 48 hours of the procedure. For infratentorial lesions, no biopsy was performed, given the risks involved and WBRT was given within 48 hours of randomization.

Results The results of this RCT are presented along four axes: *survival*, *recurrence*, *quality of life*, and *complications*.

Survival The Sx + WBRT group had a significantly longer median overall survival (Sx + WBRT – 40 weeks vs WBRT alone – 15 weeks, $p < 0.01$). This was supported by the multivariate analysis, where surgery and the "longer time from primary tumour to brain metastasis diagnosis" ($p < 0.04$) were associated with longer survival, whereas older age ($p < 0.01$) and leptomeningeal disease ($p < 0.02$) were related to shorter survival. An analysis according to the cause of death (neurological causes and systemic causes) was performed. For the neurological cause of death, the Sx + WBRT group had a significantly longer median overall survival (Sx + WBRT – 62 weeks vs WBRT alone – 26 weeks, $p < 0.0009$), which was confirmed in the multivariate analysis with surgery conferring a positive impact on survival ($p < 0.0008$) and leptomeningeal disease a negative impact ($p < 0.002$). For the systemic cause of death, there were no differences among groups (Sx + WBRT – 54 weeks vs WBRT alone – 23 weeks, $p = 0.26$)

Recurrence The Sx + WBRT group had better local control at the treated site when compared to the WBRT alone group. The recurrence rate was lower (Sx + WBRT – 20% vs WBRT alone – 52.17%, $p < 0.02$) and the median time to recurrence was longer (Sx + WBRT > 59 weeks vs WBRT alone 21 weeks, $p < 0.0001$). Also, surgical treatment ($p < 0.0001$) and the absence of leptomeningeal disease ($p < 0.0004$) were the only significant variables associated with a decreased recurrence in the primary metastatic site in the multivariate analysis. Surgical treatment had no impact on the development of other metastases in the brain or leptomeningeal disease. At the time of the recurrence, less than half of the patients (Sx + WBRT – 4/7 patients vs WBRT alone – 5/13 patients) received further individualized treatment.

Quality of Life Sx + WBRT produced longer maintenance of KPS > 70% in the treated population when compared with WBRT alone (Sx + WBRT – 38 weeks vs WBRT alone – 8 weeks, $p < 0.005$). This was confirmed in the multivariate analysis, where surgery was the only variable related to a longer maintenance of KPS > 70% ($p < 0.007$), whereas older age ($p < 0.02$) and disseminated disease ($p < 0.04$) were related to a shorter maintenance period.

Complications There were no significant differences in 30-day mortality (4% for both groups), morbidity (Sx + WBRT – 8% vs WBRT alone – 17%) and length of stay (Sx + WBRT – 27 days vs WBRT alone – 22 days) between the groups.

Conclusion Patients with systemic malignancy and a single brain metastasis treated with surgery followed by whole brain radiotherapy have a longer overall survival, and better local disease control, and quality of life with similar complication rates when compared with patients treated with whole brain radiotherapy alone.

Reviewer Commentary This paper had a very significant impact on the role of neurosurgical intervention in the context of metastatic disease in the brain. For the first time, in the brain metastatic field, it provided level I evidence (single-centre RCT) supporting the role of surgical resection in the management of this disease, where previous literature was populated only by observational studies and case series. Moreover, it changed the treatment paradigm from a *whole brain approach* to a *targeted approach* and highlighted the potential mutualistic relationship between surgery and radiation in the treatment of brain metastasis.

The contemporaneous application of this study, however, requires further elaboration. The definition of resectable disease has changed since this study was published, with the advent of perioperative neuro-monitoring and mapping techniques,[1] the improvement in access to deep-seated lesions (tubular retractor surgery, endoscopic assisted surgery),[2] and the development of safer techniques for image-guided biopsy of infratentorial lesions (robot-assisted).[3] The ubiquitous utilization of both pre- and postoperative MRI imaging has increased the accuracy of oligometastatic and leptomeningeal disease diagnosis before surgery and the assessment of residual disease after resection. Lastly, there is a bias in the data presented in this study towards the non-small-cell lung primary (Sx + WBRT – 72% and WBRT alone – 83%) and supratentorial disease (Sx + WBRT – 72% and WBRT alone – 74%), which restricts the generalization to other aetiologies and locations.

The approach to metastatic disease in the brain treatment has dramatically changed in the last 30 years since this publication, with revolutions in all the pillars of diagnosis and treatment.

New imaging techniques provide a more accurate non-invasive diagnosis of brain metastasis and tumour recurrence during follow-up. This is particularly the case with the new recommendations for the use of amino acid positron emission tomography

(PET) radiotracers by the Response Assessment in Neuro-Oncology (RANO) group[4] – [11C]-MET, [18F]-FET and [18F]-FDOPA – as a radiological tool for the delineation of brain metastasis extension, for the assessment of response to therapy, and for the differentiation between tumour progression and radionecrosis.[5]

The better understanding of the structure-function duality has empowered surgical teams to develop safer approaches and move forward the limits of resectability with the development of minimally invasive approaches. Furthermore, functional and intra-operative physiological assessment techniques are expanding the number of patients in the surgical cohort, with their impact on survival, recurrence, and quality of life, with an acceptable complication profile.[2]

The emergence of targeted therapies and immunotherapy that followed the discovery of driver mutations and immune mechanisms has altered the therapy landscape of oligometastatic disease, particularly when target mutations are identified (e.g. crizotinib in ALK (anaplastic lymphoma kinase)-positive or osimertinib in EGFR (epidermal growth factor receptor) T790M mutant lung cancer)[6] or the immune system can be modulated (e.g. ipilimumab and nivolumab in melanoma).[7]

Finally, stereotactic radiosurgery (SRS) has increasingly relegated WBRT to a secondary, "salvage therapy" role in many patients. SRS currently has two main indications in the brain metastatic disease therapy: primary or adjuvant treatment. SRS is non-inferior to surgical resection in patients with one to two metastases with suitable volume (< 4 cm) in terms of long-term local control, with a suggestion of better control in the short term compared to surgery (when the benefit over surgery decreases over time).[8] Two RCTs aimed to address this question in a similar way – Sx + WBRT vs SRS + WBRT[9] and Sx + WBRT vs SRS alone[10] – but struggled with recruitment and therefore, the conclusions and real-world applicability are limited, as highlighted in a recent review.[11] Thus, the decision on optimal therapy for patients suited to both modalities remains dependent on the experience of the treating team and patient preference. Recent evidence supports better local control with postoperative SRS after the surgical resection of up to three metastases[12] and longer cognitive-decline free survival when compared with WBRT, without the compromise of local control and overall survival.[13] Novel lines of research are focused on the potential benefit of neoadjuvant administration of SRS, investigating the potential benefit in terms of better treatment delineation and decreased leptomeningeal disease and radionecrosis.[14]

Summary Patchell et al.'s paper paved the way for a new era in the surgical treatment of brain metastatic disease. The current therapy landscape, however, has expanded to include a wide range of options, from targeted oral therapies to localized SRS. In parallel, surgery has also evolved, becoming more minimally invasive and safer due to better techniques of function preservation. Therefore, surgery continues to provide a valuable resource in the management of brain metastatic disease, particularly when addressing large and symptomatic or otherwise adjuvant-resistant metastasis.

REFERENCES

1. De Witt Hamer PC, Robles SG, Zwinderman AH, Duffau H, Berger MS. Impact of intraoperative stimulation brain mapping on glioma surgery outcome: a meta-analysis. J Clin Oncol. 2012;30(20):2559–2565. doi:10.1200/JCO.2011.38.4818
2. Sinha S, Kalyal N, Gallagher MJ, Richardson D, Kalaitzoglou D, Abougamil A, Silva M, Oviedova A, Patel S, Mirallave-Pescador A, Bleil C, Zebian B, Gullan R, Ashkan K, Vergani F, Bhangoo R, Pedro Lavrador J. Impact of preoperative mapping and intraoperative neuromonitoring in minimally invasive parafascicular surgery for deep-seated lesions. World Neurosurg. 2024;181:e1019–e1037. doi:10.1016/j.wneu.2023.11.030
3. Bahrami E, Parvaresh M, Bahrami M, Fattahi A. An experience with frame-based stereotactic biopsy of posterior fossa lesions via transcerebellar route. World Neurosurg. 2020;136:e380–e385. doi:10.1016/j.wneu.2020.01.003
4. Galldiks N, Langen KJ, Albert NL, Chamberlain M, Soffietti R, Kim MM, Law I, Le Rhun E, Chang S, Schwarting J, Combs SE, Preusser M, Forsyth P, Pope W, Weller M, Tonn JC. PET imaging in patients with brain metastasis-report of the RANO/PET group. Neuro Oncol. 2019;21(5):585–595. doi:10.1093/neuonc/noz003
5. Urso L, Bonatto E, Nieri A, Castello A, Maffione AM, Marzola MC, Cittanti C, Bartolomei M, Panareo S, Mansi L, Lopci E, Florimonte L, Castellani M. The role of molecular imaging in patients with brain metastases: a literature review. Cancers (Basel). 2023;15(7):2184. doi:10.3390/cancers15072184
6. Shaw AT, Kim DW, Nakagawa K, Seto T, Crinó L, Ahn MJ, De Pas T, Besse B, Solomon BJ, Blackhall F, Wu YL, Thomas M, O'Byrne KJ, Moro-Sibilot D, Camidge DR, Mok T, Hirsh V, Riely GJ, Iyer S, Tassell V, Polli A, Wilner KD, Jänne PA. Crizotinib versus chemotherapy in advanced ALK-positive lung cancer. N Engl J Med. 2013;368(25):2385–2394. doi: 10.1056/NEJMoa1214886
7. Larkin J, Chiarion-Sileni V, Gonzalez R, Grob JJ, Rutkowski P, Lao CD, Cowey CL, Schadendorf D, Wagstaff J, Dummer R, Ferrucci PF, Smylie M, Hogg D, Hill A, Márquez-Rodas I, Haanen J, Guidoboni M, Maio M, Schöffski P, Carlino MS, Lebbé C, McArthur G, Ascierto PA, Daniels GA, Long GV, Bastholt L, Rizzo JI, Balogh A, Moshyk A, Hodi FS, Wolchok JD. Five-year survival with combined nivolumab and ipilimumab in advanced melanoma. N Engl J Med. 2019;381(16):1535–1546. doi:10.1056/NEJMoa1910836
8. Churilla TM, Chowdhury IH, Handorf E, Collette L, Collette S, Dong Y, Alexander BM, Kocher M, Soffietti R, Claus EB, Weiss SE. Comparison of local control of brain metastases with stereotactic radiosurgery vs surgical resection: a secondary analysis of a randomized clinical trial. JAMA Oncol. 2019;5(2):243–247. doi:10.1001/jamaoncol.2018.4610
9. Roos DE, Smith JG, Stephens SW. Radiosurgery versus surgery, both with adjuvant whole brain radiotherapy, for solitary brain metastases: a randomised controlled trial. Clin Oncol (R Coll Radiol). 2011;23(9):646–651. doi:10.1016/j.clon.2011.04.009
10. Muacevic A, Wowra B, Siefert A, Tonn JC, Steiger HJ, Kreth FW. Microsurgery plus whole brain irradiation versus Gamma Knife surgery alone for treatment of single metastases to the brain: a randomized controlled multicentre phase III trial. J Neurooncol. 2008;87(3):299–307. doi:10.1007/s11060-007-9510-4
11. Fiore G, Tariciotti L, Bertani GA, Gagliano D, D'Ammando A, Ampollini AM, Schisano L, Borsa S, Pluderi M, Locatelli M, Caroli M. Surgery vs radiosurgery for patients with localized metastatic brain disease: a systematic review with meta-analysis of randomized controlled trials. Cancers (Basel). 2023;15(15):3802. doi:10.3390/cancers15153802

12. Mahajan A, Ahmed S, McAleer MF, Weinberg JS, Li J, Brown P, Settle S, Prabhu SS, Lang FF, Levine N, McGovern S, Sulman E, McCutcheon IE, Azeem S, Cahill D, Tatsui C, Heimberger AB, Ferguson S, Ghia A, Demonte F, Raza S, Guha-Thakurta N, Yang J, Sawaya R, Hess KR, Rao G. Post-operative stereotactic radiosurgery versus observation for completely resected brain metastases: a single-centre, randomised, controlled, phase 3 trial. Lancet Oncol. 2017;18(8):1040–1048. doi:10.1016/S1470-2045(17)30414-X.
13. Brown PD, Ballman KV, Cerhan JH, Anderson SK, Carrero XW, Whitton AC, Greenspoon J, Parney IF, Laack NNI, Ashman JB, Bahary JP, Hadjipanayis CG, Urbanic JJ, Barker FG 2nd, Farace E, Khuntia D, Giannini C, Buckner JC, Galanis E, Roberge D. Postoperative stereotactic radiosurgery compared with whole brain radiotherapy for resected metastatic brain disease (NCCTG N107C/CEC·3): a multicentre, randomised, controlled, phase 3 trial. Lancet Oncol. 2017;18(8):1049–1060. doi:10.1016/S1470-2045(17)30441-2
14. Das S, Faruqi S, Nordal R, Starreveld Y, Kelly J, Bowden G, Amanie J, Fairchild A, Lim G, Loewen S, Rowe L, Wallace C, Ghosh S, Patel S. A phase III, multicenter, randomized controlled trial of preoperative versus postoperative stereotactic radiosurgery for patients with surgically resectable brain metastases. BMC Cancer. 2022;22(1):1368. doi:10.1186/s12885-022-10480-z

CHAPTER 5

Prognostic Factors for Survival in Adult Patients with Cerebral Low-Grade Glioma

Pignatti F, van den Bent M, Curran D, Debruyne C, Sylvester R, Therasse P, Afra D, Cornu P, Bolla M, Vecht C, Karim ABMF, J Clin Oncol. 2002 Apr 15;20(8):2076–2084

Reviewed by Francesco Vergani, Jose Lavrador, and Keyoumars Ashkan

Objective/Research Question The purpose of this paper was to identify prognostic factors for survival in adult patients diagnosed with a cerebral low-grade glioma (LGG). The authors used their data to derive a prognostic scoring system and validated the results using an independent data set.

Study Design Pooled analysis of patients recruited in the European Organization for Research and Treatment of Cancer (EORTC) trials 22844 and 22845. These were two large phase III trials carried out in adult patients with LGG. The trials were designed to investigate the dosage and timing of postoperative radiotherapy in LGG.

Sample Size Cox analysis was performed on 322 patients from the EORTC trial 22844 (construction set), and the results were validated on 288 patients from trial 22845 (validation set). Survival was calculated as the time from randomization until death, regardless of cause (event) or censoring at the last follow-up. Survival was estimated using the Kaplan–Meier technique. The Cox proportional hazards model was used for model selection and validation, with stratification by treatment.

Inclusion/Exclusion Criteria

- Inclusion Criteria: The maximum allowed World Health Organization (WHO) performance status at randomization was 2. Adult patients were eligible if:
  - Surgery had been carried out within 8 weeks of randomization.
  - A local histopathologic diagnosis of low-grade cerebral astrocytoma, oligodendroglioma, or mixed oligoastrocytoma according to WHO typing (1979 edition) had been made.

- Exclusion Criteria
  - Patients with totally excised small grade 1 tumors, pregnancy, gross hepatic, renal, cardiovascular, or respiratory disease, other malignancies

DOI: 10.1201/9781003416197-5

in the prior given years, or any other disease that was considered to limit 5-year survival were not eligible.
- Pilocytic astrocytomas were excluded from the dataset analysis.

Intervention or Treatment Received N/A

Results Multivariate analysis on the construction set showed that the following parameters were related to a poorer prognosis in adults with LGG: age ≥40 years, astrocytoma histology subtype (as opposed to oligodendroglioma or mixed oligoastrocytoma), largest diameter of the tumor ≥6 cm, tumor crossing the midline, and the presence of neurologic deficits before surgery. The total number of unfavorable factors present was used to determine a prognostic score. For practical purposes, a simplification was introduced, and the effect of each factor was 1 since the magnitude of the estimated coefficients of the final model in the construction set was similar across factors. This yielded a score between 0 (most favorable prognosis) and 5 (worst prognosis). The score was further categorized to identify two distinct risk groups, namely a low-risk group (score 0 to 2) and a high-risk group (score 3 to 5). The validity of the multivariate model and of the scoring system was confirmed in the validation set. Overall, median survival was between 3 and 4 years in the high-risk group and between 8 and 9 years in the low-risk group.

Conclusion In adult patients with LGG, older age, astrocytoma histology, the presence of neurologic deficits before surgery, the largest tumor diameter, and a tumor crossing the midline were important prognostic factors for survival. These factors can be used to identify low-risk and high-risk patients.

Reviewer Commentary This paper represents a landmark in attempting to define prognostic factors in patients with LGG despite a large heterogeneity in the diagnosis, treatment, and expected outcomes. Its strength is to derive clinical data from two large, multicenter trials, therefore having a cohort of more than 600 patients with homogeneous inclusion criteria and good quality follow-up. This meant that it was possible to thoroughly analyze a large series of clinical variables, including age, the presence of headache, epilepsy, neurological deficits, the size of the tumor (indicated by its largest diameter), contralateral invasion (a tumor crossing the midline), the extent of resection, and the histology subtype. After multivariate analysis, only five of these variables were included in the final model to predict outcome: age, presence of deficits before surgery, largest diameter, tumor crossing the midline, and an astrocytoma histology subtype. The prognostic score derived from this paper has had a significant impact on clinical decisions and has informed guidelines on the management of LGG.[1] For example, it became more difficult to recommend simple surveillance or "watch and wait" in newly diagnosed "high-risk" LGG patients (at a time when this was the preferred option in many centers). In addition, the age cutoff at 40 was included in the recommendations of neo-adjuvant treatment with chemo-radiotherapy following surgery for LGG, again due to the perceived high risk of tumor progression and poor outcome in this group of patients.[2] Finally, many of the risk factors identified in this paper (particularly preoperative volume, the presence of neurological deficits, and the contralateral invasion of the tumor) stood the test of time and are still useful today to guide the management of patients.

Study Limitations The main limitation of this paper is that its recommendations regarding prognostic factors are based on analyses from trials conducted before the discovery of the isocitrate dehydrogenase (IDH) mutation in 2008.[3] Since 2016, the WHO classification[4] characterizes gliomas according to their IDH status as IDH mutant (IDHmt) and IDH wild type (IDHwt). It is now understood that these two tumor categories have different biological behaviors, with IDHmt gliomas occurring at a younger age and having a better prognosis, thus representing the "true" LGG".[5] The EORTC studies included in this paper likely included both IDHmt and IDHwt tumors, and it cannot be assumed that the results described remain valid for determining a prognosis in IDHmt glioma patients (as defined in the WHO 2021 classification). In particular, the analysis done on age and histology is likely to be affected by the IDH status of the tumor. It is, in fact, reasonable to expect that in the EORTC trials, older patients (above 40) were more likely to have IDHwt gliomas compared to younger patients, therefore explaining the poorer prognosis seen in this group. In addition, the histologic diagnosis used in the paper is no longer applicable; for example, the old category of "mixed oligoastrocytoma" does not exist anymore. It is still true that astrocytomas are associated with a worse prognosis compared to oligodendrogliomas, but oligodendrogliomas need to be defined as IDHmt, 1p/19q co-deleted tumors. Another limitation is the analysis performed with regard to the extent of resection. The authors looked at the extent of resection as assessed intraoperatively by surgeons as "extensive tumor resection" (more than 90%), "limited resection" (less than 90%) or biopsy only. The association with better survival for the "extensive resection" was present in the univariate analysis, but not after multivariate analysis. It is, however, well known that the extent of resection as assessed by surgeons is unreliable and an objective measurement of postoperative tumor residuum, such as with MRIs, is required when evaluating the impact of surgery on survival.

Relevant Studies In this context, it is important for the reader to be aware of this historical paper, but to complement it with a more contemporary evaluation of prognostic factors in the IDH era. Recently, van den Bent et al.[6] have re-appraised the risk factors, tailoring their review specifically to IDHmt gliomas. Of interest, the more recent literature has given conflicting evidence regarding age as a significant prognostic factor in IDHmt gliomas. Conversely, genetic analysis may allow for better prognostication of IDH-mutant glioma patients, being even superior to histological grading. The homozygous deletion of CDKN2A/B, for example, is well recognized to be associated with poorer outcomes in IDHmt gliomas. The volume of residual tumor in IDH-mutant gliomas after surgery appears to have a major prognostic significance for outcome, something that was not investigated in the original paper of Pignatti et al. In a seminal publication, Jakola et al. demonstrated that patients with LGG had a better survival at a center where surgery for maximal debulking was offered as the initial management of LGG, as opposed to a center where biopsy followed by watchful waiting was offered instead.[7] These results have been confirmed when IDH status was considered.[8] In addition, patients with total resection (complete removal of a tumor visible on the preoperative MRI) or supratotal resection (i.e. a resection extending beyond the volume of a tumor seen on the MRI, guided by functional margins) have a better survival.[9] These insights should be used today for risk stratification and for treatment decisions. In many patients with IDH-mutant grades 2 and 3 glioma, if carefully monitored after surgery, postponing radiotherapy and chemotherapy is safe, and will not jeopardize the overall outcome of patients.[6,9,10]

Summary Pignatti et al. made a major contribution in defining prognostic factors for LGG. While many of their findings are still valid, this paper is better appreciated in the light of contemporary literature following the new definition of IDHmt gliomas.

REFERENCES

1. Weller M, van den Bent M, Preusser M, et al. EANO guidelines on the diagnosis and treatment of diffuse gliomas of adulthood. Nat Rev Clin Oncol. 2020;18(3):170–186.
2. Buckner JC, Shaw EG, Pugh SL, et al. Radiation plus procarbazine, CCNU, and vincristine in low-grade glioma. N Engl J Med. 2016;374(14):1344–1355.
3. Yan H, Parsons DW, Jin G, McLendon R, Rasheed BA, Yuan W, Kos I, Batinic-Haberle I, Jones S, Riggins GJ, Friedman H, Friedman A, Reardon D, Herndon J, Kinzler KW, Velculescu VE, Vogelstein B, Bigner DD. IDH1 and IDH2 mutations in gliomas. N Engl J Med. 2009;360(8):765–773. doi:10.1056/NEJMoa0808710
4. Louis DN, Perry A, Reifenberger G, et al. The 2016 world health organi- zation classification of tumors of the central nervous system: a summary. Acta Neuropathol. 2016;131(6):803–820.
5. Cancer Genome Atlas Research Network. Comprehensive, integrative genomic analysis of diffuse lower-grade gliomas. N Engl J Med. 2015;372(26):2481–2498. doi:10.1056/NEJMoa1402121
6. van den Bent MJ, French PJ, Brat D, Tonn JC, Touat M, Ellingson BM, Young RJ, Pallud J, von Deimling A, Sahm F, Figarella Branger D, Huang RY, Weller M, Mellinghoff IK, Cloughsey TF, Huse JT, Aldape K, Reifenberger G, Youssef G, Karschnia P, Noushmehr H, Peters KB, Ducray F, Preusser M, Wen PY. The biological significance of tumor grade, age, enhancement, and extent of resection in IDH-mutant gliomas: how should they inform treatment decisions in the era of IDH inhibitors? Neuro Oncol. 2024;26(10): 1805–1822. doi:10.1093/neuonc/noae107
7. Jakola AS, Myrmel KS, Kloster R, Torp SH, Lindal S, Unsgård G, Solheim O. Comparison of a strategy favoring early surgical resection vs a strategy favoring watchful waiting in low-grade gliomas. JAMA. 2012;308(18):1881–1888. doi:10.1001/jama.2012.12807
8. Jakola AS, Skjulsvik AJ, Myrmel KS, Sjåvik K, Unsgård G, Torp SH, Aaberg K, Berg T, Dai HY, Johnsen K, Kloster R, Solheim O. Surgical resection versus watchful waiting in low-grade gliomas. Ann Oncol. 2017;28(8):1942–1948. doi:10.1093/annonc/mdx230
9. Ng S, Rigau V, Moritz-Gasser S, Gozé C, Darlix A, Herbet G, Duffau H. Long-term autonomy, professional activities, cognition, and overall survival after awake functional-based surgery in patients with IDH-mutant grade 2 gliomas: a retrospective cohort study. Lancet Reg Health Eur. 2024;46:101078. doi:10.1016/j.lanepe.2024.101078. eCollection 2024 Nov.
10. Acharya S, Lavrador JP, Sekhon PP, Visagan R, Jung J, Gullan R, Vergani F, Bhangoo R, Ashkan K. Low-grade glioma case series: lessons learned from an evolving 10-year single-institution multidisciplinary team practice. World Neurosurg. 2021;151:e47–e57. doi:10.1016/j.wneu.2021.03.101

CHAPTER 6

Long-Term Outcomes after Supratotal Resection of Diffuse Low-Grade Gliomas: A Consecutive Series with 11-Year Follow-Up

Duffau H, Acta Neurochir (Wien). 2016 Jan;158(1):51–58.

Reviewed by Piiamaria S Virtanen, Chiara A Flores, and Angela M Richardson

Background Total or subtotal surgical resection of WHO grade II gliomas (diffuse low-grade glioma) can significantly increase survival. Moreover, supratotal resection, i.e. an extended resection with a margin beyond magnetic resonance imaging (MRI) abnormalities, could decrease the risk of malignant transformation.

Research Question/Objective To report long-term functional and oncological outcomes after the supratotal resection of a WHO grade II diffuse low-grade glioma (DLGG).

Study Design Observational retrospective single-surgeon outcomes study.

Sample Size 16 patients (7 men, 9 women with a mean age of 41.3 years, range 26–63 years).

Follow-Up Mean 132 months (range, 97–198 months) postoperatively.

Inclusion/Exclusion Criteria

- Inclusion Criteria
    - Patients who underwent supratotal resection for a supratentorial DLGG between November 1998 and June 2007 with a minimum follow-up of 8 years after surgery.
- Exclusion Criteria: N/A

DOI: 10.1201/9781003416197-6

Intervention or Treatment Received Supratotal resection of DLGG, with the extent of resection up to functional cortical and subcortical structures defined by intrasurgical electrical mapping.

Methods The extent of resection was evaluated on a postoperative fluid-attenuated inversion recovery (FLAIR)-weighted MRI. Data regarding clinicoradiological features, therapeutic management, and outcomes were analyzed.

Results Seven men and nine women (mean age, 41.3 years, range, 26–63 years) were included (seizure in 15 cases, one incidental discovery). All patients resumed a normal life after surgery (no neurological deficits, no epilepsy). The volume of the postoperative cavity was larger than the preoperative tumor volume in the 16 patients. A neuropathological examination confirmed the diagnosis of WHO grade II gliomas in all cases. No adjuvant treatment was administered after resection. The mean duration of postoperative follow-up was 132 months (range 97–198 months). There was no relapse in eight cases. Eight patients experienced tumor recurrence, with an average time to relapse of 70.3 months (range 32–105 months), but without malignant transformation. Five of them have been retreated, with a reoperation (two cases), chemotherapy (three cases), and radiotherapy (two cases). All patients continue to enjoy a normal life.

Conclusion This is the first series demonstrating the prolonged impact of supratotal resection on the malignant transformation of DLGG. These original data may suggest removing a margin around the FLAIR-weighted MRI abnormalities in a more systematic manner for DLGG, not involving eloquent structures.

Reviewer Commentary Diffuse low-grade glioma (DLGG) was broadly defined as a WHO grade II glioma before recent molecular classifications, including in the study discussed. This is a disease primarily of adults with a mean age at diagnosis of 39, a median survival of approximately 5 years, and an incidence of 1 (0.5–1.3) in 100,000 people.[1–3] DLGG has been a challenging pathology to treat, with early studies showing that gross total resection improved survival compared to biopsy, but this strategy could lead to neurologic deficits.[4] Ongoing studies focused on the role of adjuvant treatment and the importance of the extent of resection in prognosis and functional outcomes.[5] The accepted surgical management strategy then aimed for maximal safe surgical resection only up to the hyperintense MRI abnormality and not beyond it, either via circumferential or sulcus-guided resection or piecemeal resection, with preservation of eloquent brain regions. Evidence favoring more aggressive management of these tumors continued to mount, with early surgical resection demonstrating decreased progression of disease and decreased malignant transformation.[6–8] Contemporaneous studies utilized histological analysis to identify DLGG cells in the peritumoral tissue up to 20 mm beyond the radiographically defined tumor border. This led to the conclusion that FLAIR MRI signal abnormalities underestimate the spatial extent of DLGGs, suggesting that more robust resection may improve outcomes.[9–11]

Hugues Duffau's study, published in 2016 in Acta Neurochirurgica, presents the long-term functional and oncological outcomes after supratotal resection (STR) of DLGG involving presumed non-eloquent supratentorial brain regions. STR pushed the boundaries of resection further, aiming to resect tumor margins beyond the T2-weighted or FLAIR MRI signal abnormality of the tumor, i.e. a margin of a peritumoral normal-appearing brain outside the radiographically defined tumor border.[12] Duffau defines STR as the "complete removal of any signal abnormalities with a volume of the postoperative cavity larger than the preoperative tumor volume".[13] Prior studies had suggested that STR may delay malignant transformation, in a short-term (3 years) follow-up study of 15 patients with DLGG who underwent STR.[7,8,13] STR also prevented the disease progression in another study by Duffau's group.[13,14] The study discussed here includes long-term data with a mean 11-year follow-up period of a consecutive series of 16 patients with a mean age of 41.3 years who underwent STR for DLGG to prevent tumor recurrence and malignant transformation. The extent of tumor resection was determined by a comparison of preoperative tumor volume to the volume of the surgical cavity on a 3-month postoperative MRI. To achieve safe STR, each operation, except one, in the series was performed awake with intraoperative functional brain mapping using cortical and subcortical electrical stimulation.[13]

This study served as the impetus for continued assessments of STR of noneloquent supratentorial DLGG in terms of improved survival and outcomes.[13] The noneloquent brain regions considered suitable for STR include those outside the cortical primary motor, somatosensory, speech, and language areas and the insula, and those that reside outside and not within or immediately adjacent to essential white matter tracts or central gray matter nuclei. While the goal of resecting a larger peritumoral tissue margin is advantageous within noneloquent areas, the risk of breaching eloquent areas with increasingly larger margins must be considered.[15] While transient neurological deficits were observed in nine patients (two with supplementary motor area syndrome, nine with language disorder), all patients recovered fully and returned to preoperative functional status.[13] The low incidence of significant postoperative deficits and the complete lack of permanent neurological deficits reported in the study indicate the safety of the approach. In Duffau's study, all 15 patients with preoperative seizures experienced improvement in epilepsy (11 with no antiepileptic drug [AED] use, four with a reduction in AEDs).[13] Later, other studies confirmed that STR in DLGG patients with seizures improves seizure control without negative effects on cognition, and improves patients' overall quality of life.[16,17]

This study represents a landmark in neuro-oncology as it challenges the traditional boundaries of glioma surgery and sets forth a crucial paradigm shift for modern neurosurgical practice by advocating a more aggressive surgical approach in the management of DLGG, which has historically been more conservative, aiming to control symptoms and minimize operative risks. This study advocates for STR as a more radical surgical approach with the potential to improve disease control, survival rates, and long-term outcomes without compromising patient safety or quality of life. This study presents compelling evidence in support of STR by demonstrating a dramatic risk reduction of malignant transformation with delay in the use of adjuvant chemotherapy and radiotherapy. No patients received adjuvant treatment postoperatively. Fifty percent of patients experienced tumor recurrence with an average time to relapse of 70.3 months.[13] Recurrences occurred at the margin of the surgical cavity, providing further evidence that local therapies have the potential to improve outcomes. Systematic reviews and meta-analyses support the conclusion that both extent of resection (EOR) and postsurgical residual volume are independent prognostic factors for improved outcomes and overall survival.[12,13]

These findings have influenced neurosurgical decision-making and informed discussions about treatment options with patients and their families, with suspected continued increased adoption of STR for DLGG in the correctly selected patients. Subsequent reviews and studies further validated and expanded upon these findings. Kreatsoulas et al. performed a systematic review, which found that while STR has a low incidence of postoperative neurologic deficits and is suitable for both asymptomatic and symptomatic DLGG patients, the overall published literature still consists of low- to moderate-quality evidence in support of STR for DLGG with the aim of improving progression-free survival and seizure control, and that larger clinical trials are necessary to better define the role of STR for the surgical resection of DLGG.[18] Ius et al. reported good outcomes with STR in patients with DLGG, including improved survival and no death events in patients who underwent STR (EOR > 100%) as compared to patients who underwent resection with EOR = 100% or EOR < 100%.[15] Rossi et al., focused primarily on IDH-mutated DLGGs, had a median follow-up of 6.8 years and demonstrated a prolonged progression-free survival (PFS) and longer overall survival (OS) in the STR subgroup, regardless of DLGG molecular subtype and tumor grade. Only six patients (5.4%) who underwent supratotal resection experienced tumor progression, as compared to 100% in the partial, 95.9% in the subtotal, and 82.4% in the total resection group.[19] Likewise, the STR group demonstrated longer malignant progression-free survival (MPFS) and a lower incidence of adjuvant therapies.[19]

Duffau and colleagues have since then extensively described the other nuances of successful STR for DLGG, focusing on functional mapping and connectome-guided STR to achieve optimal resection outcomes and brain plasticity profiling to support therapeutic decision-making.[17,20–22] Utilizing these techniques, neurosurgeons may continue to push the boundaries safely in the care of patients with DLGG.

The main limitation of the described study, as the author acknowledges, is the small sample size, which is attributed to tumor involvement of eloquent structures upon diagnosis, preventing safe supratotal resection. This is a single-surgeon series, so these results may not be generalizable to others who do not have the necessary equipment and support. Additionally, molecular typing was not completed on these tumors since this was not standard of care when the surgeries discussed were performed.

In conclusion, Duffau's research represents a significant contribution to the field of neurosurgery, presenting compelling evidence that supports the adoption of STR in well-selected cases of DLGG. This landmark study represents requisite reading for neurosurgeons aiming to enhance their understanding of glioma management and to improve patient outcomes. The findings have not only influenced clinical practice but also spurred further research into optimizing surgical strategies for DLGG. As the field continues to evolve, studies such as this will remain foundational in guiding evidence-based practice and improving patient care.

REFERENCES

1. Claus EB, Black PM. Survival rates and patterns of care for patients diagnosed with supratentorial low-grade gliomas: data from the SEER program, 1973-2001. Cancer. 2006;106(6):1358–1363. doi:10.1002/cncr.21733
2. Pignatti F, van den Bent M, Curran D, Debruyne C, Sylvester R, Therasse P, Afra D, Cornu P, Bolla M, Vecht C, Karim AB, European Organization for R, Treatment of Cancer Brain Tumor Cooperative G, European Organization for R, Treatment of Cancer Radiotherapy Cooperative G. Prognostic factors for survival in adult patients with cerebral low-grade glioma. J Clin Oncol. 2002;20(8):2076–2084. doi:10.1200/JCO.2002.08.121
3. Bauchet L. Epidemiology of diffuse low-grade gliomas. In: Duffau H, editor. Diffuse Low-Grade Gliomas in Adults. London: Springer; 2013.
4. Steiger HJ, Markwalder RV, Seiler RW, Ebeling U, Reulen HJ. Early prognosis of supratentorial grade 2 astrocytomas in adult patients after resection or stereotactic biopsy. An analysis of 50 cases operated on between 1984 and 1988. Acta Neurochir (Wien). 1990;106(3-4):99–105. doi:10.1007/BF01809449
5. Peraud A, Ansari H, Bise K, Reulen HJ. Clinical outcome of supratentorial astrocytoma WHO grade II. Acta Neurochir (Wien). 1998;140(12):1213–1222. doi:10.1007/s007010050241
6. Jakola AS, Myrmel KS, Kloster R, Torp SH, Lindal S, Unsgard G, Solheim O. Comparison of a strategy favoring early surgical resection vs a strategy favoring watchful waiting in low-grade gliomas. JAMA. 2012;308(18):1881–1888. doi:10.1001/jama.2012.12807
7. Mandonnet E, Delattre JY, Tanguy ML, Swanson KR, Carpentier AF, Duffau H, Cornu P, Van Effenterre R, Alvord EC, Jr., Capelle L. Continuous growth of mean tumor diameter in a subset of grade II gliomas. Ann Neurol. 2003;53(4):524–528. doi:10.1002/ana.10528
8. Pallud J, Mandonnet E, Duffau H, Kujas M, Guillevin R, Galanaud D, Taillandier L, Capelle L. Prognostic value of initial magnetic resonance imaging growth rates for World Health Organization grade II gliomas. Ann Neurol. 2006;60(3):380–383. doi:10.1002/ana.20946
9. Kelly PJ, Daumas-Duport C, Kispert DB, Kall BA, Scheithauer BW, Illig JJ. Imaging-based stereotaxic serial biopsies in untreated intracranial glial neoplasms. J Neurosurg. 1987;66(6):865–874. doi:10.3171/jns.1987.66.6.0865
10. Pallud J, Varlet P, Devaux B, Geha S, Badoual M, Deroulers C, Page P, Dezamis E, Daumas-Duport C, Roux FX. Diffuse low-grade oligodendrogliomas extend beyond MRI-defined abnormalities. Neurology. 2010;74(21):1724–1731. doi:10.1212/WNL.0b013e3181e04264
11. Zetterling M, Roodakker KR, Berntsson SG, Edqvist PH, Latini F, Landtblom AM, Ponten F, Alafuzoff I, Larsson EM, Smits A. Extension of diffuse low-grade gliomas beyond radiological borders as shown by the coregistration of histopathological and magnetic resonance imaging data. J Neurosurg. 2016;125(5):1155–1166. Epub 20160226. doi:10.3171/2015.10.JNS15583

12. Xia L, Fang C, Chen G, Sun C. Relationship between the extent of resection and the survival of patients with low-grade gliomas: a systematic review and meta-analysis. BMC Cancer. 2018;18(1):48. Epub 20180106. doi:10.1186/s12885-017-3909-x
13. Duffau H. Long-term outcomes after supratotal resection of diffuse low-grade gliomas: a consecutive series with 11-year follow-up. Acta Neurochir (Wien). 2016;158(1):51–58. Epub 20151103. doi:10.1007/s00701-015-2621-3
14. Yordanova YN, Moritz-Gasser S, Duffau H. Awake surgery for WHO Grade II gliomas within "noneloquent" areas in the left dominant hemisphere: toward a "supratotal" resection. Clinical article. J Neurosurg. 2011;115(2):232–239. Epub 20110506. doi:10.3171/2011.3.JNS101333
15. Ius T, Angelini E, Thiebaut de Schotten M, Mandonnet E, Duffau H. Evidence for potentials and limitations of brain plasticity using an atlas of functional resectability of WHO grade II gliomas: towards a "minimal common brain". Neuroimage. 2011;56(3):992–1000. Epub 20110321. doi:10.1016/j.neuroimage.2011.03.022
16. Raiyani V, Singh S, Sardhara J, Mehrotra A, Mani V, Paliwal VK, Pal L, Kumar A, Dikshit P, Maurya VP, Verma PK, Behari S. Seizure outcome after lesionectomy with or without concomitant anteromedial temporal lobectomy for low-grade gliomas of the medial temporal lobe. Asian J Neurosurg. 2021;16(3):518–524. Epub 20210914. doi:10.4103/ajns.AJNS_496_20
17. Silva M, Vivancos C, Duffau H. The concept of Peritumoral Zone in diffuse low-grade gliomas: oncological and functional implications for a connectome-guided therapeutic attitude. Brain Sci. 2022;12(4). Epub 20220415. doi:10.3390/brainsci12040504
18. Kreatsoulas D, Damante M, Gruber M, Duru O, Elder JB. Supratotal surgical resection for low-grade glioma: a systematic review. Cancers (Basel). 2023;15(9). Epub 20230426. doi:10.3390/cancers15092493
19. Rossi M, Gay L, Ambrogi F, Conti Nibali M, Sciortino T, Puglisi G, Leonetti A, Mocellini C, Caroli M, Cordera S, Simonelli M, Pessina F, Navarria P, Pace A, Soffietti R, Ruda R, Riva M, Bello L. Association of supratotal resection with progression-free survival, malignant transformation, and overall survival in lower-grade gliomas. Neuro Oncol. 2021;23(5):812–826. doi:10.1093/neuonc/noaa225
20. Duffau H. Functional mapping before and after low-grade glioma surgery: a new way to decipher various spatiotemporal patterns of individual neuroplastic potential in brain tumor patients. Cancers (Basel). 2020;12(9). Epub 20200913. doi:10.3390/cancers12092611
21. Duffau H. A personalized longitudinal strategy in low-grade glioma patients: predicting oncological and neural interindividual variability and its changes over years to think one step ahead. J Pers Med. 2022;12(10). Epub 20221001. doi:10.3390/jpm12101621
22. Ng S, Duffau H. Brain plasticity profiling as a key support to therapeutic decision-making in low-grade glioma oncological strategies. Cancers (Basel). 2023;15(14). Epub 20230720. doi:10.3390/cancers15143698

CHAPTER 7

The Recurrence of Intracranial Meningiomas after Surgical Treatment

Simpson D, J Neurol Neurosurg Psychiatry. 1957 Feb;20(1):22–39

Reviewed by Abdurrahman I Islim and Omar N Pathmanaban

Objective/Research Question Donald Simpson aimed to investigate the risk of a symptomatic recurrence after surgery for a meningioma and to assess related factors.

Study Design Retrospective study using two cohorts: Oxford (April 1938–December 1954) and London (1928–1938).

Sample Size 339 patients (242 patients from Oxford and 97 from London).

Follow-Up Greater than 5 years for 175 patients (51.6%) and greater than 10 years for 105 patients (31%). Twenty-eight (8.3%) patients were followed up for more than 20 years.

Inclusion/Exclusion Criteria

- Inclusion Criteria
  - Patients with an intracranial meningioma were included.
- Exclusion Criteria
  - Patients with a spinal meningioma or a primary orbital meningioma were excluded.

Intervention or Treatment Received Surgical resection or biopsy.

Results 55 cases developed a symptomatic recurrence (16.2%). However, accounting for early deaths and patients lost to follow-up, Simpson estimated the risk of a symptomatic recurrence to be 21%. The average time between surgery and recurrence was 5 years. Simpson proposed a system to classify the extent of resection by the surgeon intraoperatively. This went from grade I, a macroscopically complete resection with excision of dural attachment,

DOI: 10.1201/9781003416197-7

any abnormal bone, and excision of the wall of the sinus where applicable (e.g. wall of the superior sagittal sinus for a parasagittal meningioma), to grade V, which was defined as a simple decompression or a biopsy. Grade II was the removal of any obvious intra- and extradural disease with coagulation of the dural origin of the tumor. Grade III was a complete resection of the intradural tumor without removal or coagulation of the tumor's dural attachment, and without resection of any extradural components such as invaded sinus or bone. Grade IV was a partial resection with a residual intradural tumor. After a complete resection involving any intradural or extradural components (grades I–II), the risk of recurrence was 12.7% compared to 41.7% after an incomplete resection (grades III–V). Simpson noted venous sinus invasion (15% of cases), bone invasion (20% of cases), and brain invasion (3.7% of cases) to be related to recurrence. He also noted that tumors which recurred did not have a distinct histological appearance; some tumors showed signs of dedifferentiation and increased mitoses, while others had a benign histological appearance. This was also observed in cases where a complete resection was achieved.

Paper Significance and Impact Simpson's 1957 description of surgically managed meningioma remains relevant to this day. Despite the paper predating the availability of computerized tomography (CT)/magnetic resonance imaging (MRI) and the WHO classification, the principles of his extent of meningioma resection grading system are still applicable. The varied clinical behavior of residual meningioma has continued to push the boundaries of molecular discovery and novel classification systems until the present day.

Several studies have been published over the last 20 years assessing the ongoing relevance of Simpson's grading system. In studies of 492 patients and 901 patients, the risk of long-term recurrence increased in a stepwise fashion with the increase in the Simpson grade and the authors recommended its ongoing use.[1,2] With the scale being a subjective intraoperative measure by the surgeon, a limitation acknowledged by Simpson himself, several authors advocate for abandoning Simpson's grading system and instead using objective measures of postoperative residual tumor, based on contrast-enhanced MRI or positron emission tomography (PET),[3] which were, of course, unavailable at the time of the original paper. An example of this is the Copenhagen grading system.[4] In this system, the study authors developed a system based on the presence of tumor cells in biopsies from the margins, and whether any tumor is detectable on a postoperative Gallium-68 DOTATATE PET-CT scan, which is highly sensitive and specific for meningioma. Again, it is worth noting that Simpson's assessments aimed to provide a tool (albeit subjective) for assessing the completeness of resection at a time when objective imaging biomarkers were not available. With MRI ubiquitously available now, in developed health systems, a contrast MRI will always be available to objectively evaluate the extent of resection. Nonetheless, the principles of the Simpson grading system and its emphasis on aggressive surgery, where safe, remain relevant. Moreover, more advanced molecular imaging, such as the use of Gallium-68 radiotracers, is not universally available and health economic evaluation and practical applicability across diverse health systems will likely continue to favor simple grading systems.

The other aspect of meningiomas that Simpson noted was their heterogeneous behavior after a seemingly complete resection, despite histologically benign features. Advanced molecular platforms have now revealed that some non-malignant WHO grade I meningiomas have molecular features, such as 1p and 22q loss, a TERT (telomerase reverse transcriptase) promoter mutation, or a CDKN2A/B homozygous deletion, which would indicate a more likely aggressive clinical course. Likewise, anaplastic (WHO grade III) and atypical (WHO grade II) meningiomas may clinically behave in an indolent manner and studies have shown that these lack the above molecular features.[5] Notably, even in the era of multimodal molecular stratification, the importance of the Simpson grade I or II excision stands the test of time in conferring a lower risk of recurrence.[6]

Study Limitations

- A historic and retrospective study which preceded the era of CT and MRI, the concepts of microsurgical and endoscopic neurosurgery, and the WHO classification of meningiomas.
- Data was included from two centers, Oxford and London. The Oxford dataset was described as complete; however, the London dataset was not, due to factors such as World War II.
- It is likely that not all tumors in the cohorts were meningiomas. Some of the tumors included may have been solitary fibrous tumors, based on the descriptions provided.
- Simpson described the risk of symptomatic recurrence; however, current practice and literature assess the risk of radiological recurrence. Radiologically recurrent meningiomas do not always become symptomatic.[7]
- The Simpson classification relies on a surgeon's intraoperative subjective assessment of resection. Imaging advances can play a prominent role in overcoming this limitation. MRI is the routine standard of care, but molecular imaging, most notably the Gallium-68 DOTATATE PET-CT scan, is now used in classification systems such as that proposed by the Copenhagen group.[4]

Relevant Studies

- Simon, M., Gousias, K. Grading meningioma resections: the Simpson classification and beyond. *Acta Neurochir* 166, 28 (2024). https://doi.org/10.1007/s00701-024-05910-9.[1]
- Rapoport, BI, McDermott, M. W., & Schwartz, T. H. (2021). Letter to the Editor. Time to move beyond the Simpson scale in meningioma surgery. Journal of Neurosurgery, 135(2), 661–662. https://doi.org/10.3171/2020.12.JNS204213.[3]

- Mathiesen, T., Haslund-Vinding, J., Skjøth-Rasmussen, J., Poulsgaard, L., Fugleholm, K., Mirian, C., Daniela Maier, A., Santarius, T., Rom Poulsen, F., Andrée Larsen, V., Winther Kristensen, B., Scheie, D., Law, I., & Ziebell, M. (2022). Letter to the Editor. Copenhagen grading of meningioma. Journal of Neurosurgery, 136(5), 1506–1508. https://doi.org/10.3171/2021.10.JNS204467.[8]

Summary Almost 70 years ago, Simpson demonstrated the importance of achieving a complete resection of a meningioma and introduced a system to assess this intraoperatively by the surgeon. The principles of this still stand today. However, more objective assessment systems have been developed considering new imaging, and histological and molecular advances. The heterogeneous behavior of meningioma can now be explained by molecular discoveries, which enable better prediction of tumor behavior and prognosis.

REFERENCES

1. Gousias K, Schramm J, Simon M. The Simpson grading revisited: aggressive surgery and its place in modern meningioma management. J Neurosurg. 2016 Sep;125(3):551–60. doi: 10.3171/2015.9.JNS15754. Epub 2016 Jan 29. PMID: 26824369.
2. Przybylowski CJ, Hendricks BK, Frisoli FA, et al. Prognostic value of the Simpson grading scale in modern meningioma surgery: Barrow Neurological Institute experience. J Neurosurg. 2020 Oct 23;135(2):515–523. doi: 10.3171/2020.6.JNS20374. PMID: 33096534.
3. Letter to the Editor. Time to move beyond the Simpson scale in meningioma surgery. J Neurosurg. 2021;135(2) Journals [Internet]. [cited 2024 Oct 28]. Available from: https://thejns.org/view/journals/j-neurosurg/135/2/article-p661.xml
4. Haslund-Vinding J, Skjoth-Rasmussen J, Poulsgaard L, et al. Proposal of a new grading system for meningioma resection: the Copenhagen Protocol. Acta Neurochir (Wien). 2022;164(1):229–238.
5. Sahm F, Aldape KD, Brastianos PK, et al. cIMPACT-NOW Update 8: Clarifications on molecular risk parameters and recommendations for WHO grading of meningiomas. Neuro Oncol. 2025 Feb 10;27(2):319-330. doi: 10.1093/neuonc/noae170. PMID: 39212325; PMCID: PMC11812049.
6. Wang JZ, Patil V, Landry AP, et al. Molecular classification to refine surgical and radiotherapeutic decision-making in meningioma. Nat Med. 2024;1–11.
7. Gillespie CS, Richardson GE, Mustafa MA, et al. volumetric growth and growth curve analysis of residual intracranial meningioma. Neurosurgery. 2023;92(4):734.
8. Mathiesen T, Haslund-Vinding J, Skjøth-Rasmussen J, et al. Letter to the Editor. Copenhagen grading of meningioma. Journal of Neurosurgery. 2022;136(5):1506–1508. https://doi.org/10.3171/2021.10.JNS204467

CHAPTER 8

Phase I/II Study of Resection and Intraoperative Cesium-131 Radioisotope Brachytherapy in Patients with Newly Diagnosed Brain Metastases

Wernicke AG, Yondorf MZ, Peng L, Trichter S, Nedialkova L, Sabbas A, Kulidzhanov F, Parashar B, Nori D, Clifford Chao KS, Christos P, Kovanlikaya I, Pannullo S, Boockvar JA, Stieg PE, Schwartz TH, J Neurosurg. 2014 Aug;121(2):338–348

Reviewed by Ken Virgin and Jignesh Tailor

Background Resected brain metastases have a high rate of local recurrence without adjuvant therapy. Adjuvant whole-brain radiotherapy (WBRT) has been the standard of care with a local control rate >90%. However, WBRT is delivered over 10–15 days, which can delay other therapy and is associated with acute and long-term toxicities. Permanent cesium-131 (Cs-131) implants can be used at the time of metastatic resection, thereby avoiding the need for any additional therapy.

Research Question/Objective The authors evaluated the safety, feasibility, and efficacy of a novel therapeutic approach with permanent Cs-131 brachytherapy at the resection for brain metastases.

Study Design Prospective cohort study.

Sample Size 24 patients with a newly diagnosed metastasis to the brain were accrued to a prospective protocol between 2010 and 2012. There were 10 frontal, 7 parietal, 4 cerebellar, 2 occipital, and 1 temporal metastases. Histology included lung cancer (16), breast cancer (2), kidney cancer (2), melanoma (2), colon cancer (1), and cervical cancer (1).

Follow-Up The median follow-up was 19.3 months (range 12.89–29.57 months).

DOI: 10.1201/9781003416197-8

Inclusion/Exclusion Criteria

- Inclusion Criteria
  - A metastatic tumor, for which surgery was indicated to relieve mass effect, to reduce symptoms, to obtain pathology for diagnostic purposes, or based on a size >2.5 cm.
  - Patients had to have an Eastern Cooperative Oncology Group (ECOG)/ Zubrod Performance Status) of 0, 1, or 2 and an expected survival of ≥6 months.

- Exclusion Criteria
  - Tumor proximity to the chiasm or brainstem (increasing the risk of radiation treatment).
  - Small-cell carcinoma metastatic to the brain.
  - Pregnancy or an unwillingness to practice a form of birth control such as abstinence or oral contraceptives.

Intervention or Treatment Received Patients underwent maximally safe resection of lesions. The extent of resection and whether surgery was performed en bloc or piecemeal was noted intraoperatively and from postoperative magnetic resonance imaging obtained within 48 hours of surgery.

At the time of resection, the size of the removed tumor (maximum diameter and volume), its location (supratentorial vs infratentorial), and its relationship to the pia mater (pial vs nonpial) were noted. Also, at the time of resection, Cs-131 stranded seeds (IsoRay) with an activity of 3–5 mCi were inserted with a planned dose of 80 Gy to a depth of 5 mm from the surface of the resection cavity. The volume implant was precalculated based on preoperative data on tumor size and an institutional physics nomogram and was adjusted in real time for the resulting intracavitary volume of the resected metastasis.

The 10-cm, suture-stranded Cs-131 seeds (0.5-cm interseed spacing) were delivered in strings of 10 seeds per string, subsequently cut into smaller lengths per the nomogram, and placed as a permanent volume implant along the cavity in a tangential pattern to maintain a 7- to 10-mm spacing between seeds. As a result, the cavity was lined with the seeds in a pattern like barrel staves or parallel tracks. The seeds were then covered with Surgicel (Ethicon) to prevent seed migration and alteration of dosimetry, and Tisseel (Baxter) was used to line the cavity to limit cavity shrinkage and further prevent seed dislodgement. Within 24–48 hours postimplant, the patient underwent computerized tomography scanning to determine dose distribution.

Primary Endpoint Local (resection cavity) freedom from progression (FFP): defined as the absence of new nodular contrast enhancement 5 mm or less from the resection cavity.

Secondary Endpoints

- Regional FFP: Defined as new or increased contrast enhancement more than 5 mm from the resection cavity.
- Distant FFP: Defined as new or increased contrast enhancement elsewhere in the brain.
- Median survival.
- Overall survival (OS).
- Toxicity.

Results The median age was 65 years (range 45–84 years). The median size of resected tumors was 2.7 cm (range 1.5–5.5 cm), and the median volume of the resected tumors was 10.31 cm^3 (range 1.77–87.11 cm^3). The median number of seeds used was 12 (range 4–35), with a median activity of 3.82 mCi per seed (range 3.31–4.83 mCi) and total activity of 46.91 mCi (range 15.31–130.70 mCi).

Local FFP was 100%. There was one adjacent leptomeningeal recurrence, resulting in a one-year regional FFP of 93.8% (95% CI, 63.2–99.1%). One-year distant FFP was 48.4% (95% CI, 26.3–67.4%).

Median OS was 9.9 months (95% CI, 4.8 months, upper limit not estimated) and 1-year OS was 50.0% (95% CI, 29.1–67.8%).

Complications included a cerebrospinal fluid leak (1), seizure (1), and infection (1). There was no radiation necrosis.

Conclusion The use of post-resection permanent Cs-131 brachytherapy implants resulted in no local recurrences and no radiation necrosis. This treatment was safe, well-tolerated, and convenient for patients, resulting in a short radiation treatment course, high response rate, and minimal toxicity.

Reviewer Commentary Brachytherapy occupies a curious place in the history of neuro-oncology: a technique that is both old and, at times, forgotten. The concept of placing radioactive material directly into brain tumors dates back more than a century, with early reports of intracranial brachytherapy appearing as early as 1914, when Frazier described implantation of radioactive material into a glioma.[1] Over the ensuing decades, neurosurgeons and radiation oncologists explored multiple isotopes and delivery strategies, driven by a simple but compelling idea: deliver a high dose of radiation to tumor tissue while sparing the surrounding brain.

Throughout the latter half of the twentieth century, iodine-125 (I-125) became the dominant radioisotope used for intracranial brachytherapy, followed by palladium-103 (Pd-103) in selected settings.[2,3] These isotopes allowed permanent implantation and relatively conformal dose delivery, and early single-institution series reported encouraging local control. However, enthusiasm was tempered by variability in outcomes and, critically, by concerns regarding radiation necrosis, which emerged as a significant and sometimes devastating complication.[4,5]

Two landmark randomized controlled trials crystallized this ambivalence. Laperriere and colleagues[6] and Selker and colleagues[7] evaluated I-125 brachytherapy in malignant gliomas and demonstrated no clear survival advantage compared with standard external beam approaches. Moreover, brachytherapy demonstrated higher rates of radiation necrosis, which overshadowed any potential benefits of the technique. While these studies were methodologically rigorous and influential, they were conducted in an era preceding modern imaging, molecular classification, and refined surgical techniques. Moreover, they relied on I-125, an isotope characterized by a long half-life and prolonged low-dose radiation exposure, features now understood to contribute substantially to delayed radiation necrosis. As a result, brachytherapy gradually receded from routine neuro-oncologic practice.

The study by Wernicke et al. marks a pivotal turning point in this narrative. This work introduced cesium-131 (Cs-131), a novel radioisotope with fundamentally different physical and radiobiological properties. Cs-131 has a shorter half-life (9.7 days), a higher dose rate, and more rapid dose deposition, with approximately 90% of the therapeutic dose delivered within the first month.[8] These characteristics translate into several practical advantages: reduced exposure to normal brain tissue, a lower risk of radiation necrosis, and earlier initiation of systemic therapy.

In their prospective phase I/II experience, Wernicke and colleagues demonstrated excellent local control following resection and intraoperative Cs-131 implantation for newly diagnosed brain metastases, notably without any observed cases of radiation necrosis.[9] This finding is particularly striking when contrasted with the historical I-125 series and reinforces the notion that prior failures of brachytherapy may have reflected the limitations of isotope selection rather than the concept itself. The study was limited by the small sample size and lack of long-term data beyond 20 months. However, several other groups have reported similar experiences with Cs-131, namely a significant reduction in the degree of radiation necrosis and safety.

Study Limitations As an early phase I/II study, this work has several expected limitations. The cohort was small, single-institution, and non-randomized, with outcomes likely influenced by careful patient selection and uniformly achieved gross total resection. While the absence of radiation necrosis is encouraging, longer follow-up and larger, comparative studies are needed to confirm the durability of local control and late toxicity. Importantly, these limitations do not diminish the study's impact but rather explain why it served as a catalyst for subsequent multicenter and randomized trials rather than a definitive practice changing study on its own.

Relevant Studies This study marked a turning point that renewed interest in post-resection brachytherapy and helped bring the technique back into contemporary neurosurgical practice. By demonstrating the feasibility and safety of Cs-131–based intraoperative radiation, it directly informed the development of surgically implanted platforms such as GammaTile, a collagen-based Cs-131 delivery system designed for use at the time of tumor resection.[10] GammaTile is now being evaluated in multiple prospective clinical trials, including the ROADS phase III randomized trial in brain metastases, the GESTALT trial integrating GammaTile into standard therapy for newly diagnosed glioblastoma, and the BRIDGES trial comparing GammaTile-based treatment paradigms with conventional care.[11] Collectively, these efforts reflect a clear resurgence of post-resection brachytherapy as a viable and evolving strategy in modern neuro-oncology.

Looking forward, the implications extend beyond adult neuro-oncology. Pediatric brain tumors present a particularly compelling opportunity for intracranial brachytherapy. External beam radiation and proton beam therapy, while effective, are associated with profound and lasting neurocognitive sequelae in children.[12] In addition, delays inherent to referral and treatment at specialized centers can allow local recurrence or progression during critical windows. Localized, immediate radiation delivery at the time of surgery offers a potential strategy to mitigate both toxicity and delay.

In this context, the re-emergence of Cs-131 brachytherapy represents more than a technical advance; it reflects a philosophical shift toward precision, timing, and tissue preservation. Building on this foundation, we will be leading a phase I clinical trial of GammaTile brachytherapy following resection of recurrent pediatric brain tumors at Indiana University School of Medicine, Riley Hospital for Children.

Taken together, the work by Wernicke et al. stands as a landmark, not because it introduces brachytherapy to neurosurgery, but because it shows how revisiting an old idea with new tools can meaningfully change the field.

REFERENCES

1. Frazier CH. Intracranial tumors treated by radium implantation. Ann Surg. 1914;60:465–475.
2. Schulder M, Black PM, Shrieve DC, Alexander E III, Loeffler JS. Permanent low-activity iodine-125 implants for cerebral metastases. J Neurooncol. 1997;33:213–221.
3. Schwarz SB, Thon N, Nikolajek K, Niyazi M, Tonn JC, Belka C. Iodine-125 and palladium-103 brachytherapy for brain tumors — a review. Radiat Oncol. 2012;7:30.
4. Huang K, Sneed PK, Kunwar S, et al. Surgical resection and permanent iodine-125 brachytherapy for brain metastases. J Neurooncol. 2009;91:83–93.
5. Gutin PH, Phillips TL, Wara WM, et al. Brachytherapy of recurrent malignant brain tumors with removable high-activity iodine-125 sources. Journal of Neurosurgery. 1984;60(1):61–68.
6. Laperriere NJ, Leung PM, McKenzie S, et al. Randomized study of brachytherapy in malignant glioma. Int J Radiat Oncol Biol Phys. 1998;41:1005–1011.

7. Selker RG, Shapiro WR, Burger P, et al. The Brain Tumor Cooperative Group randomized trial of I-125 brachytherapy. Neurosurgery. 2002;51:343–357.
8. Ravi A, Keller BM, Pignol JP. A comparison of postimplant dosimetry for Pd-103 versus Cs-131 seeds. Med Phys. 2011;38:6046–6052.
9. Wernicke AG, Yondorf M, Peng L, et al. Phase I/II study of resection and intraoperative cesium-131 brachytherapy in brain metastases. J Neurosurg. 2014;121:338–348.
10. Garcia MA, Turner A, Brachman DG. The role of GammaTile in the treatment of brain tumors: a technical and clinical overview. J Neurooncol. 2024;166(2):203–212.
11. Chen AM, Chang S, Pouliot J, et al. Advances in intracranial brachytherapy platforms. Neuro Oncol. 2018;20:149–158.
12. Merchant TE, Pollack IF, Loeffler JS. Brain tumors across the age spectrum: biology, therapy, and late effects. Lancet Oncol. 2010;11:83–94.

CHAPTER 9

Natural History of Asymptomatic Colloid Cysts of the Third Ventricle

Pollock BE, Huston J, J Neurosurg. 1999 Sep;91(3):364–369

Reviewed by Bruce E Pollock

Research Question/Objective Determine the natural history of patients with incidentally discovered colloid cysts of the third ventricle.

Study Design Retrospective review of patients diagnosed with asymptomatic colloid cysts at the Mayo Clinic, Rochester, Minnesota, between 1974 and 1998.

Sample Size 58 patients.

Follow-Up Mean follow-up was 79 months (range 7–268 months) after diagnosis of a colloid cyst; the number of patients followed at 2, 5, and 10 years after diagnosis was 40, 28, and 14, respectively.

Inclusion/Exclusion Criteria

- Inclusion Criteria
    - The inclusion criteria were: 162 patients diagnosed with a colloid cyst of the third ventricle between 1974 and 1998.
    - Considered asymptomatic with respect to the colloid cyst at the time of diagnosis.
    - Managed non-operatively with observation and serial neuroimaging rather than immediate surgical treatment.

- Exclusion Criteria
    - 94 patients (58%) were excluded because they were either symptomatic from the cyst and underwent surgical resection or had previously undergone a surgical procedure for their cyst.
    - 3 patients were excluded from the study because they died within 6 months of unrelated causes.
    - 7 patients were lost to follow-up.

Intervention Observation with serial neuroimaging.

DOI: 10.1201/9781003416197-9

Results Symptomatic progression related to the cyst was 0%, 0%, and 8% at 2, 5, and 10 years, respectively. No patient died suddenly during the follow-up interval. Two of 34 patients (6%) with imaging follow-up (6%) had either cyst growth ($n = 1$) or developed hydrocephalus ($n = 1$) at a mean of 41 months after diagnosis (range 4–160 months).

Conclusion Patients diagnosed with asymptomatic colloid cysts can be managed safely with observation and serial neuroimaging. If a patient becomes symptomatic, the cyst is enlarging, or the patient develops hydrocephalus, prompt neurosurgical intervention is necessary to prevent neurologic decline from these benign tumors.

Author/Reviewer Commentary At the time we wrote "Natural History of Asymptomatic Colloid Cysts of the Third Ventricle",[1] I had recently joined the Department of Neurological Surgery at the Mayo Clinic, Rochester, Minnesota. Although the bulk of my practice involved stereotactic radiosurgery, I was required to participate in the care of a wide variety of neurologic conditions, including basic spine, trauma, and adult tumors. In this context, I was periodically consulted to see a patient with a colloid cyst, and I struggled to provide the best advice for patients who were asymptomatic, and this lesion was discovered incidentally.

Up to that point, observation of patients diagnosed with incidental colloid cysts was rarely recommended because of the fear of acute neurological deterioration secondary to ventricular obstruction. Little and MacCarty reported that four of 38 patients (11%) with colloid cysts seen at the Mayo Clinic between 1929 and 1973 presented with a sudden deterioration and death.[2] Mathiesen et al. reported 37 patients with colloid cysts managed at the Karolinska Institute, Stockholm, Sweden, between 1984 and 1995.[3] Five patients were admitted in a comatose state, and two died despite emergency ventriculostomy. Four of seven patients who were initially observed became symptomatic and required surgical resection 6–37 months after their diagnosis. They concluded that most younger patients would become symptomatic during their lifetime and that expectant surgical resection is the preferred management strategy. Conversely, Kondziolka and Lunsford recommended observation in six asymptomatic patients with small colloid cysts (<7 mm in diameter) evaluated between 1984 and 1995 at the University of Pittsburgh.[4] The patients remained asymptomatic in follow-up from 3 to 7 years after diagnosis. Based on their experience, they felt that observation with serial imaging is possible for asymptomatic patients with small cysts and normal ventricular size.

Based on the paucity of information available to guide treatment decisions for these patients, I asked my friend, John Huston III, if the radiology department could provide a list of all the patients diagnosed at the Mayo Clinic with colloid cysts. The answer was yes, and he provided me with the names and clinic numbers of 162 patients imaged between January 1974 and June 1998 with third ventricular colloid cysts. The clinical histories and available imaging were reviewed, and patients without recent follow-up were contacted by telephone to determine their clinical status and most recent neuroimaging.

Surprisingly, only one patient (2%) had progressive symptoms related to the colloid cyst. The patient was a 57-year-old woman who, 8.4 years after diagnosis, had developed enlarged ventricles even though the cyst itself was unchanged in appearance and she remained asymptomatic. Surgical resection of the colloid cyst was recommended, but the patient refused. Five months later, the patient developed acute obstructive hydrocephalus, and despite the emergent placement of bilateral external ventricular drains, which were later converted to ventriculoperitoneal shunts, the patient sustained a significant brainstem injury. She died 4 years later in a nursing home, more than 13 years after she was diagnosed with a colloid cyst. The 2-, 5-, and 10-year incidence of cyst-related symptoms was 0%, 0%, and 8%, respectively. Importantly, no patient died suddenly during the follow-up interval. Consequently, we concluded that it is safe to observe patients diagnosed with asymptomatic colloid cysts. If a patient becomes symptomatic, the cyst is enlarging, or the patient develops hydrocephalus, prompt neurosurgical intervention is necessary to prevent neurologic decline from these benign tumors.

Study Limitations This study had several limitations that may affect the accuracy of its conclusions. First, the physical films of patients were available for review only for studies performed after 1988. As a result, we depended on radiology reports to characterize the cysts for scans done before that time. Second, 42 patients (72%) underwent computerized tomography alone, so that the initial cyst size may not be precise, and the magnetic resonance imaging (MRI) characteristics were not available for all patients. Third, the mean age of patients at the time of colloid cyst diagnosis was 57 years, so a mean follow-up of 6.6 years may be inadequate for this group whose life expectancy approaches three decades. Last, many patients (41%) did not have any imaging follow-up, so potential cyst growth or changes in the imaging characteristics could not be evaluated in those patients.

Relevant Studies After the publication of this paper, we proposed a theory on the natural history of third ventricular colloid cysts.[5] We compared 87 patients with cyst-related symptoms having surgery to 68 asymptomatic patients who were managed conservatively. Recursive partitioning was used to examine the association of patient and tumor characteristics with the development of cyst-related symptoms. Multivariate analysis found that younger patient age, cyst size, ventricular dilatation, and increased signal on T2-weighted MRI correlated with cyst-related symptoms. Our theory put forward the concept that symptom development relates to the interaction of three factors: the rate of cyst growth, the development of cerebrospinal fluid (CSF) obstruction, and the fact that most colloid cysts stop enlarging over time. For patients with slow cyst growth, if the cyst stops enlarging before causing CSF obstruction, the patient remains asymptomatic and can be managed conservatively. In a subset of patients, cyst growth is gradual and then stops before causing sudden CSF blockage, although the ventricles may become enlarged due to the elastic properties of the brain changing over time, shifting the intracranial pressure-volume curve to the right. A steady state is subsequently re-established, allowing the intracranial pressure to remain normal despite the ventricles being enlarged. Again, observation with serial neuroimaging is generally safe for this group of patients. Alternatively, if cyst growth is rapid or continues slowly over time, CSF flow from the lateral ventricles becomes blocked and the patient develops cyst-related symptoms and requires surgery.

In 2016, Beaumont and colleagues performed a retrospective review of 163 patients with colloid cysts managed at Washington University, St. Louis, Missouri, from 1996 to 2014, and developed the Colloid Cyst Risk Score (CCRS).[6] Fifty-seven patients with incidental cysts were followed with surveillance neuroimaging (mean follow-up 5.1 years). Five patients with incidental cysts (8.8%) progressed and underwent resection. No patient with an incidental, asymptomatic colloid cyst experienced acute obstructive hydrocephalus or sudden neurological deterioration in the absence of antecedent trauma. The five risk factors for symptomatic colloid cysts (age at presentation [<65 years], presence of headache, cyst diameter ≥7 mm, cyst hyperintensity on fluid-attenuated inversion recovery [FLAIR] MRI, and cyst location in an anatomical risk zone I [defined as within the foramen of Monro at the anterior margin of the third ventricle]) were combined into a simple 5-point grading scale (the CCRS). The CCRS provided statistically significant stratification of symptomatic patients across the five CCRS levels, ranging from 5.9% in CCRS 2 to 96.0% in CCRS 5.

More recently, Velicu et al. from King's College Hospital, London, UK, reviewed 82 colloid cyst patients (asymptomatic, $n = 60$) treated between 2009 and 2019.[7] No asymptomatic patient experienced acute neurologic decline during a mean follow-up of 58 months. Logistic regression analysis found three risk factors for symptomatic colloid cysts: T1-weighted MRI hyperintense/mixed signal appearance, location in risk zone I (as defined by Beaumont et al.[6]), and a volume >236.49 mm^3. They concluded that few asymptomatic colloid cysts showed progression requiring surgery, with no instances of acute deterioration or fatal events, thereby supporting a conservative approach for this group of patients.

REFERENCES

1. Pollock BE, Huston III J. Natural history of asymptomatic colloid cysts of the third ventricle. J Neurosurg. 1999;91:364–369.
2. Little JR, MacCarty CS. Colloid cysts of the third ventricle. J Neurosurg. 1974;39:230–235.
3. Mathiesen T, Grane P, Lindgren L, Lindquist C. Third ventricle colloid cysts: a consecutive 12-year series. J Neurosurg. 1997;86:5–12.
4. Kondziolka D, Lunsford LD. Management of colloid cysts. Cont Neurosurg. 1994;16(9):1.
5. Pollock BE, Schreiner SA, Huston III J. A theory on the natural history of colloid cysts of the third ventricle. Neurosurgery. 2000;46:1077–1083.
6. Beaumont TL, Limbrick DD, Rich KM, Wippold FJ, Dacey RG. Natural history of colloid cysts of the third ventricle. J Neurosurg. 2016;125:1420–1430.
7. Velicu MA, Rossmann K, Vahedi A, Lavrador JP, Vergani F, Bhangoo R, Gullan R, Booth T, Ashkan K. On natural history and management of colloid cysts: Time to rethink? World Neurosurg. 2023;170:e188–e199.

CHAPTER 10

Surgical Risk as Related to Time of Intervention in the Repair of Intracranial Aneurysms

Hunt WE, Hess RM, J Neurosurg. 1968 Jan;28(1):14–20

Reviewed by Matthew Tobin and Brad Bohnstedt

Research Question/Objective Does early vs late surgical intervention in ruptured intracranial aneurysms affect patient outcome?

Study Design Retrospective review.

Sample Size 275 patients with aneurysmal subarachnoid hemorrhage over a 12-year period.

Intervention or Treatment Received Patients were classified according to surgical risk based on a modified Botterell's classification:

- Grade I: Asymptomatic, or minimal headache and slight nuchal rigidity.
- Grade II: Moderate to severe headache, nuchal rigidity, no neurological deficit other than cranial nerve palsy.
- Grade III: Drowsiness, confusion, or mild focal deficit.
- Grade IV: Stupor, moderate to severe hemiparesis, possibly early decerebrate rigidity and vegetative disturbances.
- Grade V: Deep coma, decerebrate rigidity, moribund appearance.

Results In patients admitted at a good neurological grade (I–II), overall mortality was 20%, decreasing to 14% among those who underwent surgery; nearly all non-operative deaths were due to early rebleeding. Operative mortality was strongly grade-dependent, at 1.4% for grade I and 22% for grade II patients, with most grade II deaths attributable to cerebral infarction from vasospasm and meningeal inflammation. In patients admitted at grade III, early surgery was associated with high mortality (40%). A delayed treatment strategy allowed 55% of these patients to improve to grades I–II before surgery, substantially lowering operative risk. In this group, cerebral infarction was the predominant cause of death, while rebleeding was less frequent.

DOI: 10.1201/9781003416197-10

Conclusion This review of 275 patients with intracranial aneurysms identified neurological grade, meningeal reaction, and associated systemic disease as the key determinants of surgical risk. Aneurysm surgery was associated with very low mortality in patients without significant meningeal inflammation, neurological deficit, or major comorbidity. Meningeal reaction alone substantially increased operative risk. Early surgical intervention was most beneficial for patients presenting in good neurological condition (grades I–II) to reduce the risk of rebleeding, whereas patients presenting in poorer condition benefited from initial conservative management, allowing neurological improvement before surgery and thereby reducing operative mortality.

Author/Reviewer Commentary The article "Surgical Risk as Related to Time of Intervention in the Repair of Intracranial Aneurysms" addresses a pivotal question in the field of neurosurgery: how does the timing of surgical intervention influence outcomes for patients with intracranial aneurysms? Intracranial aneurysms, particularly those that have ruptured, can lead to life-threatening hemorrhagic strokes and significant neurological impairment. Given these serious implications, timely surgical intervention is essential for minimizing complications and improving survival rates. This review will critically evaluate the article's findings and implications and how they have shaped aneurysm treatment over recent decades.

The authors conducted a retrospective analysis to examine surgical outcomes for patients' ruptured intracranial aneurysms, specifically focusing on how the timing of surgical repair affects these outcomes. To do this, Hunt and Hess utilized their updated grading system for patients presenting with aneurysmal subarachnoid hemorrhage, which was based on a prior classification by Botterell et al.[1,2] The study categorized the timing of intervention into early vs delayed treatment. Early treatment was defined as treatment within 24 hours for grade I or II patients, while late treatment was defined as treatment at the time when higher-grade patients (grades III–V) became grade I–II patients. By comparing patient outcomes across these categories, the authors assess the rates of complications, rebleeding, and overall survival associated with different timings of surgical intervention.

The major finding of this work was that surgical intervention for ruptured aneurysms at the early timepoint, i.e. within 24 hours, portends a survival benefit to low-grade subarachnoid hemorrhage patients. Additionally, increased morbidity and mortality in those patients not operated on largely correlated with either higher early rebleeding rates or with complications related to delayed cerebral ischemia from vasospasm. The experience of Hunt and Hess suggests that in the lower-grade patients, the risk of complications was higher in those patients presenting with signs and symptoms of meningeal reaction, which can lead to worse surgical outcomes.

Furthermore, Hunt and Hess show that a large proportion of higher-grade patients eventually make it to the lower-grade categories after an initial period of conservative management to mitigate early rebleeding or the sequelae of the initial hemorrhage. Key findings from the study suggest that earlier intervention correlates with significantly reduced complication rates and improved survival, especially for those with ruptured aneurysms. The authors advocated for a shift in the thought process for the treatment of these patients, suggesting that treatment of ruptured aneurysms should occur more expeditiously compared to previous thought patterns.

Study Limitations While the benefit of early intervention was shown, there are some key limitations in the original paper. One such limitation is that there was not a standardized definition for the delayed treatment group. While the early treatment group was defined within 24 hours, the delayed group consisted of all patients who originally presented as high grade on admission but eventually became lower-grade patients. The timeframe in which patients improved from high grade to low grade was not well characterized, which could introduce some level of bias in the data for the delayed surgery group.

One significant limitation was that the original paper did not discuss or control for confounding factors, which we now know play a significantly large role in deciding on the role for the treatment of ruptured aneurysms. Considerations including, for instance, patient age, patient comorbidities, and the characteristics of the aneurysm, were not well addressed. All of these factors, which we now know contribute to patient outcomes, were not well described in the original paper. While specific individual aneurysm characteristics were excluded, Hunt and Hess did subcategorize patients into those in which extracranial vessel sacrifice was required vs those patients that only had intracranial procedures done. These two different surgical modalities alone could very well contribute to differing patient outcomes and this was perhaps illustrated by the higher mortality in those patients who had some form of vessel sacrifice compared to those in which just the aneurysm alone was treated.

An additional limitation of the study was that there was no longitudinal data presented on patient outcome beyond the index hospitalization. While the in-hospital mortality data is critical, of equal importance is how these patients did long-term and what sort of functional outcomes they had. Because of the lack of long-term data, the paper may fail to capture the lasting effects of surgical timing on a patient's overall health outcome. While the paper contributes valuable insights into the timing of surgical interventions for intracranial aneurysms, the limitations must be carefully considered when interpreting its findings.

Relevant Studies While the above limitations should not be discounted, more recent work has gone on to show similar results compared to the original study, indicating that earlier management of ruptured intracranial aneurysms decreases overall morbidity and mortality.[3–5] However, modern neurosurgical practice has evolved considerably since the publication of Hunt and Hess's study. With the rapid evolution of endovascular therapy options, these approaches are increasingly employed to secure ruptured aneurysms compared to open surgical treatments. Further, data such as that from the International Subarachnoid Aneurysm Trial (ISAT) suggest more favorable mortality outcomes for the endovascular management of ruptured aneurysms.[3]

Advances in microsurgical techniques, endovascular therapy, and neurocritical care have transformed the management of intracranial aneurysms. Current guidelines often advocate for early intervention in good-grade patients (those with minimal neurological deficits) while still acknowledging the potential benefits of delayed surgery in specific clinical scenarios, such as poor-grade patients or those with significant medical comorbidities.

Furthermore, the introduction of endovascular techniques, such as coil embolization and flow diversion, has provided an alternative to open surgical repair, allowing for earlier and potentially safer intervention in patients previously deemed high-risk for surgery. Studies comparing outcomes of surgical vs endovascular treatment have shown favorable results for the latter, particularly in reducing the risk of rebleeding and overall morbidity.[3] Additionally, newer studies have shown that not all high-grade patients are doomed to poor outcomes, with up to 50% of high-grade patients having favorable outcomes.[6,7] As such, there has been some new data suggesting that the original Hunt and Hess grading scale be recategorized into a "modified Hunt and Hess grading scale" which also incorporates a patient's presenting Glascow Coma Scale into the grade, with the aim of trying to incorporate the degree of brainstem dysfunction on presentation.[8]

The original Hunt and Hess paper is a seminal work in the field of neurosurgery and established, early on, that the early treatment of ruptured intracranial aneurysms leads to improved outcomes for these patients. This study on the timing of surgical intervention for intracranial aneurysms remains a cornerstone in the field of neurosurgery. Its findings catalyzed a reevaluation of surgical timing, emphasizing the risks associated with early intervention and shaping subsequent clinical practices. However, the evolution of diagnostic and therapeutic technologies necessitates a contextual understanding of their conclusions. Modern neurosurgery continues to build upon the foundational work of Hunt and Hess, integrating new evidence and techniques to optimize patient outcomes in the treatment of intracranial aneurysms.

Summary In summary, the original Hunt and Hess paper represents a landmark contribution that fundamentally shaped the evaluation and management of patients with aneurysmal subarachnoid hemorrhage. While the study's historical significance is undeniable, ongoing research and clinical advancements ensure that the management of intracranial aneurysms remains a dynamic and continually improving field, always striving to balance the risks and benefits of surgical intervention to achieve the best possible patient outcomes.

REFERENCES

1. Botterell EH, Lougheed WM, Scott JW, Vandewater SL. Hypothermia, and interruption of carotid, or carotid and vertebral circulation, in the surgical management of intracranial aneurysms. J Neurosurg. 1956;13(1):1–42.
2. Hunt WE, Meagher JN, Barnes JE. The management of intracranial aneurysm. J Neurosurg. 1962;19:34–40.
3. Molyneux AJ, Kerr RS, Yu LM, et al. International subarachnoid aneurysm trial (ISAT) of neurosurgical clipping versus endovascular coiling in 2143 patients with ruptured intracranial aneurysms: a randomised comparison of effects on survival, dependency, seizures, rebleeding, subgroups, and aneurysm occlusion. Lancet. 2005;366(9488):809–817.
4. Kassell NF, Torner JC, Haley EC, Jr., Jane JA, Adams HP, Kongable GL. The International Cooperative Study on the Timing of Aneurysm Surgery. Part 1: Overall management results. J Neurosurg. 1990;73(1):18–36.
5. Phillips TJ, Dowling RJ, Yan B, Laidlaw JD, Mitchell PJ. Does treatment of ruptured intracranial aneurysms within 24 hours improve clinical outcome? Stroke. 2011;42(7): 1936–1945.
6. Komotar RJ, Schmidt JM, Starke RM, et al. Resuscitation and critical care of poor-grade subarachnoid hemorrhage. Neurosurgery. 2009;64(3):397–410; discussion 410–391.
7. Wartenberg KE. Critical care of poor-grade subarachnoid hemorrhage. Curr Opin Crit Care. 2011;17(2):85–93.
8. Al-Mufti F, Dicpinigaitis AJ, Bowers CA, et al. Prognostication following aneurysmal subarachnoid hemorrhage: the modified hunt and hess grading scale. Stroke Vasc Interv Neurol. 2024;4(5):e001349.

Chapter 11

International Subarachnoid Aneurysm Trial (ISAT) of Neurosurgical Clipping versus Endovascular Coiling in 2,143 Patients with Ruptured Intracranial Aneurysms: A Randomized Trial

Molyneux A, Kerr R, Stratton I, Sandercock P, Clarke M, Shrimpton J, Holman R; International Subarachnoid Aneurysm Trial (ISAT) Collaborative Group, Lancet. 2002 Oct; 360(9342):1267–1274

Reviewed by Richard Kerr

Research Question/Objective To compare the safety and efficacy of a policy of endovascular detachable coil treatment of ruptured intracranial aneurysms, with a policy of standard treatment using open surgery and direct clipping.

Study Design Prospective randomized multicenter clinical trial.

Sample Size 2,143 patients randomly assigned to either neurosurgical clipping (n = 1,070) or endovascular treatment with detachable platinum coils (n = 1,073).

Follow-Up Patients were followed up at 2 months, 12 months and yearly thereafter using the modified Rankin Scale. Data was collected with a validated method using a postal questionnaire with a Euroqol health state questionnaire, and questions concerning employment status, further hospital admissions and episodes of rebleeding.

Inclusion/Exclusion Criteria

- Inclusion Criteria
  - Confirmed a subarachnoid hemorrhage (SAH) within the last 28 days.
  - Intracranial aneurysm considered to be responsible for the bleed.
  - Clinical state that justified treatment by either surgery or coiling.
  - Aneurysm judged to be suitable for either treatment method based on the angiographic anatomy.
  - Uncertainty as to how the aneurysm should be treated.
  - Appropriate informed consent or assent was obtained according to criteria laid down by the local ethics committee.

DOI: 10.1201/9781003416197-11

- Exclusion criteria
  - SAH occurred more than 28 days before randomization.
  - Patient unsuitable for one or both treatments.
  - Consent refused.
  - Patient participating in another trial of SAH treatment.

Intervention or Treatment Received Most patients received their allocated treatments (95.3%). Nine patients allocated to endovascular treatment crossed over to surgery, and 38 allocated to neurosurgery crossed over to endovascular treatment. However, the analysis was performed according to the intention-to-treat principle.

Results The trial aimed to recruit 2,500 patients but was stopped early by the steering committee, having been advised of the interim results. The results showed that 23.7% of the patients allocated to endovascular treatment were dependent or dead at 1 year compared to 30.6% of those allocated to surgery. This represents a relative and absolute risk reduction of 22.6% and 6.9%, respectively, for patients in this randomized cohort allocated to endovascular treatment.

Conclusion The results indicate that for the patients with ruptured intracranial aneurysms eligible for either treatment randomized in this trial, endovascular treatment was significantly more likely to result in survival free of disability at 1 year when compared to open surgery. However, long-term follow-up was vital to ensure the durability of benefit. The data at 1 year indicated that the risk of further bleeding was low with either treatment, but more frequent with endovascular coiling.

Author/Reviewer Commentary This was a pragmatic trial, examining a relatively new form of treatment for patients following aneurysmal SAH. It was an opportunity to critically examine the safety and efficacy of this novel therapy, and thus to try to establish the role of this when considering treatment of this acute and potentially devastating condition. A small trial had already been published from Finland that suggested endovascular therapy may provide an advantage,[1,2] but ISAT was the first large multicenter randomized trial to address this question. We conducted a small pilot feasibility study initially, but the formal trial started in 1997. The trial results firmly indicated that for the patients randomized (of good grade with small anterior circulation aneurysms), endovascular therapy did confer a significant advantage, and certainly in the UK, it resulted in many more patients being treated with coils rather than open surgery.

The publication of ISAT was met with significant criticism around the applicability of the results to all patients admitted after SAH, as only 20% of those screened were randomized in the study; concerns were expressed about the long-term durability and the risk of requiring further treatment and/or suffering a rebleed, and the possible positive impact that neurovascular subspecialists would have on the surgical outcomes.

These concerns were summarized in position statements from various national societies.[3,4]

The applicability of ISAT to all patients after SAH was a continuing concern, as well as the issue of neurosurgical vascular subspecialists, and to answer this question, a North American trial was designed based on one center, but with all patients admitted into the trial. The Barrow Ruptured Aneurysm Trial (BRAT) published the 1-year results in 2012,[5] these showing the same outcome that had been identified in ISAT. Those treated endovascularly had fewer poor outcomes than those treated surgically.

A meta-analysis[6] of the 3 published trials followed, concluding that "On the basis of the analysis of the 3 high-quality prospective controlled trials available, there is strong evidence to indicate that endovascular coil embolization is associated with better outcomes compared with surgical clipping in patients amenable to either therapeutic strategy". A subsequent Cochrane review[7] published in 2018 also concluded that "if the aneurysm is considered suitable for both neurosurgical clipping and endovascular coiling, coiling is associated with a better outcome".

That trend has continued and now endovascular treatment is considered by some to be 'the mainstay' of treatment, especially with the advances in coil and other device technology.[8] However, there have been advances in surgical techniques as well and published guidance from the American Heart and Stroke associations on the management of ruptured aneurysms[9] suggests that a team-based approach is crucial, concluding that "balancing the goal of securing the ruptured aneurysm with risk of intervention is based on patient and aneurysm characteristics and should be determined by specialists with expertise in endovascular and surgical treatments".

Study Limitations The patients randomized were predominantly those with small (<10 mm) anterior circulation aneurysms and of good grade. Few posterior circulation aneurysms were included or those of poor grade, and there was an underrepresentation of middle cerebral lesions.

Follow-up was limited and, as has been indicated, a long-term review is crucial to establish durability. Other aspects, such as the risk of epilepsy, assessments of delayed ischemia, rebleeding rates, neuropsychological impact and long-term mortality associated with SAH, all needed to be addressed.

Relevant Studies A discussion of studies that came before or after the discussed article that are of relevance and provide additional context.

A follow-up of patients randomized was crucial to establish durability. Further results from ISAT were published in 2005[10] and 2015,[11] this 18-year follow-up of the UK cohort confirming that at 10 years, the probability of disability-free survival remained significantly greater after endovascular therapy.

A follow-up analysis of the BRAT study was published in 2013,[12] 2015,[13] and 2019,[14] the final study considering the outcome of only the saccular aneurysms treated at this one center, concluding that there was no significant difference in terms of the modified Rankin Scale outcomes or death.

Other relevant studies include analysis of the risk of seizures,[15] a comparison of the neuropsychological impact[16] and a study of the required retreatment rates.[17]

REFERENCES

1. Vanninen R, Koivisto T, Saari T, et al. Ruptured intracranial aneurysms: acute endovascular treatment with electrolytically detachable coils—a prospective randomized study. Radiology. 1999;211:325–365.
2. Koivisto T, Vanninen R, Hurskainen H, et al. Outcomes of early endovascular versus surgical treatment of ruptured cerebral aneurysms: a prospective randomized study. Stroke. 2000;31:2369–2377.
3. Derdeyn CP, Barr JD, Berenstein A, Connors JJ, Dion JE, Duckwiler GR, Higashida RT, Strother CM, Tomsick TA, Turski P. The International Subarachnoid Aneurysm Trial (ISAT): a position statement from the executive committee of the American society of interventional and therapeutic neuroradiology and the American society of neuroradiology. AJNR Am J Neuroradiol. 2003;24(7):1404–1408.
4. Raabe A, Schmiedek P, Seifert V, Stolke D. German society of neurosurgery section on vascular neurosurgery: position statement on the International Subarachnoid Hemorrhage Trial (ISAT). Zentralbl Neurochir. 2003;64(3):99–103.
5. McDougall CG, Spetzler RF, Zabramski JM, et al. The barrow ruptured aneurysm trial. J Neurosurg. 2012;116:135–144.
6. Lanzino G, Murad MH, d'Urso PI, Rabinstein AA. Coil embolization versus clipping for ruptured intracranial aneurysms: a meta-analysis of prospective controlled published studies. AJNR Am J Neuroradiol. 2013;34(9):1764–1768.
7. Lindgren A, Vergouwen MD, van der Schaaf I, Algra A, Wermer M, Clarke MJ, Rinkel GJ. Endovascular coiling versus neurosurgical clipping for people with aneurysmal subarachnoid haemorrhage. Cochrane Database Syst Rev. 2018;8:CD003085.
8. Deshmukh AS, Priola SM, Katsanos AH, Scalia G, Alves AC, Srivastava A, Hawkes C. The management of intracranial aneurysms: current trends and future directions. Neurol Int. 2024;16(1):74–94.
9. Hoh BL, Ko NU, Amin-Hanjani S, Chou SH-Y, Cruz-Flores S, Dangayach NS, Derdeyn CP, Welch BG. 2023 guideline for the management of patients with aneurysmal subarachnoid hemorrhage: a guideline from the American Heart Association/American Stroke Association. Stroke. 2023;54(7):e314–e357.
10. Molyneux AJ, Kerr RSC, Yu L-M, Clarke M, Sneade M, Yarnold JA, Sandercock P; International Subarachnoid Aneurysm Trial (ISAT) Collaborative Group. International Subarachnoid Aneurysm Trial (ISAT) of neurosurgical clipping versus endovascular coiling in 2143 patients with ruptured intracranial aneurysms: a randomised comparison of effects on survival, dependency, seizures, rebleeding, subgroups, and aneurysm occlusion. Lancet. 2005;366(9488):809–817.
11. Molyneux AJ, Birks J, Clarke A, Sneade M, Kerr RSC. The durability of endovascular coiling versus neurosurgical clipping of ruptured cerebral aneurysms: 18-year follow-up of the UK cohort of the International Subarachnoid Aneurysm Trial (ISAT). Lancet. 2015;385(9969):691–697.
12. Spetzler RF, McDougall CG, Albuquerque FC, Zabramski JM, Hills NK, Partovi S, Nakaji P, Wallace RC. The barrow ruptured aneurysm trial: 3-year results. J Neurosurg. 2013;119(1):146–157.

13. Spetzler RF, McDougall CG, Zabramski JM, Albuquerque FC, Hills NK, Russin JJ, Partovi S, Nakaji P, Wallace RC. The barrow ruptured aneurysm trial: 6-year results. J Neurosurg. 2015;123(3):609–617.
14. Spetzler RF, McDougall CG, Zabramski JM, Albuquerque FC, Hills NK, Nakaji P, Karis JP, Wallace RC. Ten-year analysis of saccular aneurysms in the Barrow Ruptured Aneurysm Trial. J Neurosurg. 2019;132(3):771–776.
15. Hart Y, Sneade M. Birks J, Rischmiller J, Kerr R, Molyneux A. Epilepsy after subarachnoid hemorrhage: the frequency of seizures after clip occlusion or coil embolization of a ruptured cerebral aneurysm. Results from the International Subarachnoid Aneurysm Trial. J Neurosurg. 2011;115(6):1159–1168.
16. Scott RB, Eccles F, Molyneux AJ, Kerr RSC, Rothwell PM, Carpenter K. Improved cognitive outcomes with endovascular coiling of ruptured intracranial aneurysms: neuropsychological outcomes from the International Subarachnoid Aneurysm Trial (ISAT). Stroke. 2010;41(8):1743–1747.
17. Campi A, Ramzi N, Molyneux AJ, Summers PE, Kerr RSC, Sneade M, Yarnold JA, Rischmiller J, Byrne JV. Retreatment of ruptured cerebral aneurysms in patients randomized by coiling or clipping in the International Subarachnoid Aneurysm Trial (ISAT). Stroke. 2007;38(5):1538–1544.

CHAPTER 12

International Study of Unruptured Intracranial Aneurysms Investigators (ISUIA 2) Unruptured Intracranial Aneurysms: Natural History, Clinical Outcome, and Risks of Surgical and Endovascular Treatment

Wiebers DO, et al., Lancet. 2003 Jul 12;362(9378):103–110

Reviewed by Daniel C Walsh

Research Question/Objective The management of unruptured intracranial aneurysms is controversial. Investigators from the International Study of Unruptured Intracranial Aneurysms aimed to assess the natural history of unruptured intracranial aneurysms and to measure the risk associated with their repair.

Study Design Centres in the USA, Canada, and Europe enrolled patients for the prospective assessment of unruptured aneurysms.

Sample Size 4,060 patients were assessed: 1,692 did not have aneurysmal repair, 1,917 had open surgery, and 451 had endovascular procedures.

Intervention or Treatment Received Investigators recorded the natural history in patients who did not have surgery, and assessed morbidity and mortality associated with the repair of unruptured aneurysms by either open surgery or endovascular procedures.

Results Five-year cumulative rupture rates for patients who did not have a history of subarachnoid haemorrhage with aneurysms located in an internal carotid artery, anterior communicating or anterior cerebral artery, or middle cerebral artery were 0%, 2.6%, 14.5%, and 40% for aneurysms less than 7 mm, 7–12 mm, 13–24 mm, and 25 mm or greater, respectively, compared with rates of 2.5%, 14.5%, 18.4%,

DOI: 10.1201/9781003416197-12

and 50%, respectively, for the same size categories involving posterior circulation and posterior communicating artery aneurysms. These rates were often equalled or exceeded by the risks associated with surgical or endovascular repair of comparable lesions. A patient's age was a strong predictor of surgical outcome, and the size and location of an aneurysm predicted both surgical and endovascular outcomes.

Conclusion Many factors are involved in the management of patients with unruptured intracranial aneurysms. Site, size, and group-specific risks of the natural history should be compared with site, size, and age-specific risks of repair for each patient.

Reviewer Commentary The publication of the ISUIA 2 manuscript in 2003[1] was, in fact, the latest and much-anticipated work from collaborators determined to better understand the natural history of unruptured intracranial aneurysms. The interpretations of this data stoked some controversy, which continues to this day. I recall a dinner with the neurosurgeon spouse of someone working on the project who shared that they had agreed never to discuss it at the family table for the sake of harmony. Yet it remains a seminal piece of work in the cerebrovascular field and a popular subject for study when developing critical appraisal skills as a neurosurgical trainee.

The ISUIA project came partly in response to the proliferation of good-quality, cross-sectional imaging, which resulted in diagnoses of aneurysms that would have previously never come to light. The ranks of the "worried well" continue to swell and if there is a hope to reassure them, the natural history of an unruptured aneurysm needs to be precisely understood, while the consequences of a ruptured intracranial aneurysm are so severe as to make deciding to treat one simplicity itself in most cases.

The first ISUIA study[2] had retrospective as well as prospective components. The size and location of an aneurysm, as well as any preceding history of rupture, were confirmed as significant factors influencing the risk of bleeding. However, the relatively short follow-up limited conclusions about the balance between risks and benefits of treatment. ISUIA 2 set out to examine that issue in more depth. The treatment paradigm was shifting in favour of endovascular methods while the studies were underway, with much attendant controversy. The issue of whether treatment might be worse than the disease in many cases was a thorny subject.

PAPER SIGNIFICANCE AND IMPACT

Not All Small Aneurysms Are Comparable ISUIA 2 provided evidence in support of unruptured intracranial aneurysms having a quite distinct natural history from their ruptured relatives. The significance of ISUIA 2 was that, for the first time, natural history data from prospectively identified aneurysms was reported. That removed the risk of selection bias inherent in a retrospective study.

Furthermore, this data reinforced that the prior rupture of a separate aneurysm conferred a more adverse natural history than might otherwise have been expected and was reported as group 2. However, survivors who had suffered a poor outcome from a previous rupture, defined as having a modified Rankin score of 4 or 5, were excluded from the study and the numbers were significantly less than in group 1.

ISUIA 2 has been frequently and incorrectly cited as demonstrating a rupture risk of 0% for small anterior circulation aneurysms in patients without a previous history of aneurysmal subarachnoid haemorrhage. That stems from the decision to report the 5-year cumulative rupture risk as 0 in Table 12.1. The observed rate of rupture was 0.1% per annum. The correct interpretation of those data, therefore, would be to acknowledge that the natural history would be more benign than the procedural morbidity of any treatment and would remain so for several years. If further confirmation that small aneurysms should not be represented as having no risk of bleeding were needed, it could be found in the SUAVe[3] study, which observed a rate of bleeding of 0.54% overall in aneurysms less than 5 mm in size, followed for 6–10 years, a finding that broadly endorsed the ISUIA 2 data.

How confident should one be in that 0.1% figure? Conservatively treated patients were subject to 6,544 patient years of follow-up. The mean duration of follow-up for conservatively managed patients was 4.1 years, although with a standard deviation of 2 years, reflecting significant variance (see the "Study Limitations" section below).

What is more, aneurysm size may be a dynamic variable. At the time of the ISUIA 2 study, data was relatively sparse on the likelihood that an aneurysm would increase in size over time and on the precise implications of such a change. This should bring into question the rationale for offering treatment of small unruptured anterior circulation aneurysms.

A potential explanation is that small acutely ruptured aneurysms have an inherently different natural history from the cohort captured by the ISUIA studies. Is it possible that short-lived, inherently fragile small aneurysms grow quickly and rupture, accounting for those cases seen in acute practice? On the other hand, incidentally

Table 12.1 5-Year Cumulative Rupture Rates According to Size and Location of Unruptured Aneurysm.

	<7 mm		**7–12 mm**	**13–24 mm**	**>25 mm**
	Group 1	Group 2			
Cavernous carotid artery *n* = 210	0	0	0	3.0%	6.4%
AC/MC/IC (*n* = 1037)	0	1.5%	2.6%	14.5%	40%
Post-P comm (*n* = 445)	2.5	3.4%	14.5 %	18.4%	50%

Abbreviations: AC, anterior communicating or anterior cerebral artery; IC, internal carotid artery (not cavernous carotid artery); MC, middle cerebral artery; Post-P comm, vertebrobasilar, posterior cerebral arterial system, or the posterior communicating artery.

Source: From Wiebers DO, et al. Lancet. 2003 Jul 12;362(9378):103–10. doi: 10.1016/s0140-6736(03)13860-3. PMID: 12867109.

discovered small aneurysms, as encountered in observational studies, could reflect an inherently stable cohort with these growing slowly, if at all.

Risks of Treatment This study also brought into focus the procedural morbidity associated with treating unruptured aneurysms (Figure 12.1). Although the largest aneurysms might have the most adverse natural history, it was clear that under conditions prevailing at the time of the ISUIA 2 study, any benefit of treatment of the largest and most dangerous aneurysms could be offset by the associated procedural morbidity. Some would argue that the relatively low morbidity associated with coiling of small aneurysms justifies their treatment[4] but with larger datasets confirming a small but significant risk associated with treatment, even the most interventional of healthcare systems have had reason to reflect.[5,6]

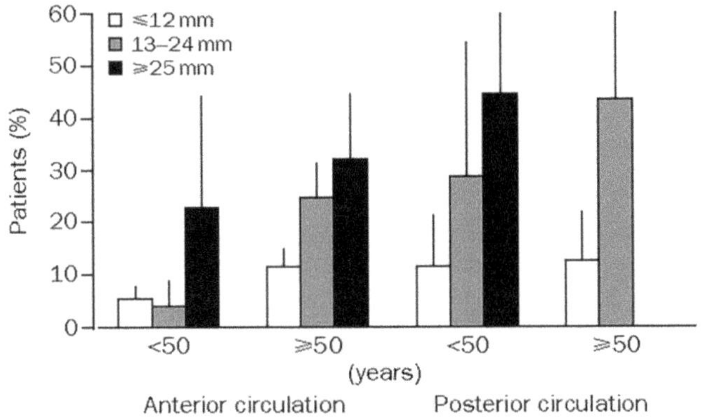

Figure 12.1 Poor surgical outcomes at one year by age, site, and size of aneurysm. (Poor outcome is death, a Rankin Score between 3 and 5, or impaired cognitive status. Bars show a 95% confidence interval.)

Unintended Consequences? Once ISUIA and other studies confirmed larger or posterior circulation aneurysms as being at significantly higher risk, it made it ethically difficult to deny treatment to patients with these aneurysms for the sake of further, longer-term natural history studies and making a randomized controlled trial comparing observation with intervention of larger aneurysms less likely in the future.[7]

Endovascular treatment options for unruptured aneurysms have also proliferated, creating a difficulty with the programmed obsolescence of novel devices, each iteration of which promises to resolve any shortcoming of the previous generation. Adequately powered comparative studies are prevented by a lack of community equipoise relating to treatment, which precludes long-term evaluation of the "site, size, and age-specific risks of repair" that the ISUIA 2 authors envisaged their work pointing towards.

Study Limitations ISUIA 2 attracted criticism for a selection bias, some of it resulting from the earlier ISUIA 1 study. Small aneurysms were more likely to be excluded from treatment on the basis that they were considered to have a relatively benign natural history.

Another potential weakness was the possibility of missing very small aneurysms if relying on cross-sectional angiography for diagnosis.[8,9] Once recruited to the study, all patients underwent catheter angiography to confirm the presence, size, and number of aneurysms. It is possible, therefore, that larger aneurysms were disproportionately represented in the sample.

There was a significant crossover of patients to receive treatment from the conservative arm, although the motivations for that decision were unclear. More than 500 patients were censored from analysis as they underwent treatment during follow-up.

Attrition under follow-up was also significant, with only 21% of patients overall reaching 4 years of follow-up.

A decision to analyze posterior communicating artery aneurysms as part of the posterior circulation group was justified on embryological grounds. That is logical for true aneurysms of the posterior communicating artery or perhaps in the presence of a foetal circulation. Most of what are termed posterior communicating artery aneurysms arise from the posterior carotid wall adjacent to the posterior communicating branch. Are they truly so different to anterior choroidal or superior hypophyseal aneurysms? While subsequent small studies have suggested a uniquely high risk of rupture and particular haemodynamic stresses in the communicating segment, this remains a contentious point.[10–13]

Relevant Studies The size and location of an intracranial aneurysm remain the justification for most management decisions around the globe. There has been increasing recognition that the natural history of an aneurysm is significantly impacted by genetic influences and haemodynamic factors but the tools to reliably personalize risk for the individual remain elusive.

Efforts to synthesize the effects of other risk factors for aneurysmal rupture still very much rely on the ISUIA 2 conclusion. Decision support tools, such as the PHASES[14,15] and Unruptured Intracranial Aneurysm Treatment Score (UIATS)[16] systems, still weigh the same factors most significantly as emerged from ISUIA 2. There remains substantial inconsistency in the application of such tools, such that they have not supplanted reference to ISUIA 2 in daily practice.[17–19] Efforts to integrate morphological characteristics into prognostic estimations remain difficult to quantify on an individual basis.[20,21] Practice guidelines today still rely on a lower level of evidence than all would prefer, and ISUIA 2 retains a position as an important piece of the jigsaw.[22]

Conclusion The ISUIA project made an interesting cameo during an important legal case before the High Court of Justice of England and Wales in 2015. This case,[23] and its subsequent appeal,[24] had important ramifications for the disclosures of expert witnesses during medical negligence proceedings in the United Kingdom, but more interesting to the present reader will be how ISUIA 1, when relied upon to argue that treatment would not in retrospect have been offered for a small unruptured aneurysm, was considered to have been rejected by the neurosurgical community.

Although the matter was not explored in depth in court, the judgement and subsequent appeal gave significant credence to neurosurgical editorialising to the effect that the "1998 ISUIA paper was not generally accepted in the neurosurgical community as scientifically unbiased and reliable". A harsh reading.

During the appeal, it was accepted that treatment would likely have been offered. The advent of ISUIA 2 in 2003 should have confirmed expectant management as a reasonable management alternative, and no compelling evidence has emerged to the contrary since.

Happily, as the judgement did not turn on this question, the outcome was unaffected but it is a salutary reminder that impassioned opinion sometimes carries farther than reasoned observation.

REFERENCES

1. Wiebers D, Whisnant J, Huston J, et al. Unruptured intracranial aneurysms: natural history, clinical outcome, and risks of surgical and endovascular treatment. Lancet. 2003;362:103–110.
2. Unruptured intracranial aneurysms–risk of rupture and risks of surgical intervention. N Engl J Med. 1998;339(24):1725–1733. doi:10.1056/NEJM199812103392401
3. Sonobe M, Yamazaki T, Yonekura M, Kikuchi H. Small unruptured intracranial aneurysm verification study: SUAVe study, Japan. Stroke. 2010;41(9):1969–1977. doi:10.1161/STROKEAHA.110.585059
4. Beneš V, Mitchell P, Molyneux AJ, Renowden SA. Endovascular coiling in 131 patients with low complication rate justifies treating most unruptured intracranial aneurysms. Cent Eur Neurosurg. 2010 Feb;71(1):1–7. doi: 10.1055/s-0029-1220938. PMID: 20198740.
5. Malhotra A, Wu X, Forman HP, Matouk CC, Gandhi D, Sanelli P. Management of tiny unruptured intracranial aneurysms: a comparative effectiveness analysis. JAMA Neurol. 2018;75(1):27–34. doi:10.1001/JAMANEUROL.2017.3232
6. Johnston SC. Leaving tiny, unruptured intracranial aneurysms untreated: why is it so hard? JAMA Neurol. 2018;75(1):13–14. doi:10.1001/JAMANEUROL.2017.2559
7. Raymond J, Guillemin F, Proust F, et al. Unruptured intracranial aneurysms: a critical review of the International Study of Unruptured Intracranial Aneurysms (ISUIA) and of appropriate methods to address the clinical problem. Interv Neuroradiol. 2008;14(1):85. doi:10.1177/159101990801400111
8. White PM, Wardlaw J. Unruptured intracranial aneurysms: prospective data have arrived. Lancet. 2003;362(9378):90–91. doi:10.1016/S0140-6736(03)13891-3
9. Wardlaw JM, White PM. The detection and management of unruptured intracranial aneurysms. Brain. 2000;123(2):205–221. doi:10.1093/brain/123.2.205

10. Arrambide-Garza FJ, Alvarez-Lozada LA, de León-Gutiérrez H, et al. Fetal-type posterior cerebral artery and association of rupture in posterior communicating artery aneurysms: A systematic review and meta-analysis. Clin Neurol Neurosurg. 2023;231. doi:10.1016/J.CLINEURO.2023.107815
11. Xu ZH, Kim BS, Lee KS, Choi JH, Shin YS. Morphological and clinical risk factors for the rupture of posterior communicating artery aneurysms: significance of fetal-type posterior cerebral artery. Neurol Sci. 2019;40(11):2377–2382. doi:10.1007/S10072-019-03991-4
12. Matsukawa H, Fujii M, Akaike G, et al. Morphological and clinical risk factors for posterior communicating artery aneurysm rupture. J Neurosurg. 2014;120(1):104–110. doi:10.3171/2013.9.JNS13921
13. Chien A, Lau V, Yi Q, Chang W. Posterior communicating artery aneurysms demonstrate faster interval growth than other growing aneurysms. Neuroradiol J. 2017;31(3):288. doi:10.1177/1971400917709621
14. Backes D, Vergouwen MDI, Groenestege ATT, et al. PHASES score for prediction of intracranial aneurysm growth. Stroke. 2015;46:1221–1226.
15. Greving JP, Wermer MJH, Brown RD, et al. Development of the PHASES score for prediction of risk of rupture of intracranial aneurysms: a pooled analysis of six prospective cohort studies. Lancet Neurol. 2014;13(1). doi:10.1016/S1474-4422(13)70263-1
16. Etminan N, Brown RD, Beseoglu K, et al. The unruptured intracranial aneurysm treatment score: A multidisciplinary consensus. Neurology. 2015;85(10):881. doi:10.1212/WNL.0000000000001891
17. Kailaya-Vasan A, Frantzias J, Kailaya-Vasan J, Anderson IA, Walsh DC. Current decision support tools fail to agree or predict therapeutic decisions in a single cohort of unruptured intracranial aneurysms. Acta Neurochir (Wien). 2022;164(3):771–779. doi:10.1007/S00701-021-04852-W
18. Rutledge C, Raper DMS, Jonzzon S, et al. Sensitivity of the Unruptured Intracranial Aneurysm Treatment Score (UIATS) in the elderly: retrospective analysis of ruptured aneurysms. World Neurosurg. 2021;152:e673–e677. doi:10.1016/J.WNEU.2021.06.021
19. Molenberg R, Aalbers MW, Mazuri A, et al. The Unruptured Intracranial Aneurysm Treatment Score as a predictor of aneurysm growth or rupture. Eur J Neurol. 2020;28(3):837. doi:10.1111/ENE.14636
20. Backes D, Rinkel GJE, Greving JP, et al. ELAPSS score for prediction of risk of growth of unruptured intracranial aneurysms. Neurology. 2017;88(17):1600–1606.
21. van Kammen MS, Greving JP, Kuroda S, et al. External validation of the ELAPSS score for prediction of unruptured intracranial aneurysm growth risk. J Stroke. 2019;21(3):340. doi:10.5853/JOS.2019.01277
22. Etminan N, de Sousa DA, Tiseo C, et al. European Stroke Organisation (ESO) guidelines on management of unruptured intracranial aneurysms. Eur Stroke J. 2022;7(3):V.
23. EXP v Barker [2015] EWHC 1289 (QB) (07 May 2015). Accessed March 9, 2025. https://www.bailii.org/cgi-bin/format.cgi?doc=/ew/cases/EWHC/QB/2015/1289.html&query=(EXP+OR+Respondent+OR+(Claimant)+OR+-+OR+-+OR+DR+OR+CHARLES+OR+SIMON+OR+BARKER)
24. EXP v Barker [2017] EWCA Civ 63 (10 February 2017). Accessed March 9, 2025. https://www.bailii.org/ew/cases/EWCA/Civ/2017/63.html

CHAPTER 13

Effect of Oral Nimodipine on Cerebral Infarction and Outcome after Subarachnoid Haemorrhage: British Aneurysm Nimodipine Trial

Pickard JD, Murray GD, Illingworth R, Shaw MD, Teasdale GM, Foy PM, Humphrey PR, Lang DA, Nelson R, Richards P, Sinar J, Bailey S, Skene A ,
BMJ. 1989 Mar 11;298(6674):636–642

Reviewed by Ramez Wadie Kirollos

Objective/Research Question To determine the efficacy of oral nimodipine in reducing cerebral infarction and poor functional outcomes after subarachnoid haemorrhage (SAH).

Study Design This was a double-blinded, placebo-controlled, randomised trial with an intention-to-treat analysis. The multicentre study involved four regional neurosurgical units from the United Kingdom (Southampton, Glasgow, London, and Liverpool).

Sample Size The recruitment period was from June 1985 to September 1987, with 554 patients included in the final analysis.

Inclusion/Exclusion Criteria

- Inclusion Criteria
  - Patients more than 18 years old.
  - Within 96 hours from SAH onset.
  - Diagnosis confirmed with lumbar puncture, computer tomography scan (angiography was not necessary for recruitment into the trial).

- Exclusion Criteria
  - Young patient less than 18 years old.
  - Late presentation beyond 96 hours of onset.
  - Pregnancy, major medical comorbidities (cardiac, renal, hepatic, or lung disease).
  - SAH causing coma in the week preceding the most recent SAH.
  - Lack of informed consent.

DOI: 10.1201/9781003416197-13

Intervention or Treatment Received Placebo or nimodipine given at 60 mg every 4 hours orally or via nasogastric tube for 21 days, initiated within 96 hours of SAH ictus.

Methods The outcomes measured included the incidence of cerebral infarction, ischaemic neurological deficits, and functional outcomes using the Glasgow Coma Scale (GCS) at 3 months follow-up. Patients were monitored clinically and radiologically, as necessary, for deterioration defined by focal neurological deficit or more than 1 point worsening in the GCS for more than 6 hours. Deterioration was classified as either rebleed, cerebral ischaemia, cerebral infarction, or others. Poor functional outcomes were defined as death or severe disability.

Results Patients given nimodipine had a 22% incidence of cerebral infarction compared to 34% in patients given a placebo. This corresponds to a significant reduction of cerebral infarction by 34% (95% confidence interval [CI], 13–50%). The nimodipine and placebo groups had a 20% and 33% incidence of poor functional outcomes, respectively. This demonstrates a reduction of poor functional outcomes by 40% (95% CI, 20–55%). There were no differences in mortality or adverse effects between the two groups.

Conclusion Enteral nimodipine, given at 60 mg every 4 hours, for 21 days, is well tolerated and prophylactically reduces the rate of cerebral infarctions and poor functional outcomes at 3 months for patients with aneurysmal SAH.

REVIEWER COMMENTARY

Application/Significance/Impact Delayed cerebral ischaemia is a significant predictor of poor outcome after an aneurysmal SAH, with related infarction shown to be associated with an almost five-fold increase in the likelihood of an unfavourable outcome at 1 year.[1] This article was classified as a landmark paper because of its contributions to the treatment and the understanding of the pathogenesis of delayed cerebral ischaemia, and the eventual inclusion of nimodipine as part of the standard of care in various SAH guidelines.[2,3]

As the largest double-blinded placebo-controlled trial looking at the effect of oral nimodipine in SAH at that time, this article established not only the appropriate route, dose, and duration of nimodipine, but also the treatment intent (prophylactic, rather than therapeutic) with which the medication should be utilised. This was accomplished by contrasting against prior similar but smaller controlled[4–6] and uncontrolled studies that looked at intravenous preparations and at different dosages (unpublished Bayer trial 3247/3293). These studies demonstrated that intravenous and oral forms of administration had similar areas under the curve and that a higher dose at 90 mg every four hours did not show additional benefit compared with the 60 mg dosing.

A large meta-analysis was eventually published in 2007, including 16 trials and over 3,000 patients. That article demonstrated that oral nimodipine administration conferred a relative risk of 0.67 of poor outcomes in SAH. It concluded that "the evidence for nimodipine is not beyond all doubt but given the potential benefits and modest risks of this treatment, oral nimodipine is currently indicated in patients with aneurysmal SAH", further reinforcing the place of nimodipine in the medical management for this condition.[7]

Today, knowledge on delayed cerebral ischaemia has progressed significantly, including a formal definition,[8] and an improved understanding of its various contributory pathogenetic processes.[9] At the time of this study, it was a relatively unknown phenomenon with no clear evidence of either. This study provided subtle yet robust clues about its mechanism. The original intent in using calcium channel antagonists such as nimodipine was to reduce cerebral vasospasm and, by extension, delayed cerebral ischaemia. However, nimodipine had a disproportionately larger effect on poor functional outcomes compared to that on cerebral infarctions. Furthermore, there was a reduced rate of cerebral infarctions despite there being no less cerebral vasospasm. This strongly hinted that vasospasm, although important, is not the only contributor to poor outcomes after SAH, and that the mechanism of nimodipine did not directly impact vasospasm. This unaccounted-for contributor led to cerebral infarctions and poor functional outcomes separately, and ultimately shaped our modern understanding of the pathogenesis of delayed cerebral ischaemia.

Study Limitations Because the article was published more than three decades ago, some temporally based limitations impact its validity but not necessarily its applicability. One of the main limitations is the relatively low number of proven aneurysms in the entire series (368 aneurysms in 554 patients, 66.4%). Another limitation is the slightly different clinical grading of SAH applied in the study compared to that which is commonly used today, the World Federation of Neurosurgical Society (WFNS) grading scale (clinical grading used: grade I, GCS 15, neurologically intact apart from cranial nerve palsy; grade II, GCS 15, neurologically intact apart from cranial nerve palsy but with neck stiffness and/or headache; grade III, GCS 13–14, with or without neurological deficit; grade IV, GCS 8–12, with or without neurological deficit; grade V, GCS 3–7, with or without abnormal posturing. WFNS grading scale: grade I, GCS 15; grade II, GCS 13–14, without focal neurological deficit; grade III, GCS 13–14, with focal neurological deficit; grade IV: GCS 7–12; grade V: GCS 3–6). This, in addition to newer evidence showing that radiological grading, such as the modified Fisher scale, affects the incidence of Delayed Cerebral Ischemia (DCI), was not sufficiently factored into the analysis. Finally, the treatment of aneurysmal SAH has evolved significantly over the years. The progression of surgical techniques, the increasing use of endovascular treatment, particularly in the posterior circulation, and a superior understanding of blood pressure control and fluid status have all led to improved overall functional outcomes. Although it is difficult to quantify, these might alter the manner in which nimodipine interacts with the disease process.

The diagnosis and classification of SAH and delayed cerebral ischaemia have improved significantly through the years, with better pathogenic understanding and access to faster and more accurate radiological imaging and techniques, including computed tomography angiography and perfusion scans. Its management, as well, has progressed, further contributing to improved outcomes. The principle of prophylactic enteral nimodipine, to be administered early, before the onset of delayed cerebral ischaemia, remains conclusive and relevant.

Relevant Studies Contemporary research has shed light on various aspects of nimodipine in the context of SAH. Nimodipine-related neuroprotective effects have been well documented despite a lack of understanding of the exact pathways. Prior hypotheses included effects on vasospasm, which was not demonstrated in this landmark article. A recent attempt at deriving its mechanism of action used a murine model and focused on microcirculatory dysfunction.[10] The middle cerebral artery was perforated via an endovascular approach and intraperitoneal nimodipine was administered. Subsequent 2-photon microscopy revealed significantly reduced posthaemorrhagic microvasospasm in the nimodipine-treated group compared to the control, without affecting global microarterial constriction.

Current evidence for enteral nimodipine requires dosing every four hours with a risk of hypotension. In addition, plasma, brain, and cerebrospinal fluid nimodipine concentrations were found in a study to be lower than the median effective dose. Nimodipine administered in a locoregional manner, into the subarachnoid space, would theoretically overcome these limitations. A randomised, double-blinded, placebo-controlled trial, NEWTON-2, where a single-dose sustained-release formulation administered via an external ventricular drain was conceived.[11] Unfortunately, a planned interim analysis revealed that the study was unlikely to achieve its primary endpoint, and the study was halted. This was a disappointing development as a previous study using another calcium channel antagonist, nicardipine, implanted locally during surgery, demonstrated a promising reduction in DCIs.[12] Currently, the only "locally administered" form of nimodipine having a clear, though temporary effect on vasospasm and cerebral perfusion, remains to be intraarterial.[13]

Authors have previously speculated that the negative aneurysmal SAH trials might have been related to the poor sensitivity of outcome measures, selection of patients with a low DCI risk[14] or that the effects of nimodipine might have been large, diluting the relatively smaller effects of other interventions. Regardless, the search for further preventative and therapeutic treatment options for DCI continues.

Acknowledgement The author wishes to acknowledge the contribution of Jia Xu Lim, FRCS (SN), Shu Kiat Chan, MBBS, Adriel Z Leong, FRCS (SN), and Felicia Hui Zhuang Chua, FRCS (SN) in the preparation of this chapter.

REFERENCES

1. Veldeman M, Rossmann T, Haeren R, et al. Delayed cerebral infarction after aneurysmal subarachnoid hemorrhage. Neurology. 2024;103:e209607.
2. Subarachnoid haemorrhage caused by a ruptured aneurysm: diagnosis and management. London: National Institute for Health and Care Excellence (NICE). 2022 Nov 23 (NICE Guideline, No. 228).
3. Hoh BL, Ko NU, Amin-Hanjani S, et al. 2023 guideline for the management of patients with aneurysmal subarachnoid hemorrhage: a guideline from the American Heart Association/American Stroke Association. Stroke. 2023;54:e314–e370.
4. Allen GS, Ahn HS, Preziosi TJ, et al. Cerebral arterial spasm - a controlled trial of nimodipine in patients with subarachnoid hemorrhage. N Eng J Med. 1983;308:619–624.
5. Philippon J, Grob R, Dagreou F, Guggiari M, Rivierez M, Viars P. Prevention of vasospasm in subarachnoid haemorrhage. A controlled study with nimodipine. Acta Neurochir (Wien). 1986;82:110–114.
6. Neil-Dwyer G, Mee E, Dorrance D, Lowe D. Early intervention with nimodipine in subarachnoid haemorrhage. Eur Heart J. 1987;8:41–47.
7. Dorhout Mees SM, Rinkel GJ, Feigin VL, Algra A, van den Bergh WM, Vermeulen M, et al. Calcium antagonists for aneurysmal subarachnoid haemorrhage. Cochrane Database Syst Rev. 2007;2007:CD000277.
8. Vergouwen MD; Participants in the International Multi-Disciplinary Consensus Conference on the Critical Care Management of Subarachnoid Hemorrhage. Vasospasm versus delayed cerebral ischemia as an outcome event in clinical trials and observational studies. Neurocrit Care. 2011;15:308–311.
9. Budohoski KP, Guilfoyle M, Helmy A, et al. The pathophysiology and treatment of delayed cerebral ischaemia following subarachnoid haemorrhage. J Neurol Neurosurg Psychiatry. 2014;85:1343–1353.
10. Schwarting J, Harapan BN, Lin X, Plesnila N, Terpolilli NA. Nimodipine reduces microvasospasms after experimental subarachnoid hemorrhage. Stroke 2020;54: 2666–2670.
11. Carlson AP, Hanggi D, Wong GK, Etminan N, Mayer SA, Aldrich F, et al. Single-dose intraventricular nimodipine microparticles versus oral nimodipine for aneurysmal subarachnoid hemorrhage. Stroke. 2020;51:1142–1149.
12. Kasuya H, Onda H, Sasahara A, Takeshita M, Hori T. Application of nicardipine prolonged-release implants: analysis of 97 consecutive patients with acute subarachnoid hemorrhage. Neurosurgery. 2005;56:895–902.
13. Hanggi D, Turowski B, Beseoglu K, Yong M, Steiger HJ. Intra-arterial nimodipine for severe cerebral vasospasm after aneurysmal subarachnoid hemorrhage: influence on clinical course and cerebral perfusion. Am J Neuroradiol. 2008;29:1053–1060.
14. Carlson AP, Hanggi D, Macdonald R, Shuttleworth CW. Nimodipine reappraised: an old drug with a future. Curr Neuropharmacol. 2020;18:65–82.

Chapter 14

A Proposed Grading System for Arteriovenous Malformations

Spetzler RF, Martin NA, J Neurosurg. 1986 Oct;65(4):476–483

Reviewed by Robert F Spetzler

Objective/Research Question To propose a simple system that weighs the important features of an individual arteriovenous malformation (AVM) and thus grades the lesion according to its degree of surgical difficulty.

Study Design N/A

Sample Size N/A

Inclusion/Exclusion Criteria N/A

Follow-Up N/A

Intervention or Treatment Received N/A

Results N/A

Conclusion If this scale, in its simplicity, proves to predict operative morbidity in other series, it will provide a useful tool for decision-making in the management of patients with AVMs. As a further benefit, it will facilitate a comparison of AVM treatment results between series or between techniques.

Paper Description An important factor in making a recommendation for treatment of a patient with arteriovenous malformations (AVMs) is to estimate the risk of surgery for that patient. A simple, broadly applicable grading system that is designed to predict the risk of morbidity and mortality attending the operative treatment of specific AVMs is proposed. The lesion is graded based on size, pattern of venous drainage, and neurological eloquence of the adjacent brain. All AVMs fall into one of six grades. Grade I malformations are small, superficial, and located in the noneloquent cortex; grade V lesions are large, deep, and situated in neurologically critical areas; and grade VI lesions are essentially inoperable AVMs. The retrospective application of this grading scheme to a series of surgically

DOI: 10.1201/9781003416197-14

excised AVMs has demonstrated its correlation with the incidence of postoperative neurological complications. The application of a standardized grading scheme will enable a comparison of results between various clinical series and between different treatment techniques, and will assist in the process of management decision-making.[1]

Author/Reviewer Commentary As a young cerebrovascular neurosurgeon with an intense interest in arteriovenous malformations (AVMs), it became apparent to me that comparing the success of treating these complex lesions was difficult because of their incredible heterogeneity. The risks associated with the treatment of a small superficial AVM in the frontal cortex were completely different from those associated with the treatment of a large deep AVM in the thalamus. The frustration of making sense of these challenging lesions led me to consider ways to stratify AVMs into categories with similar risks associated with their surgical obliteration.

My first fellow, Neil Martin, and I sat down and listed all the factors that we thought had a role in determining the complexity of these lesions and the risks associated with their surgical treatment. Factors such as the number of feeding arteries, the degree and location of draining veins, anatomical location, the age of the patient, and the patient's general health were all considered.

A rational AVM grading system needed to be simple, easy to use, and have reliable predictive value for assessing surgical risk. We were convinced that, as an example, deep venous drainage automatically increased the risk of surgery because some portion of the lesion was deep and anatomically more difficult to remove. The size of an AVM was easily identified as a risk factor. Eloquence also made sense as a risk factor because the surgical risk involved in removing a lesion from the speech area was obviously greater than that involved in removing a lesion from the nondominant temporal lobe, for example.

By dividing size into three categories, we emphasized the progressive risk associated with increasing AVM size. We chose categories of less than 3 cm, 3–6 cm, and greater than 6 cm and gave these categories 1, 2, and 3 points, respectively, to establish a grading system. Deep venous drainage is easily identified on diagnostic studies and automatically emphasizes the increased surgical risk associated with deep venous drainage. An AVM received 1 point if deep venous drainage was present and no points if there was no deep drainage. Similarly, an AVM received 1 point if located in the eloquent brain and no points if not.

Thus, when a small AVM was located in the noneloquent brain and was superficial without any deep drainage, the lowest number of points would be 1, based on size. Alternatively, a large AVM more than 6 cm in diameter with deep drainage and located in the eloquent brain would have the maximum number of points: 3 for size, 1 for deep drainage, and 1 for eloquence, giving a maximum of 5 points. Applying this grading system to a retrospective series, followed by a prospective series of AVMs treated at our own institution, verified the robustness of the grading system in predicting surgical risk.[1–5]

Relevant Studies Many series reported in the literature used the grading system and verified its reliability in predicting surgical risk.[1–5] Lawton et al. thoughtfully added additional risk factors that further refined the grading system.[6,7] Unfortunately, this refinement further divides these uncommon lesions into additional categories, making it difficult to accumulate sufficient numbers in each group for statistical analysis. Indeed, we have gone in the opposite direction; in presenting our AVM experience at multiple conferences, I have generally combined the grade I and II AVMs into a single category, grade A, because of their similar outcomes; kept grade III separate, as grade B; and then combined grade IV and V AVMs into grade C, again because of similar outcomes.[8] The advantage of this recategorization is that it provides an even more simplified system, and having only three grades results in a much greater number of lesions in each grade, allowing for more robust statistical analyses.[5] This simplified grading scale was published with Francisco Ponce, who was my chief resident at the time.[8] The venerable surgeon Michael Morgan, with his large AVM experience, adopted this new grading system with good results.[5]

In general, based on our experience and that of others, we have recommended surgical resection for all grade I and II (grade A) AVMs, multimodality treatment for grade III (grade B) AVMs, and no treatment unless there are multiple hemorrhages or progressive neurological deficit for grade IV and V (grade C) AVMs.

We have been gratified by the wide acceptance of these grading systems for these difficult lesions. Obviously, we want to emphasize that any grading system is only one tool in our armamentarium to help guide us in providing the best recommendation for our patients and their families. The selection process is the essence of the art of medicine.[9,10]

REFERENCES

1. Spetzler RF, Martin NA. A proposed grading system for arteriovenous malformations. 1986. J Neurosurg. 2008;108(1):186–193.
2. Hamilton MG, Spetzler RF. The prospective application of a grading system for arteriovenous malformations. Neurosurgery. 1994;34(1):2–6; discussion 6–7.
3. Gallardo F, Martin C, Chang L, et al. [Usefulness of Gradation Scales in the Surgical Treatment of Cerebral Arteriovenous Malformations]. Surg Neurol Int. 2019; 10(Suppl 1):S46–S57.
4. Simons M, Morgan MK, Davidson AS. Cohort studies, trials, and tribulations: systematic review and an evidence-based approach to arteriovenous malformation treatment. J Neurosurg Sci. 2018;62(4):444–453.
5. Morgan MK, Davidson AS, Assaad NNA, Stoodley MA. Critical review of brain AVM surgery, surgical results and natural history in 2017. Acta Neurochir (Wien). 2017;159(8):1457–1478.
6. Lawton MT, Kim H, McCulloch CE, et al. A supplementary grading scale for selecting patients with brain arteriovenous malformations for surgery. Neurosurgery. 2010;66(4): 702–713; discussion 713.
7. Catapano JS, Frisoli FA, Nguyen CL, et al. Intermediate-grade brain arteriovenous malformations and the boundary of operability using the supplemented Spetzler-Martin grading system. J Neurosurg. 2022;136(1):125–133.

8. Spetzler RF, Ponce FA. A 3-tier classification of cerebral arteriovenous malformations. Clinical article. J Neurosurg. 2011;114(3):842–849.
9. Burkhardt JK, Winkler EA, Catapano JS, et al. Surgical selection and outcomes among elderly patients with brain arteriovenous malformations. Neurosurg Focus. 2020;49(4):E9.
10. Han PP, Ponce FA, Spetzler RF. Intention-to-treat analysis of Spetzler-Martin grades IV and V arteriovenous malformations: natural history and treatment paradigm. J Neurosurg. 2003;98(1):3–7.

Chapter 15

Early Decompressive Surgery in Malignant Infarction of the Middle Cerebral Artery: A Pooled Analysis of Three Randomized Controlled Trials

Vahedi K, Hofmeijer J, Juettler E, Vicaut E, George B, Algra A, Amelink GJ, Schmiedeck P, Schwab S, Rothwell PM, Bousser M-G, van der Worp HB, Hacke W, for the DECIMAL, DESTINY, and HAMLET Investigators, Lancet Neurol. 2007 Mar;6(3):P215–P222

Reviewed by Fezaan A Kazi and Rabia Qaiser

Research Question/Objective This study aimed to determine whether decompressive surgery within 48 hours of stroke onset reduces mortality and improves functional outcomes in patients with malignant infarction of the middle cerebral artery (MCA).

Study Design The study was a pooled analysis of individual patient data from three European randomized controlled trials (RCTs): DECIMAL, DESTINY, and HAMLET. These trials shared a similar design and primary outcome measures, allowing for combined data analysis.

Sample Size A total of 93 patients were included in the pooled analysis, with 51 patients assigned to the decompressive surgery group and 42 patients assigned to the control group.

Follow-Up Patients were followed for a duration of 12 months post-randomization to assess mortality and functional outcomes based on the modified Rankin Scale (mRS).

Inclusion/Exclusion Criteria

- Inclusion Criteria
  - All included trials used similar inclusion and exclusion criteria, differing only in age limits and allowable time from symptom onset. Eligible patients had clinical deficits consistent with MCA infarction, a National Institutes of Health Stroke Scale (NIHSS) score >15, and a decreased level of consciousness (NIHSS item 1a ≥1). Imaging criteria required infarction involving ≥50% of the MCA territory or an infarct volume >145 cm³ on diffusion-weighted magnetic resonance imaging.

DOI: 10.1201/9781003416197-15

  - Age eligibility ranged from 18–55 years in DECIMAL and 18–60 years in DESTINY and the pooled DECIMAL/DESTINY/HAMLET analysis. Time from symptom onset to enrollment was <24 hours in DECIMAL, <36 hours in DESTINY, and <45 hours in HAMLET.

- Exclusion criteria
  - Exclusion criteria included a pre-stroke modified Rankin Scale score of ≥2, bilaterally fixed dilated pupils, contralateral ischemia, space-occupying hemorrhagic transformation (PH2), life expectancy <3 years, significant comorbidities, coagulopathy, contraindications to anesthesia, and pregnancy.

Intervention or Treatment Received The decompressive surgery group underwent hemicraniectomy with duraplasty within 48 hours of stroke onset. The procedure involved removing a large bone flap (minimum 12 cm), with additional temporal bone removed so that the floor of the middle cerebral fossa could be reached. Then a dural patch, consisting of pericranium or a commercially available dura substitute, was placed, and cranioplasty was performed after at least 6 weeks. The control group received the best medical management according to established guidelines for acute ischemic stroke and space-occupying brain edema.

Results In a pooled analysis of 93 patients, decompressive surgery was associated with substantial improvements in survival and functional outcomes compared with medical management alone. A significantly greater proportion of surgically treated patients achieved an mRS score of ≤4 (75% vs 24%) and ≤3 (43% vs 21%), as well as overall survival (78% vs 29%). These effects corresponded to a number needed to treat of two for survival regardless of functional outcome, two for survival with mRS ≤4, and four for survival with mRS ≤3. Importantly, the benefit of decompressive surgery was consistent across all three included trials.

Conclusion The study concluded that early decompressive surgery significantly reduces mortality without increasing the number of very severely disabled survivors in patients with malignant MCA infarction.

Reviewer Commentary The study provides strong evidence supporting early decompressive surgery in malignant MCA infarction in patients aged 60 years or younger within 48 hours of stroke onset. This is a procedure that has since trended toward becoming the standard of care in most neurosurgical practices. The pooled analysis of three separate RCTs increases statistical power and confirms findings from prior non-randomized studies, which lends confidence to clinical decision-makers in choosing surgical management. Studies since then have also shown that patients who undergo surgery have better long-term quality of life compared to those receiving conservative management, despite the increased potential for moderate disability in older patients.[1–3] This is particularly relevant given the initial concerns that increased survival would come at the cost of severe disability. The surgical approach has since become standard practice in many centers worldwide. The lack of generalizability in early studies, largely due to strict inclusion criteria, remains an important consideration, but the accumulating evidence has led to a broader acceptance and refinement of patient selection criteria. Future studies should focus on long-term cognitive and functional outcomes, especially in older patients, to optimize decision-making for both patients and clinicians.

However, while mortality was reduced, some survivors remained functionally dependent following surgery, highlighting the potential debilitating effects of major surgery on long-term health outcomes and quality of life. There is a definite need for further research into patient selection and long-term quality of life outcomes, to better target which patients can demonstrate the most benefit from undergoing early surgical management.

Study Limitations Some limitations include minor baseline differences between the individual trials, such as variations in stroke severity at randomization and differences in systolic blood pressure between groups, which may have influenced outcomes. The absence of blinded outcome assessment in all trials introduces the possibility of observer bias, potentially affecting the accuracy of functional outcome evaluations. The study's generalizability is limited, as participants were capped at 60 years, leaving uncertainty about the procedure's effectiveness in older populations. Additionally, the effect of surgery beyond 48 hours remains unclear, as patients treated outside this window were excluded, making it difficult to determine whether later intervention would yield similar benefits. Variability in neuroimaging criteria across trials also presents a limitation, as differences in infarct volume and location assessment may have affected patient selection and subsequent outcomes. Finally, while the study establishes mortality reduction, long-term quality-of-life assessments beyond 12 months were not included, limiting insight into the sustained impact of decompressive surgery on functional independence.

Relevant Studies Early non-randomized studies suggested that decompressive hemicraniectomy reduced mortality in malignant cerebral infarction but provided limited data on long-term functional outcomes. These early reports raised particular concern regarding the benefit of surgery in older patients. For example, Uhl et al. reported that only 12% of patients older than 50 years who underwent hemicraniectomy survived with functional independence, while 37% died or were left severely disabled.[4] Similarly, Gupta et al. found that 80% of patients older than 50 years who underwent hemicraniectomy were either severely disabled or died.[5]

Subsequent randomized studies challenged these conclusions. Notably, the DESTINY II trial in 2014 demonstrated a survival benefit from early decompressive hemicraniectomy in patients older than 60 years.[6] More recent literature has further shown that surgical intervention can confer meaningful quality-of-life benefits in this population. For instance, Rauen et al. reported significantly higher long-term quality-of-life scores in patients older than 60 years at 10-year follow-up after surgery compared with those managed conservatively.[1]

Future research should continue to emphasize long-term follow-up, patient-centered quality-of-life outcomes, and optimal surgical timing in order to further refine patient selection criteria.

REFERENCES

1. Rauen K, Reichelt L, Probst P, Schäpers B, Müller F, Jahn K, Plesnila N. Decompressive craniectomy is associated with good quality of life up to 10 years after rehabilitation from traumatic brain injury. Crit Care Med. 2020;48(8):1157–1164. doi:10.1097/CCM.0000000000004387
2. Hamamoto Filho PT, Gonçalves LB, Koetz NF, Silvestrin AML, Alves Júnior AC, Rocha LA, Módolo GP, de Avila MAG, Martin LC, Neugebauer H, Zanini MA, Bazan R. Long-term follow-up of patients undergoing decompressive hemicraniectomy for malignant stroke: quality of life and caregiver's burden in a real-world setting. Clin Neurol Neurosurg. 2020;197:106168. doi:10.1016/j.clineuro.2020.106168
3. Waqas M, Malik N, Shamim MS, Nathani KR, Abbasi SA. Quality of life among patients undergoing decompressive craniectomy for traumatic brain injury using Glasgow Outcome Scale Extended and Quality of Life After Brain Injury Scale. World Neurosurg. 2018;116:e783–e790. doi:10.1016/j.wneu.2018.05.092
4. Uhl E, Kreth FW, Elias B, Goldammer A, Hempelmann RG, Liefner M, Nowak G, Oertel M, Schmieder K, Schneider GH. Outcome and prognostic factors of hemicraniectomy for space occupying cerebral infarction. J Neurol Neurosurg Psychiatry. 2004;75(2):270–274.
5. Gupta R, Connolly ES, Mayer S, Elkind MS. Hemicraniectomy for massive middle cerebral artery territory infarction: a systematic review. Stroke. 2004;35(2):539–543. Epub 2004 Jan 5. doi:10.1161/01.STR.0000109772.64650.18
6. Jüttler E, Unterberg A, Woitzik J, et al. Hemicraniectomy in older patients with extensive middle-cerebral-artery stroke. N Engl J Med. 2014;370(12):1091–100. doi:10.1056/NEJMoa1311367

CHAPTER 16

Benefit of Carotid Endarterectomy in Patients with Symptomatic Moderate or Severe Stenosis: North American Symptomatic Carotid Endarterectomy Trial (NASCET)

Barnett HJM, Taylor DW, Eliasziw M, Fox AJ, Ferguson GG, Haynes RB, Rankin RN, Clagett GP, Hachinski VC, Sackett DL, Thorpe KE, Meldrum HE, Spence JD, N Engl J Med. 1998 Nov 12;339(20):1415–1425

Reviewed by Alice L Hung and Judy Huang

Research Question/Objective This is a prospective multicenter randomized controlled trial that compared the outcomes following endarterectomy vs medical therapy in patients with symptomatic moderate (less than 70%) carotid stenosis.

Study Design Patients who were eligible for the study were enrolled between December 1987 and December 1996. They were randomized to the medical arm or surgical arm using a centralized computer-generated algorithm.

Sample Size A total of 2,267 patients were randomized to either the medical or surgical groups. After panel review, 41 patients were excluded for having greater than 70% stenosis (24 patients), no stenosis on angiography (11 patients), no ischemic event (3 patients), no informed consent (2 patients), and no available information (1 patient). Of the 2,226 patients who remained, 1,118 were in the medical group and 1,108 in the surgical group. Furthermore, of the 2,226 total patients, 858 had high-moderate stenosis (50–69%), while 1,368 had low-moderate stenosis (less than 50%). In the low-moderate group, 425 patients had mild stenosis (less than 30%). The authors noted that these patients were included in the analysis, but excluding them did not affect the results.

Of note, 21 patients within the surgical group did not undergo surgery (withdrew consent, medical complications, or surgeon's preference). In the medical group, 200 underwent endarterectomy (88 progressed to greater than 70% stenosis, 34 had

DOI: 10.1201/9781003416197-16

another ipsilateral stroke, and 78 were per the request of the patient/physician). It was noted that censoring the crossover did not affect the findings of the study.

Follow-Up Patients were followed up at 1, 3, 6, 9, and 12 months with neurological assessments, then every 4 months after the first year. Brain imaging was obtained when there were suspected cerebral ischemic events. Ultrasound was performed after 1 month and then yearly. Angiography was repeated if noninvasive imaging was concerning for worsening stenosis.

Inclusion/Exclusion Criteria

- Inclusion Criteria – To be eligible, patients must have had:
  - An ischemic event (a transient ischemic attack or a nondisabling stroke) on the side of the carotid stenosis within 180 days.
  - Angiographic evidence of 30% or more carotid stenosis and no other significant tandem lesions or complete occlusion.

- Exclusion Criteria
  - No informed consent.
  - No correlating carotid stenosis on angiography.
  - Distal/intracranial carotid stenosis worse than the proximal lesion or complete carotid occlusion.
  - Non-atherosclerotic carotid disease.
  - No symptoms localizing to the side of the carotid stenosis.
  - A large cerebral infarct that compromised function on that side of the brain.
  - Comorbidity with a life expectancy of less than 5 years.
  - Concurrent cardiac illness that might have been associated with a cardioembolic event.
  - Prior ipsilateral carotid endarterectomy.

While patients older than 80 were excluded from the first phase of the NASCET trial, they were included in this study.

Intervention or Treatment Received Medical therapy in both groups consisted of antithrombotic medication (i.e. aspirin), antihypertensive medications, and lipid-lowering medications. Specific surgical techniques used for endarterectomy were left to the discretion of each surgeon.

Results The 5-year treatment failure rate, as defined as any stroke (disabling or nondisabling) ipsilateral to the carotid stenosis (primary outcome), was 22.2% in the medical therapy group versus 15.7% for the surgical therapy group in patients with high-moderate stenosis ($p = 0.045$). This translated to a 6.5% absolute risk reduction and 15 patients needed to be treated to prevent one ipsilateral stroke within 5 years. The difference between the medical and surgical groups for the low-moderate stenosis group was not statistically significant ($p = 0.16$). Secondary analysis, looking at any stroke, any disabling stroke, any stroke or death from any cause, and any disabling stroke or death from any cause, all showed a similarly significant difference between the medical and surgical groups in the high-moderate stenosis subgroup, and no statistically significant difference in the low-moderate stenosis subgroup (Table 2[1]).

Furthermore, the study demonstrated that the difference between the medical and surgical groups was most significant in the severe carotid stenosis group, decreased for the high-moderate stenosis group, and was no longer significant in the low-moderate stenosis group (Figure 1[1]).

In both the high-moderate and severe stenosis (>70%) groups, the risk of stroke on the side of stenosis decreased to 2% per year within the first 10 days after surgery, as compared to 3% per year after 2 to 3 years in the medical group (Figure 2[1]). There was no difference between the medical and surgical groups in the causes of death and distribution of stroke in all patients with moderate carotid stenosis.

The study also found seven factors associated with increased risk of perioperative stroke and death: carotid occlusion on the opposite side, carotid disease on the left, less than 650 mg aspirin daily, no prior myocardial infarction/angina, lesion on computerized tomography or magnetic resonance imaging ipsilateral to the carotid stenosis, diabetes mellitus, and diastolic pressure greater than 90 mmHg. Increased benefit following surgery was correlated with male sex, recent stroke, recent hemispheric symptoms, and taking more than 650 mg aspirin daily.

Conclusion Carotid endarterectomy reduced the risk of stroke within the first 2 to 3 years compared to medical management in select patients with high-moderate (50–70%) symptomatic carotid stenosis. There was no benefit of endarterectomy in patients with mild-moderate symptomatic carotid stenosis. Patient comorbidities such as diabetes, high blood pressure, and contralateral carotid disease should also be considered in weighing the risks and benefits of carotid endarterectomy.

Study Limitations The study cautioned against overzealous adaptation of carotid endarterectomy for the management of carotid stenosis. It emphasized that the surgeons performing endarterectomy in this study were all well-experienced, thereby reducing the complication rate as compared to surgeons with less experience. Furthermore, the measurement of carotid stenosis should also be considered carefully, as different methods of calculation could lead to overestimation of the degree of stenosis as compared to the methods used in this study.

Reviewer Commentary In the late 1970s and 1980s, there was a rise in the number of carotid endarterectomies that were performed. However, this was also accompanied by an increase in the complication rate, leading to large randomized controlled trials looking at the benefits of carotid endarterectomy and appropriate indications.[2] One of the major clinical trials that was launched was the North American Symptomatic Carotid Endarterectomy Trial (NASCET), which randomized patients with symptomatic carotid stenosis to the medical management arm and the endarterectomy arm. The groups were further stratified by severe stenosis (70–99% stenosis) and moderate stenosis (30–70% stenosis). The trial was ended early for the group with severe stenosis after results demonstrated statistically significant benefit in the surgical group, namely a 17% absolute risk reduction of ipsilateral stroke within the first 24 months in the surgical group versus the medical group, and a 10.6% absolute risk reduction for the next 2 years.[3,4] The trial continued for the moderate stenosis group, and more patients were accrued. This study described the findings of patients with moderate carotid stenosis in the NASCET trial.

In this study, the results demonstrated a 6.5% absolute risk reduction in the surgical group compared to the medical management group for patients with high-moderate (50–70%) stenosis. There was no significant difference in the low-moderate stenosis (30–50%) group. Furthermore, the study also identified risk factors such as hypertension, diabetes mellitus, left-sided carotid disease, and contralateral carotid occlusion, which increased the risk of perioperative mortality. The authors concluded that while there may be a benefit of carotid endarterectomy in patients with high-moderate stenosis, caution must be exercised.[1]

Another large multicenter randomized controlled trial conducted around this period was the European Carotid Surgery Trial (ECST). In this study, patients with carotid stenosis and an ischemic event in the same distribution within the past 6 months were enrolled and randomized to the surgical and medical arms. Results demonstrated a significant benefit of surgical intervention in those with 80% or greater stenosis.[5] However, it should be noted that due to the differences in calculation of carotid stenosis between the NASCET and ECST studies, the cutoffs in degrees of carotid stenosis to achieve surgical benefit are not interchangeable (Figure 1).[6]

Despite differences in measurement, both trials found that patients with high-grade symptomatic carotid stenosis derive benefit from carotid endarterectomy compared to medical therapy alone. Following the publication of these findings, there was a rise in the number of carotid endarterectomies performed in the 1990s for patients with symptomatic disease. A higher percentage of patients receiving surgery had greater than 70% stenosis, and the overall perioperative neurologic complications rate has decreased.[7] Overall, there has been a reduction in the percentage of inappropriate surgery since the publication of the randomized trials.[8,9] The NASCET study marked a defining moment in the management of carotid stenosis, establishing our current guidelines in the selection of appropriate surgical candidates.

REFERENCES

1. Barnett HJ, Taylor DW, Eliasziw M, et al. Benefit of carotid endarterectomy in patients with symptomatic moderate or severe stenosis. North American Symptomatic Carotid Endarterectomy Trial Collaborators. N Engl J Med. 1998;339(20):274–275. doi:10.1056/NEJM199811123392002
2. Chassin MR. Appropriate use of carotid endarterectomy. N Engl J Med. 1998;339(20): 1169–1179. doi:10.1056/NEJM199811123392010
3. North American symptomatic carotid endarterectomy trial. Methods, patient characteristics, and progress. Stroke. 1991;22(6):711–720. doi:10.1161/01.STR.22.6.711
4. HJM B, DW T, RB H, et al. Beneficial effect of carotid endarterectomy in symptomatic patients with high-grade carotid stenosis. N Engl J Med. 1991;325(7):445–453. doi:10.1056/NEJM199108153250701
5. Randomised trial of endarterectomy for recently symptomatic carotid stenosis: final results of the MRC European Carotid Surgery Trial (ECST). Lancet. 1998;351(9113): 1379–1387. doi:10.1016/S0140-6736(97)09292-1
6. Rothwell PM, Gibson RJ, Slattery J, Sellar RJ, Warlow CP. Equivalence of measurements of carotid stenosis. A comparison of three methods on 1001 angiograms. European Carotid Surgery Trialists' Collaborative Group. Stroke. 1994;25(12):2435–2439. doi:10.1161/01.STR.25.12.2435
7. Brittenden J, Murie JA, Jenkins AM, Ruckley C V, Bradbury AW. Carotid endarterectomy before and after publication of randomized controlled trials. Br J Surg. 1999 Feb;86(2): 206–10. doi: 10.1046/j.1365-2168.1999.01027.x. PMID: 10100788.
8. Halm EA, Tuhrim S, Wang JJ, Rojas M, Hannan EL, Chassin MR. Has evidence changed practice? Appropriateness of carotid endarterectomy after the clinical trials. Neurology. 2007;68(3):187–194. doi:10.1212/01.WNL.0000251197.98197.E9
9. Easton JD. History of carotid endarterectomy then and now: personal perspective. Stroke. 2014;45(6). doi:10.1161/STROKEAHA.113.003501. Epub 2014 Jan 7. PMID: 24399374.

Chapter 17

Trial of Early Minimally Invasive Removal of Intracerebral Hemorrhage (ENRICH)

ENRICH Investigators, Pradilla G, Ratcliff JJ, Hall AJ, Saville BR, Allen JW, Paulon G, McGlothlin A, Lewis RJ, Fitzgerald M, Caveney AF, Li XT, Bain M, Gomes J, Jankowitz B, Zenonos G, Molyneaux BJ, Davies J, Siddiqui A, Chicoine MR, Keyrouz SG, Grossberg JA, Shah MV, Singh R, Bohnstedt BN, Frankel M, Wright DW, Barrow DL, N Engl J Med. 2024 Apr 11;390(14):1277–1289

Reviewed by Aditya Kondajji and Mark Bain

Research Question/Objective Previous studies investigating conventional craniotomy for the evacuation of intracerebral hemorrhages (ICHs) have largely demonstrated improvement in mortality, but not functional outcome, when compared to medical care alone. ENRICH aims to determine how functional outcomes for minimally invasive hematoma evacuation plus guideline-based medical management compare to standard management alone for lobar and anterior basal ganglia ICH.

Study Design Prospective, multicenter, adaptive, randomized trial with endpoint adjudication.

Sample Size 300 total patients, 150 within the surgical group, 150 within the control group.

Follow-Up Follow-up occurred at 30, 90, and 180 days with audio-recorded structured interviews.

Inclusion/Exclusion Criteria

- Inclusion Criteria
  - Aged 18–80 years with acute, spontaneous, supratentorial ICH
  - ICH volume of 30–80 mL
  - Glasgow Coma Scale score between 5 and 14
  - National Institutes of Health Stroke Scale (NIHSS) score of more than 5
  - Modified Rankin Scale (mRS) score before hemorrhage of 0–1
  - If surgery could be performed within 24 hours of the last known well time

DOI: 10.1201/9781003416197-17

- Exclusion Criteria
  - Uncorrectable coagulopathy
  - The need for long-term anticoagulation that must be initiated within 5 days of the initial ICH
  - The presence of intraventricular hemorrhage (IVH) involving more than 50% of either lateral ventricle
  - Primary thalamic or infratentorial hemorrhage
  - The presence of a secondary cause of hemorrhage (e.g. ruptured aneurysm, AVM)
  - A very poor neurologic exam (i.e. fixed dilated pupils bilaterally, extensor posturing), or a very good neurologic exam (NIHSS <5)

Intervention or Treatment Received Minimally invasive craniotomy via trans-sulcal, para-fascicular approach using the NICO BrainPath system and hematoma evacuation through suction and the NICO Myriad system.

Results The primary efficacy endpoint was a utility-weighted mRS score at 180 days, with higher scores indicating better outcomes. At interim analysis after recruitment of 175 patients, the futility criteria were met for anterior basal ganglia hemorrhages (posterior probability of meaningful effect of 0.177, threshold of 0.2), and recruitment subsequently only included lobar hemorrhages. The utility-weighted mRS score at 180 days was 0.458 for the surgery group and 0.374 for the control group, for a difference of 0.084 (95% Bayesian credible interval, 0.005 to 0.163; posterior probability of superiority of 0.981, threshold of 0.975). The benefit of surgery was not assumed to be equal across hemorrhage locations; for anterior basal ganglia hemorrhage, the between-group difference was −0.013 (95% Bayesian credible interval, −0.147 to 0.116) and for lobar hemorrhage, the between-group difference was 0.127 (95% Bayesian credible interval, 0.035 to 0.219).

Conclusion The results suggest that minimally invasive surgical evacuation for lobar supratentorial intracerebral hemorrhage through a trans-sulcal, para-fascicular approach results in better weighted disability scores when compared to medical management alone.

Author/Reviewer Commentary The role of surgery in the management of supratentorial ICH remains a topic of great interest and debate. ENRICH's extensive inclusion and exclusion criteria, in conjunction with a highly standardized surgical technique, suggest that the functional benefit seen in the study is likely to only be reproducible in limited patients and in institutions with access to NICO's equipment.

This is the strictest interpretation of the data. In a broader perspective, ENRICH highlights two key aspects for the neurosurgeon managing an ICH: patient selection and an understanding of neuroanatomy when deciding a surgical trajectory.

No significant meaningful benefit was seen in surgical intervention for anterior basal ganglia hemorrhages. This is perhaps due to the consolidation of numerous white matter fibers as they approach the deep gray nuclei, resulting in dense, "high-risk" territories in which surgical manipulation may only serve to further dissect the remaining intact axons. In this sense, although evacuation may ameliorate secondary inflammation near the basal ganglia, it is possible that iatrogenic trauma may disrupt residual functioning parenchyma, resulting in a reduced ability to rehabilitate from the initial hemorrhagic insult.

For patients with lobar hemorrhage, functional benefit was demonstrated when compared to standard management alone. It is important to highlight that with a median ICH volume size of 54 mL in the surgical group, the residual median volume after surgery was 7 mL, representing a 73% median reduction in volume. This significant reduction in hematoma volume is partially attributable to the nature of the port system utilized; the cone shape allows displacement of white matter fibers rather than transection, particularly when the trajectory is planned in parallel with white matter tracts. Additionally, surgeons can manipulate the port under visualization in a rotary fashion, allowing for a more complete circumferential evacuation that can better reduce the injurious inflammatory response secondary to ICH.[1]

Beyond addressing the neurotoxicity of the hemorrhage, surgical evacuation treats the mass effect of the hematoma itself. Particularly for larger hemorrhages or those involving the temporal lobe, the space-occupying lesion of the hematoma and its associated cerebral edema may necessitate decompressive hemicraniectomy. Although it was an exploratory endpoint in ENRICH, it is notable that five (3%) patients within the surgical group vs 30 (20%) patients within the control group required surgical decompression. It is known that surgical decompression improves mortality.[2] Thus, although the study focused on functional outcomes, the mortality benefit seen in ENRICH would likely have been greater had the study truly compared surgery against medical management alone.

Study Limitations There are a few important limitations to ENRICH. First, the study exclusively enrolled ICH volumes of 30–80 mL, which were measured by the [length × width × height]/2 method. As such, the results of the study cannot be applied to hemorrhages less than or exceeding these volumes. External validity is further limited by strict exclusion criteria (e.g. presence of mechanical heart valve, end-stage renal disease, limited IVH) and by surgical superiority only being demonstrated for lobar hemorrhages. Furthermore, hemorrhage patterns may vary, and the formula is best suited for ellipsoid hematomas; thus, the true hemorrhage volume may differ from what is calculated. This latter point was addressed in the study by having two neuroradiologists adjudicate the computerized tomography hemorrhage volumes. ENRICH was also sponsored by NICO, the manufacturer of the BrainPath and Myriad devices used in this study, and while NICO was not involved in trial design or data collection, it is important to acknowledge that other devices from separate manufacturers were not included.

Relevant Studies Several studies laid the groundwork to investigate the impact of surgical intervention on morbidity and mortality in the setting of ICH. There is level C evidence to suggest that supratentorial hematoma evacuation through conventional craniotomy offers a mortality benefit.[2] In 2005, the Surgical Trial in Intracerebral Hemorrhage (STICH I) studied the utility of early surgery within 24 hours of randomization for supratentorial ICH measuring at least 2 cm in diameter.[3] Of note, there was no standardization of surgical approach which included burr hole, endoscopy, and stereotaxy. The true time-to-surgery from symptom onset was approximately 30 hours, making it unclear if these patients may have benefited from earlier surgical intervention. Furthermore, the study did note a mortality benefit for lobar hemorrhages without IVH; patients with deep-seated hemorrhage or with the presence of IVH fared more poorly compared to medical management alone.

This subgroup analysis ultimately prompted STICH II, published 8 years later, which specifically explored surgical intervention within 48 hours of symptom onset via craniotomy for lobar hemorrhages, without IVH, ranging from 10 to 100 mL in volume.[4] STICH II was more homogenous in terms of the surgical intervention offered, with 98% of patients within the early surgery group undergoing craniotomy. When compared to ENRICH, STICH II was far less selective in enrollment and included patients with pre-hemorrhage mRS scores of 2–4. At its conclusion, STICH II ultimately did not show a benefit in functional outcomes with surgical intervention but did show a mortality benefit, consistent with the subgroup analysis of STICH I.

Minimally Invasive Surgery Plus Recombinant Tissue Plasminogen Activator (rt-PA) for Intracerebral Hemorrhage Evacuation (MISTIE) III served as another important stepping stone in the surgical management of both deep and lobar supratentorial ICH, utilizing minimally invasive catheter aspiration followed by irrigation with thrombolysis.[5] Ultimately, in comparison to medical management alone, there was no benefit in functional outcomes. While MISTIE III sought to minimize parenchymal trauma through a catheter-based approach, it is important to note that the trajectory of the catheter was based on the long-axis of the hematoma, as opposed to considered white matter tracts. Additionally, as the authors themselves highlight, round hematomas may have required multiple catheter trajectories to adequately evacuate.

When considering the outcomes of the STICH and MISTIE trials, the surgical methodology and outcomes of ENRICH become clear: lobar hemorrhages can be safely treated, with improvements in functional outcomes, through a minimally invasive approach, respecting white matter tracts while having the freedom to perform a more complete evacuation via a trans-sulcal port.

REFERENCES

1. Zhu H, Wang Z, Yu J, et al. Role and mechanisms of cytokines in the secondary brain injury after intracerebral hemorrhage. Prog Neurobiol. 2019;178:101610.
2. Greenberg SM, Ziai WC, Cordonnier C, et al. 2022 Guideline for the management of patients with spontaneous intracerebral hemorrhage: a guideline from the American Heart Association/American Stroke Association. Stroke. 2022;53(7):e282–e361.
3. Mendelow AD, Gregson BA, Fernandes HM, et al. Early surgery versus initial conservative treatment in patients with spontaneous supratentorial intracerebral haematomas in the International Surgical Trial in Intracerebral Haemorrhage (STICH): a randomised trial. Lancet. 2005;365(9457):387–397.
4. Mendelow AD, Gregson BA, Rowan EN, Murray GD, Gholkar A, Mitchell PM. Early surgery versus initial conservative treatment in patients with spontaneous supratentorial lobar intracerebral haematomas (STICH II): a randomised trial. Lancet. 2013;382(9890):397–408.
5. Hanley DF, Thompson RE, Rosenblum M, et al. Efficacy and safety of minimally invasive surgery with thrombolysis in intracerebral haemorrhage evacuation (MISTIE III): a randomised, controlled, open-label, blinded endpoint phase 3 trial. Lancet. 2019;393(10175):1021–1032.

Chapter 18

Randomized Trial of Cerebrospinal Fluid Shunt Valve Design in Pediatric Hydrocephalus

Drake JM, Kestle JR, Milner R, Cinalli G, Boop F, Piatt J Jr, Haines S, Schiff SJ, Cochrane DD, Steinbok P, MacNeil N, Neurosurgery. 1998 Aug;43(2):294–303

Reviewed by Eisha Christian

Objective Forty percent of standard cerebrospinal fluid shunts implanted for the treatment of pediatric hydrocephalus fail within the first year. Two new shunt valves designed to limit excess flow, particularly in upright positions, were studied to compare treatment failure rates with those for standard differential pressure valves.

Methods 344 hydrocephalic children (aged from birth to 18 years) undergoing their first cerebrospinal fluid shunt insertion were randomized at 12 North American or European pediatric neurosurgical centers. Patients received one of three valves, i.e. a standard differential-pressure valve; a Delta valve (Medtronic PS Medical, Goleta, California), which contains a siphon-control component designed to reduce siphoning in upright positions, or an Orbis-Sigma valve (Cordis, Miami, Florida), with a variable-resistance, flow-limiting component. Patients were monitored for a minimum of 1 year. Endpoints were defined as shunt failure resulting from shunt obstruction, over-drainage, loculations of the cerebral ventricles, or infection. Outcome events were assessed by blinded independent case review.

Results 150 patients reached an endpoint; shunt obstruction occurred in 108 (31.4%), over-drainage in 12 (3.5%), loculated ventricles in two (0.6%), and infection in 28 (8.1%). Sixty-one percent were shunt failure-free at 1 year and 47% at 2 years, with a median shunt failure-free duration of 656 days. There was no difference in shunt failure-free duration among the three valves ($P = 0.24$).

Conclusion Cerebrospinal fluid (CSF) shunt failure, predominantly from shunt obstruction and infection, remains a persistent problem in pediatric hydrocephalus. Two new valve designs did not significantly affect shunt failure rates.

DOI: 10.1201/9781003416197-18

Research Question/Objective This study was designed to assess the differences in failure rate at 1 year between three shunt valve types.

Study Design Multicenter randomized trial.

Sample Size 344 patients.

Follow-Up 3, 12, 24, and 36 months.

Inclusion/Exclusion Criteria

- Inclusion Criteria
  - Age ≤18
  - Newly diagnosed hydrocephalus diagnosed with computerized tomography, magnetic resonance imaging, or ultrasound
  - Initial ventriculoperitoneal shunt insertion

- Exclusion Criteria
  - Previous indwelling CSF shunt
  - Active abdominal or CSF infection
  - Leptomeningeal tumor spread
  - Marked prematurity with risk of skin erosion from hardware
  - Systemic disorders
  - Septated loculations requiring multiple shunts
  - Dandy–Walker malformation
  - Arachnoid cyst causing hydrocephalus
  - Inability to be monitored for 1 year

Intervention or Treatment Received Ventriculoperitoneal shunt insertion with one of three valve types: standard differential pressure valve, Delta valve (additional siphon-control device to limit flow in upright position), Orbis-Sigma valve (limits flow by progressively narrowing flow orifice with increasing pressure).

Results Primary endpoint (**shunt failure at 1 year**) was met by 150 (43.6%) patients. There were no differences among the three shunt valve groups: 61% of patients were free of shunt failure at 1 year and 47% at 2 years.

The key results pertaining to secondary endpoints included the following:

- There were no deaths related to shunt failure.
- There was no difference in surgical complications between the three valves.
- Valve design seemed to have an impact on the type of shunt malfunction (there were no failures from over-drainage with the Orbis-Sigma valve) and the site of obstruction (there were fewer ventricular catheter obstructions with the Orbis-Sigma valve). However, the Orbis-Sigma valve had an increased rate of valve occlusion compared to the standard and Delta valves.
- There was no difference in hospital stay between the three valves.

Conclusion There was no difference in shunt failure rates at the 1-year follow-up between the standard differential pressure, Delta, and Orbis-Sigma valves.

Relevant Studies The shunt design trial remains one of the few randomized device trials in neurosurgery, and the first to evaluate CSF shunt valve designs. In a subsequent sequel to this trial, Kestle et al. published 3-year follow-up data, once again demonstrating that shunt valve design did not influence shunt survival.[1] In 2000, Drake et al. in *CSF Shunt 50 Years On: Past, Present, and Future*, expanded on this work by paving the way for the Hydrocephalus Clinical Research Network (HCRN), which was created to answer questions left unanswered by the original shunt design trial.[2] In this follow-up paper, the authors identified that the position of the ventricular catheter may influence shunt failure. They also suggested that additional investigation into the endoscopic placement of ventricular catheters was warranted based on their data in the original trial. They concluded that endoscopic third ventriculostomy, which had become an alternative to a CSF shunt in some patients, should be studied in a similar manner.

Sixteen years after the publication of this landmark trial, Baird et al. published a systematic review on pediatric hydrocephalus, which included 22 papers: the shunt design trial remained the only class I evidence on the effects of valve type on shunt survival.[3] This systematic review concluded that there was still insufficient evidence to demonstrate an advantage of one valve over another.

In 2016, the HCRN continued this work by publishing their findings of a multicenter prospective cohort study with 1,036 patients across six centers once again confirming no impact on valve type on shunt survival.[4] Their cohort included patients with programmable valves in addition to the original valves included in the shunt design trial. The HCRN, which can trace its roots to the shunt design trial, has gone on to publish 39 papers on a variety of topics, including shunt infection, hydrocephalus of prematurity, and endoscopic third ventriculostomy.

Study Limitations/Future Directions The shunt design trial is a landmark paper in neurosurgery in both its design and impact; however, with the evolution in valve technology, a repeat randomized study is overdue. In addition, the original trial was not powered to allow analysis for specific age groups or hydrocephalus etiology. The HCRN has continued this sentinel work with 39 papers including randomized studies on the initial shunt insertion site, but there continue to be questions left unanswered. Hall et al. in 2024 published a small retrospective series of patients with posthemorrhagic hydrocephalus of prematurity, concluding that programmable valves did not change overall shunt survival, but they did reduce the number of revisions per patient.[5] Future directions emanating from the shunt design trial and the HCRN would look at new valve types in addition to subgroup analysis, such as age and hydrocephalus etiology, as well as developmental and quality-of-life outcome measures.

REFERENCES

1. Kestle J, Drake J, Milner R, Sainte-Rose C, Cinalli G, Boop F, Piatt J, Haines S, Schiff S, Cochrane D, Steinbok P, MacNeil N. Long term follow-up data from the shunt design trial. Pediatr Neurosurg. 2000;33:230–236.
2. Drake JM, Kestle JR, Tuli S. CSF shunts 50 years on: past, present and future. Childs Nerv Syst. 2000;16(10–11):800–804. doi:10.1007/s003810000351
3. Baird LC, Mazzola CA, Auguste KI, Klimo P Jr, Flannery AM; Pediatric Hydrocephalus Systematic Review and Evidence-Based Guidelines Task Force. Pediatric hydrocephalus: systematic literature review and evidence-based guidelines. Part 5: effect of valve type on cerebrospinal fluid shunt efficacy. J Neurosurg Pediatr. 2014;14(Suppl 1):35–43. doi:10.3171/2014.7.PEDS14325
4. Riva-Cambrin J, Kestle JR, Holubkov R, Butler J, Kulkarni AV, Drake J, Whitehead WE, Wellons JC 3rd, Shannon CN, Tamber MS, Limbrick DD Jr, Rozzelle C, Browd SR, Simon TD; Hydrocephalus Clinical Research Network. Risk factors for shunt malfunction in pediatric hydrocephalus: a multicenter prospective cohort study. J Neurosurg Pediatr. 2016;17:382–390.
5. Hall BJ, Ali AMS, Hennigan D, Pettorini B. Hydrocephalus in prematurity: does valve choice make a difference? Childs Nerv Syst. 2024;40(4):1091–1098. doi:10.1007/s00381-023-06204-8

CHAPTER 19

Endoscopic Third Ventriculostomy in the Treatment of Childhood Hydrocephalus

Kulkarni AV, Drake JM, Mallucci CL, Sgouros S, Roth J, Constantini S; Canadian Pediatric Neurosurgery Study Group. J Pediatr. 2009 Aug; 155(2):254–259

Reviewed by Armaan K Malhotra and Abhaya V Kulkarni

Objective To develop a model to predict the probability of endoscopic third ventriculostomy (ETV) success in the treatment of hydrocephalus based on a child's individual characteristics.

Study Design We analyzed 618 ETVs performed consecutively on children at 12 international institutions to identify predictors of ETV success at 6 months. A multivariable logistic regression model was developed on 70% of the dataset (training set) and validated on 30% of the dataset (validation set).

Results In the training set, 305/455 ETVs (67.0%) were successful. The regression model (containing patient age, cause of hydrocephalus, and previous cerebrospinal fluid shunt) demonstrated a good fit (Hosmer–Lemeshow, $p = 0.78$) and discrimination (C-statistic = 0.70). In the validation set, 105/163 ETVs (64.4%) were successful, and the model maintained a good fit (Hosmer–Lemeshow, $p = 0.45$), discrimination (C-statistic = 0.68), and calibration (calibration slope = 0.88). A simplified ETV Success Score (ETVSS) was devised that closely approximates the predicted probability of ETV success.

Conclusion Children most likely to succeed with ETV can now be accurately identified and spared the long-term complications of cerebrospinal fluid (CSF) shunting.

Author/Reviewer Commentary Pediatric hydrocephalus remains an important worldwide contributor to morbidity, mortality, and healthcare expenditure in low-, middle-, and high-income countries alike.[1,2] In the early 2000s, the predominant modality of surgical hydrocephalus treatment was by means of CSF shunt insertion. While effective, this procedure confers risks of over-drainage, infection, and

DOI: 10.1201/9781003416197-19

obstruction, each of which necessitates repeat surgical intervention. Furthermore, the scalability of shunt insertion as a solution across low-income country healthcare systems (the predominant location for pediatric hydrocephalus patients globally) is limited by both access and the cost of implants.[3] With the emergence of endoscopy as an alternate surgical approach for the treatment of hydrocephalus, the prospect of an alternative implant-free solution was promising for surgeons, families, and patients. However, early ETV research highlighted an approximate 30% risk of ETV failure, requiring conversion to shunt insertion (with the highest risk in the initial months after treatment) as well as differential success across differing hydrocephalus etiologies.[4] This was the impetus for the development of a clinical prediction model to facilitate ETV patient selection with a goal of reducing treatment failures and patient morbidity by tailoring a surgical approach based on specific patient characteristics.

In 2009, we derived and internally validated the ETVSS through the Canadian Pediatric Neurosurgery Group initiative, extending that collaboration to include a total of three countries (Israel, the UK, and Canada).[5] To derive the ETVSS, we utilized data from patients 19 years or younger undergoing ETV for hydrocephalus across 12 participating centers between 1989 and 2006 ($n = 618$ patients). The primary study outcome was ETV success 6 months after treatment, defined by the absence of any subsequent CSF diversion procedures following ETV. A multivariable logistic regression model was iteratively constructed using backward elimination methods; the subsequent model was then validated using a random data split (internal validation) and assessed using several performance metrics. The resultant ETVSS incorporated the variables age, etiology, and the presence of a prior shunt to predict the pre operative probability of ETV success at 6 months after surgery. The scores ranged from 0 (the lowest chance of ETV success) to 90 (the highest chance of ETV success) (Figure 19.1), and approximated the percentage chance of ETV success. This prediction model quantified for the first time the component characteristics associated with ETV success and offered a probabilistic heuristic for hydrocephalus surgical decision-making.

Following the introduction of the ETVSS, there was ongoing clinical uncertainty regarding the intermediate patients, such as those with ETV success scores ranging from 40 to 60. The continuous nature of the ETVSS offered clear guidance for patients with very high or very low predicted probabilities of success; however, for those with intermediate scores, the optimal choice between ETV and shunt placement remained unclear. Further, it was also unknown whether the patients predicted to have high chances of success with ETV were the same patients with high chances of shunt success. A secondary study was therefore conducted using pooled data from pediatric patients with newly diagnosed hydrocephalus from the Shunt Design Trial and the previously described ETVSS derivation cohort to determine long-term success after ETV compared to shunt, grouped by baseline ETVSS.[6,7] The cohort was stratified into high ETVSS (≥80), moderate ETVSS (50–70) and low ETVSS (≤40) groups and patients were followed for up to 48 months, although there were very low cohort numbers at the latter follow-up time points. Using time-to-event survival methods with a time-treatment interaction

ETV SUCCESS SCORE

= Age Score + Etiology Score + Previous Shunt Score
≈ percentage probability of ETV success

SCORE	AGE	ETIOLOGY	PREVIOUS SHUNT
0	<1 MONTH	POST-INFECTIOUS	PREVIOUS SHUNT
10	1 MONTH TO <6 MONTHS		NO PREVIOUS SHUNT
20		MYELOMENINGOCELE INTRA-VENTRICULAR HEMORRHAGE NON-TECTAL BRAIN TUMOR	
30	6 MONTHS TO <1 YEAR	AQUEDUCTAL STENOSIS TECTAL TUMOR OTHER ETIOLOGY	
40	1 YEAR TO <10 YEARS		
50	≥10 YEARS		

Figure 19.1 The endoscopic third ventriculostomy success score.[5]

term (to account for time-varying hazards), we showed a declining risk of ETV failure relative to shunt failure as time from surgery increased across all strata. For the high ETVSS group, ETV failure risk was lower than shunt failure risk from very shortly after surgery and onwards. For the low and moderate ETVSS groups, shunt failure risk was lower immediately after surgery until approximately 3 to 6 months post-surgery, after which ETV failure risk appeared lower. This data corroborated the construct validity of the ETVSS and enhanced its clinical utility by contextualizing the continuous ETVSS ranges with interpretable categories corresponding to low, moderate, and high success relative to shunt insertion.

Despite multicenter data from multiple countries used to derive the original ETVSS, an important limitation of the ETVSS at inception was the lack of external validation data to demonstrate generalizability. In the years following the ETVSS publication, several groups independently externally validated the ETVSS, demonstrating concordance between failure rates and predicted ETV success, including at longer-term follow-up of 36 months in the United Kingdom and the United States.[8–10] This emerging evidence supported the robustness of the ETVSS in varied patient cohorts from differing countries and healthcare settings. As expected, the generalizability of the ETVSS has not been uniform across all countries, case mixes, and practice settings, especially when benchmarked against regression models derived from local data, which frequently exhibit overfitting.[11,12]

Most recently, 15 years following the publication of the ETVSS, the multicenter Hydrocephalus Research Network reevaluated the predictive performance of the score in a contemporary cohort with two main goals. First, they sought to challenge the age categorization and etiology groupings of the original ETVSS, and second, they sought to assess the candidacy of radiographic variables obtained from preoperative neuroimaging with the aim of improving prediction accuracy.[13] This study included 761 patients undergoing first-time ETV without prior shunt history and demonstrated stable performance of the original ETVSS. Neither age modifications, etiology modifications, nor the addition of radiographic variables meaningfully improved ETV success predictions compared to the original model. Of note, this contemporary cohort had ~70% of patients with preoperative predicted ETVSS scores ≥80, which is an increase from approximately 50% when compared to the pre-ETVSS era, suggesting a shift in ETV patient selection since the publication of the ETVSS.[7]

The ETVSS has been through the arc of a clinical prediction model, from the original derivation to the establishment of construct validity, external validation (including temporal validation), clinical utility assessment, and reevaluation using contemporary variables. It remains a robust tool to predict ETV success, which has demonstrably shifted the landscape of patient selection for pediatric hydrocephalus practitioners since its publication. Ultimately, the aim of such clinical decision support tools is to facilitate evidence-based individualized surgical decision-making and to reduce the morbidity of pediatric hydrocephalus for children around the world.

REFERENCES

1. Dewan MC, Rattani A, Mekary R, et al. Global hydrocephalus epidemiology and incidence: systematic review and meta-analysis. J Neurosurg. 2018;130(4):1065–1079. doi:10.3171/2017.10.Jns17439
2. Kahle KT, Klinge PM, Koschnitzky JE, et al. Paediatric hydrocephalus. Nat Rev Dis Primers. 2024;10(1):35. doi:10.1038/s41572-024-00519-9
3. Warf BC. Pediatric hydrocephalus in East Africa: prevalence, causes, treatments, and strategies for the future. World Neurosurg. 2010;73(4):296–300. doi:10.1016/j.wneu.2010.02.009
4. Drake JM. Endoscopic third ventriculostomy in pediatric patients: the Canadian experience. Neurosurgery. 2007;60(5):881–886; discussion 881–6. doi:10.1227/01.Neu.0000255420.78431.E7

5. Kulkarni AV, Drake JM, Mallucci CL, Sgouros S, Roth J, Constantini S. Endoscopic third ventriculostomy in the treatment of childhood hydrocephalus. J Pediatr. 2009;155(2): 254–259.e1. doi:10.1016/j.jpeds.2009.02.048
6. Drake JM, Kestle JR, Milner R, et al. Randomized trial of cerebrospinal fluid shunt valve design in pediatric hydrocephalus. Neurosurgery. 1998;43(2):294–303; discussion 303–5. doi:10.1097/00006123-199808000-00068
7. Kulkarni AV, Drake JM, Kestle JRW, Mallucci CL, Sgouros S, Constantini S. Predicting who will benefit from endoscopic third ventriculostomy compared with shunt insertion in childhood hydrocephalus using the ETV success score: clinical article. J Neurosurg Pediatr. 2010;6(4):310–315. doi:10.3171/2010.8.PEDS103
8. Durnford AJ, Kirkham FJ, Mathad N, Sparrow OC. Endoscopic third ventriculostomy in the treatment of childhood hydrocephalus: validation of a success score that predicts long-term outcome. J Neurosurg Pediatr. 2011;8(5):489–493. doi:10.3171/2011.8.Peds1166
9. Naftel RP, Reed GT, Kulkarni AV, Wellons JC. Evaluating the Children's Hospital of Alabama endoscopic third ventriculostomy experience using the endoscopic third ventriculostomy success score: an external validation study. J Neurosurg Pediatr. 2011;8(5):494–501. doi:10.3171/2011.8.Peds1145
10. García LG, López BR, Botella GI, et al. Endoscopic third ventriculostomy success score (ETVSS) predicting success in a series of 50 pediatric patients. Are the outcomes of our patients predictable? Childs Nerv Syst. 2012;28(8):1157–1162. doi:10.1007/s00381-012-1836-3
11. Yordanov S, Garnett MR, Santarius T, Holland K, Jalloh I, Jawad Naushahi M. An audit of endoscopic third ventriculostomy (ETV) in a regional paediatric neurosurgical centre assessing the accuracy and feasibility of the ETV success score. Acta Neurochir (Wien). 2022;164(6):1453–1458. doi:10.1007/s00701-022-05151-8
12. Foley RW, Ndoro S, Crimmins D, Caird J. Is the endoscopic third ventriculostomy success score an appropriate tool to inform clinical decision-making? Br J Neurosurg. 2017;31(3):314–319. doi:10.1080/02688697.2016.1229744
13. Verhey LH, Kulkarni AV, Reeder RW, et al. A re-evaluation of the endoscopic third ventriculostomy success score: a hydrocephalus clinical research network study. J Neurosurg Pediatr. 2024;33(5):417–427. doi:10.3171/2023.12.Peds23401

CHAPTER 20

Antibiotic or Silver versus Standard Ventriculoperitoneal Shunts (BASICS): A Multicentre, Single-Blinded, Randomized Trial and Economic Evaluation

Mallucci CL, Jenkinson MD, Conroy EJ, Hartley JC, Brown M, Dalton J, Kearns T, Moitt T, Griffiths MJ, Culeddu G, Solomon T, Hughes D, Gamble C; for the BASICS Study Collaborators, Lancet. 2019 Oct 26;394(10208):1530–1539

Reviewed by Michael D Jenkinson and Conor L Mallucci

Research Question/Objective To determine whether an antibiotic- or silver-impregnated ventriculoperitoneal shunt reduces early infection (within 6 months) compared to standard shunts in newly diagnosed hydrocephalus following insertion of the first de novo shunt.

Study Design Multicentre, single-blind, randomized controlled trial.

Sample Size 1,605 paediatric and adult patients.

Follow-Up Minimum of 6 months and a maximum of 2 years, depending on the time of randomization.

Inclusion/Exclusion Criteria

- Inclusion Criteria
  - Patients of any age, with hydrocephalus of any aetiology, undergoing insertion of their first ventriculoperitoneal shunt.
  - Patients with a failed endoscopic third ventriculostomy, previous external ventricular drain (EVD), or an indwelling ventricular access device.

- Exclusion Criteria – Patients were excluded if they had:
  - Active cerebrospinal fluid (CSF) or a peritoneal infection.
  - Multi-loculated hydrocephalus that needed multiple shunts or neuro-endoscopy.

DOI: 10.1201/9781003416197-20

- Ventriculoatrial or pleural shunts.
- Previous ventriculoperitoneal shunt.

Intervention or Treatment Received Patients were randomized 1:1:1 to receive standard, antibiotic, or silver shunts.

Results 1,605 patients aged 0 to 91 years were randomly assigned to either antibiotic ($n = 536$), antibiotic ($n = 538$), or silver shunt ($n = 531$). Eleven patients were excluded from the analysis (7 had an infection at insertion and 4 did not receive a shunt). Median follow-up was 22 months. 398 (25%) of the 1,594 follow-up patients had a shunt revision, of which 75 (5%) were for infection. Infection was seen in 32 (6%) of 533 standard shunts, 12 (2%) of 535 antibiotic shunts, and 31 (6%) of 526 silver shunts (cause-specific hazard ratio 0.38, 97.5% confidence interval [CI], 0.18–0.8, $p = 0.0038$) (Figure 20.1). Adverse events were non-life-threatening and mostly related to valve or catheter function in 135 (25%) standard, 127 (23%) antibiotic, and 134 (36%) silver shunts.

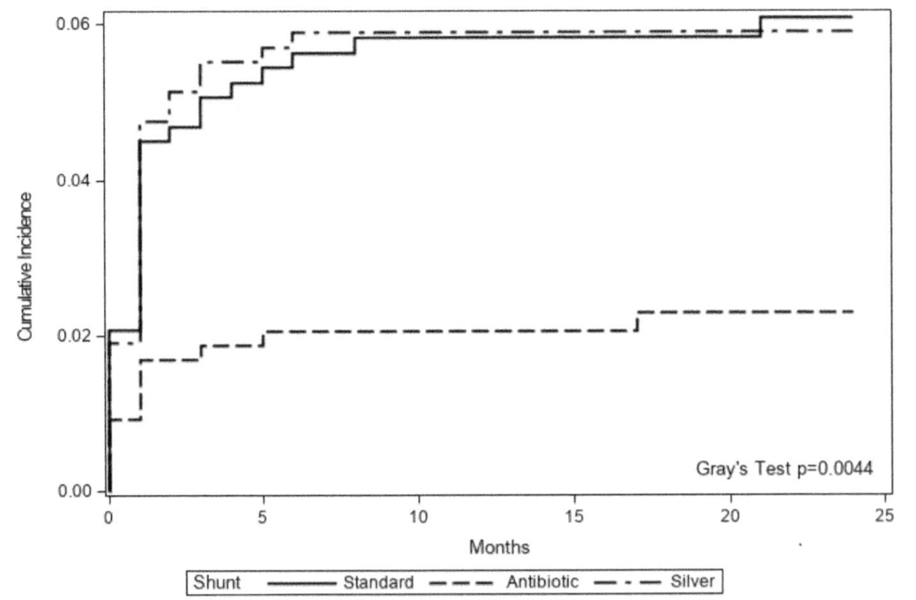

Number at risk
By shunt group

Months	0	6	12	18	24
Standard	533	441	381	315	259
Antibiotic	535	442	381	319	250
Silver	526	420	366	309	252

Figure 20.1 Cumulative incidence plot of infection by shunt type.

Conclusion The Balanced Solutions versus Saline in Intensive Care Study (BASICS) trial provides evidence to support the use of antibiotic shunts in patients undergoing insertion of their first ventriculoperitoneal shunt. Antibiotic shunts benefit patients of all ages by reducing the risk and harm of shunt infection.

Author/Reviewer Commentary Before designing and running the BASICS trial,[1] we were early adopters of antibiotic shunts, despite the lack of properly powered studies to support their use in routine clinical practice.[2] Our initial experience of 214 antibiotic shunts in the highest risk patients (neonates and children) reported a reduction in infection rates from 27% to 10.4%.[3] Data from the UK Shunt Registry reported that across all ages, there was a 3% infection rate with antibiotic shunts, compared to 4.7% in standard shunts.[4] Although this was non-randomized data, antibiotic shunt usage progressively increased in the UK neurosurgery community.

In 2011, silver-impregnated shunts were launched in the UK market with a claim to reduce infection. There was no good evidence to support their use, with only one observational study of silver shunts used to successfully treat seven patients with active CSF infection.[5] Encouragingly, in a limited-centre, randomized controlled trial of EVDs in children and adults, silver EVDs reduced infection from 21.4% (30/140) to 12.3% (17/138) ($p = 0.042$).[6] We were concerned that silver shunts would be readily adopted into routine practice based on the EVD trial, leading to a slew of unpowered, single-centre, retrospective studies, which are prone to bias.

The launch of the silver shunt provided the opportunity to test the device against standard shunts and to also test antibiotic shunts within the same clinical trial. The BASICS trial is the largest prospective randomized study of patients with shunts for hydrocephalus worldwide and was appropriately powered to detect a difference in infection rates between antibiotic, silver and standard shunts. The study had several strengths: (1) there was a central classification of infection, thereby removing the risk of bias by the treating neurosurgeon; (2) patient retention was high and withdrawal was low, therefore it was unlikely that shunt infection was missed; (3) patients were recruited across all ages and socioeconomic classes; and (5) the results have good generalizability since we did not mandate specific surgical techniques of infection control bundles. Furthermore, the health economic analysis from the perspective of the National Health Service (NHS) showed that for every infection avoided, there was a cost savings of £13,5753.

Study Limitations Ventriculo-atrial, ventriculo-pleural, and revision ventriculo-peritoneal shunts were excluded from the study, although we postulate that the results are translatable.

Relevant Studies We have undertaken a clinical and health economic impact analysis of the BASICS trial on routine shunt surgery practice and shunt infection in the UK. Using data from the UK Shunt Registry, we compared antibiotic and standard shunt use, shunt infection, and a budget impact analysis in patients undergoing insertion of their first ventriculoperitoneal shunt for hydrocephalus during the period pre-BASICS (1 January 2004 to 30 June 2013) and post-BASICS (1 January 2018 to 31 December 2021). There were 12,476 new shunt insertions and 2,482 revisions. Antibiotic shunt use increased from 36.9% in paediatrics and 20.5% in adults in 2004, to 99.2% in paediatrics and 96.8% in adults in 2021. The largest annual change in antibiotic shunt use was between 2018 and 2019 (year of BASICS publication), with a 14.9% increase in paediatrics and a 27.2% increase in adults. Compared to standard shunts, the infection rates for antibiotic shunts were significantly lower in children (5.1% versus 1.9%, $p < 0.001$) and adults (1.5% versus 0.9%, $p = 0.031$). Transitioning to antibiotic shunts is estimated to save the NHS £955,811 (95% CI, £698,332–£1,229,359) per annum. This follow-up study shows that the BASICS study has impacted clinical practice in the UK significantly, demonstrating that antibiotic shunts are the first choice for patients and that they reduce infection in routine clinical practice, saving the NHS around £1 million per year.[7] These results should be translatable on a wider global scale for patient benefit.

REFERENCES

1. Mallucci CL, Jenkinson MD, Conroy EJ, Hartley JC, Brown M, Dalton J, Kearns T, Moitt T, Griffiths MJ, Culeddu G, Solomon T, Hughes D, Gamble C; BASICS Study collaborators. Antibiotic or silver versus standard ventriculoperitoneal shunts (BASICS): a multicentre, single-blinded, randomised trial and economic evaluation. Lancet. 2019;394(10208):1530–1539. doi:10.1016/S0140-6736(19)31603-4
2. Thomas R, Lee S, Patole S, Rao S. Antibiotic-impregnated catheters for the prevention of CSF shunt infections: a systematic review and meta-analysis. Br J Neurosurg. 2012;26(2):175–184. doi:10.3109/02688697.2011.603856
3. Hayhurst C, Cooke R, Williams D, Kandasamy J, O'Brien DF, Mallucci CL. The impact of antibiotic-impregnated catheters on shunt infection in children and neonates. Childs Nerv Syst. 2008;24(5):557–562. doi:10.1007/s00381-007-0521-4
4. Richards HK, Seeley HM, Pickard JD. Efficacy of antibiotic-impregnated shunt catheters in reducing shunt infection: data from the United Kingdom Shunt Registry. J Neurosurg Pediatr. 2009;4(4):389–393. doi:10.3171/2009.4.PEDS09210
5. Izci Y, Secer H, Akay C, Gonul E: Initial experience with silver-impregnated polyurethane ventricular catheter for shunting of cerebrospinal fluid in patients with infected hydrocephalus. Neurol Res. 2009;31:234–237.
6. Keong NC, Bulters DO, Richards HK, Farrington M, Sparrow OC, Pickard JD, Hutchinson PJ, Kirkpatrick PJ. The SILVER (Silver Impregnated Line versus EVD Randomized trial): a double-blind, prospective, randomized, controlled trial of an intervention to reduce the rate of external ventricular drain infection. Neurosurgery. 2012;71(2):394–403; discussion 403–4. doi:10.1227/NEU.0b013e318257bebb
7. Bakhsh A, Fernández Méndez R, Culeddu G, Gillespie CS, Wood E, Palma M, Pickard JD, Hughes DA, Gamble C, Mallucci CL, Joannides AJ, Jenkinson MD. Clinical and health economic impact of the BASICS trial on ventriculoperitoneal shunt surgery: UK Shunt Registry analysis. J Neurosurg. 2026:1–11. Epub ahead of print. doi:10.3171/2025.8.JNS251266

Chapter 21

A Randomized Trial of Prenatal versus Postnatal Repair of Myelomeningocele (MOMS Trial)

Adzick NS, Thom EA, Spong CY, Brock JW III, Burrows PK, Johnson MP, Howell LJ, Farrell JA, Dabrowiak ME, Sutton LN, Gupta N, Tulipan NB, Alton MED, Farmer DL, N Engl J Med. 2011 Mar 17;364(11):993–1004

Reviewed by Hiba J Mustafa and Kholoud Arab

Research Question/Objective To compare outcomes in children with prenatal repair versus (vs) postnatal repair of open spina bifida (OSB).

Study Design A multicenter randomized controlled trial was conducted at three maternal-fetal surgery centers in the United States.

Sample Size The calculated sample size was 200. A total of 183 candidates were recruited from 2003 through December 2010, and the study was stopped early due to efficacy.

Inclusion/Exclusion Criteria

- Inclusion Criteria
  - Singleton pregnancies with an antenatal diagnosis of OSB.
  - The highest level of spinal dysraphism, starting at T1 to S1.
  - Evidence of hindbrain herniation.
  - Must have undergone amniocentesis confirming a normal karyotype, and the gestational age (GA) at randomization was 19.0 to 25.9 weeks.
  - Participating pregnant women had to be ≥18 years old and residents of the United States.

- Exclusion Criteria
  - A fetal anomaly unrelated to meningomyelocele.
  - Severe kyphosis.
  - Increased risk of preterm labor (a previous preterm birth or short cervix).
  - Placental abruption.
  - Previous upper uterine segment hysterotomy.

DOI: 10.1201/9781003416197-21

- Any maternal contraindications to surgical intervention.
- A body mass index of ≥35 kg/m^2.

Intervention or Treatment Received All participants underwent randomization in a 1-to-1 ratio to either prenatal or postnatal surgery. Prenatal surgery was performed through a Pfannenstiel incision laparotomy and a hysterotomy with a uterine stapler for hemostasis. The repair was performed by study-approved surgeons using standardized operative techniques and perioperative magnesium sulfate.

Follow-Up All women in the prenatal surgery group stayed locally with a support person until delivery. Women in the postnatal group went home and returned for delivery. Regardless of the group assignment, all patients enrolled in the study were scheduled for cesarean delivery at 37 weeks. Patients needing earlier delivery (due to spontaneous or medically indicated preterm delivery) were delivered by cesarean section at the study center. The same team of surgeons performed both prenatal and postnatal OSB surgeries.

Children were evaluated at 12 and 30 months of age by physical, neurological, and developmental testing. Imaging studies at 12 months were obtained, including spine radiography and magnetic resonance imaging of the head and spine. At 30 months, the functional level was assessed by videotaping motor, sensory, and distal somatosensory functions. The motor function was then adjusted according to the anatomical level previously determined at 12 months based on radiography. Independent practitioners blinded to the treatment assigned reported the results.

Outcomes were preassigned as two main primary outcomes and multiple secondary outcomes. The "Results" section details these outcomes.

Results The primary outcome was a composite measure of fetal or neonatal death, cerebrospinal fluid (CSF) shunt placement, or meeting predefined criteria for shunting as determined by an independent, blinded neurosurgeon. This outcome was assessed at 12 months of age and occurred in 68% of patients in the prenatal repair group compared with 98% in the postnatal repair group.

A second primary outcome was assessed at 30 months of age and consisted of a composite of cognitive performance, measured by the Mental Development Index of the Bayley Scales of Infant Development II, and motor function, adjusted for lesion level. Compared with postnatal repair, prenatal repair was associated with superior motor function, with children demonstrating functional motor levels that exceeded their assigned anatomical lesion level. No significant difference in cognitive scores was observed between groups.

Secondary outcomes included maternal, fetal/neonatal, and infant measures. Maternal morbidity related to prenatal surgery included pulmonary edema in 6%, significant thinning of the uterine scar in 25%, and partial or complete uterine scar dehiscence in 10%. There was no maternal mortality. Blood transfusion at delivery was required in 9% of patients in the prenatal group compared with 1% in the postnatal group. Pregnancy-related complications were more frequent following prenatal repair, including spontaneous preterm labor (38% vs 14%) and premature rupture of membranes (46% vs 8%). Other complications, such as chorioamniotic separation, oligohydramnios, and placental abruption, occurred in 26%, 21%, and 6% of cases, respectively. No differences were observed in maternal medical complications.

Prematurity was the most significant fetal and neonatal complication associated with prenatal repair, occurring in 84% of cases. The mean GA at delivery was 34 weeks in the prenatal group compared with 37 weeks in the postnatal group, with 10% of prenatal repairs resulting in delivery before 30 weeks' gestation. As a consequence, respiratory distress syndrome occurred more frequently following prenatal repair (21% vs 6%). No significant differences were observed in other complications of prematurity, including periventricular leukomalacia and necrotizing enterocolitis. Birth weight was significantly lower in the prenatal group, attributable to an earlier GA rather than impaired fetal growth.

Secondary infant outcomes assessed at 12 months demonstrated the radiographic superiority of prenatal repair with respect to Chiari II malformation. Nearly 80% of infants had no or mild hindbrain herniation, 80% had no brainstem kinking, and 54% had normal positioning of the fourth ventricle. By 12 months, only 40% of infants in the prenatal group required CSF shunting, compared with 82% in the postnatal group, representing an approximate 50% reduction.

At 30 months of age, children who underwent prenatal repair demonstrated superior motor outcomes on both the Bayley and Peabody developmental motor scales. They were more likely to walk independently or with orthotics (42% vs 21% and 29% vs 36%, respectively). Prenatal repair was also associated with more favorable motor–anatomical level concordance, with a greater proportion of children demonstrating motor function one or more levels better than their anatomical lesion (32% vs 12%) and fewer demonstrating worse motor levels (13% vs 28%). Improvements were noted across the stationary, locomotion, and object-manipulation domains. Parent-reported outcomes using the Functional Independence Measure for Children (WeeFIM) instrument also indicated superior self-care and mobility in the prenatal repair group.

Conclusion This landmark randomized clinical trial demonstrates the superiority of prenatal repair. These children are more likely to walk, with or without prostheses, and less likely to require CSF diversion. Despite the favorable outcomes, these surgeries are associated with substantial neonatal morbidities, mainly due to prematurity.

Reviewer Commentary The Management of Myelomeningocele Study (MOMS) trial is a landmark study that fundamentally altered neurosurgical management of open spina bifida by providing level I evidence that prenatal myelomeningocele repair improves key neurosurgical outcomes, including reduced CSF diversion, reversal of hindbrain herniation, and superior lesion-adjusted motor function. The trial reshaped expectations for functional recovery and established shunt dependency and motor–anatomical concordance as core neurosurgical outcome measures in this population. Beyond its immediate clinical implications, the MOMS trial transformed surgical counseling, expanded the neurosurgeon's role into prenatal decision-making, and laid the foundation for contemporary fetal surgery programs and subsequent technical innovations. Its impact is reflected in its extensive influence on the literature, with the original publication cited more than **2,000 times**, underscoring its enduring role as the definitive reference guiding neurosurgical practice in the post-MOMS era.

Study Limitations The study's strict criteria did not allow for the examination of outcomes in patients with different characteristics, such as a BMI of >30, GA beyond 26 weeks, and children with no hindbrain herniation at the time of randomization.

Relevant Studies There have been numerous studies published after the MOMS trial from different centers worldwide reporting outcomes of prenatal spina bifida repair, including CSF diversion, mobility, and urinary continence[1–28] (see Table 21.1).

An open surgery was performed in the majority of these published cases. However, multiple investigators have proposed modifications to the surgical approach with minimally invasive techniques to reduce the associated maternal morbidity. These include a percutaneous approach, laparotomy-assisted, and mini-laparotomy-assisted fetoscopic surgery. While some studies showed less favorable outcomes regarding CSF diversion with fetoscopy, others showed a comparable effect. No head-to-head comparison of both approaches has been conducted, and no definite conclusion can be reached. However, current data is promising.

Most follow-up studies found similar improved CSF diversion rates. A meta-analysis of nine studies involving 948 cases of prenatally repaired lesions found that GA at surgery of ≥25 weeks, a lateral ventricular diameter of >15 mm, myeloschisis lesions, and a lesion level of L2 or higher appeared to be strongly associated with the need for CSF diversion at 12 months of age.[29]

The ability to walk is of significant concern to OSB patients and their parents. While the MOMS trial did not provide insight into the long-term outcomes of prenatally operated children, the follow-up study (MOMS 2), reporting outcomes at school age (5.9–10.3 years), demonstrated the superiority of prenatal repair in walking with or without assistive devices (29 vs 11%). A meta-analysis of post-MOMS published data from five studies of 234 pregnancies that had prenatal OSB repair with data on ambulation found that lateral ventricular diameter of ≥15 mm, lesion level T12-L2, and preoperative severe hindbrain herniation are factors negatively associated with walking without assistance.[30]

Table 21.1 Published Studies Since the MOMS

Author	Country	N	Approach	Hydrocephalus Treatment	Ability to Walk	Urinary Continence	Major Urological Surgery
Danzer[1]	USA	54	open	n.s.	26/32 (81.2%)	n.s.	n.s.
Lee[2]	USA	11	n.s	n.s.	n.s.	3 (12%)	n.s.
Faria[3]	Brazil	6	open	2 (33.3%)	5 (83.3%)	n.s.	n.s.
Zamlynski[4]	Poland	18	open	5 (27.7%)	9 (50%)	n.a.	n.a.
Macedo[5]	Brazil	19	n.s.	n.s.	n.s.	n.s.	1 (5.3%)
Moldenhauer[6]	USA	100	open	2/83 (2.4%)	n.s.	n.s.	n.s.
Tulipan[7]	USA	183	open	40/91 (44%)	n.s.	n.s.	n.s.
Graf[8]	Germany	71	fetoscopic	32 (45.1%)	n.s.	n.s.	n.s.
Pedreira[9]	Brazil	10	fetoscopic	3/7 (42.9%)	n.s.	5/7 (71.4%)	n.s.
Elbabaa[10]	USA	55	open	30 (54.5%)	n.s.	n.s.	n.s.
Farmer[11]	USA	91	open	n.s.	39/60 (65%)	n.s.	n.s.
Moron[12]	Brazil	237	open	n.s.	n.s.	n.s.	n.s.
Pastuszka[13]	Poland	36	open	n.s.	n.s.	12 (33.3%)	n.s.
Vonzun, 2020[14]	Switzerland	49	open	16/30 (53.3%)	n.s.	n.s.	n.s.
Spoor[15]	Netherlands	93	open	65/91 (71%)	n.s.	n.s.	n.s.
Brock III[16]	USA	78	open	n.s.	n.s.	46/75 (61.3%)	12/75 (16%)
Carrabba[17]	Italy	5	fetoscopic	3 (60%)	n.s.	n.s.	n.s.
Mohrlen[18]	Switzerland	20	open	11 (55%)	n.s.	n.s.	n.s.
Flanders[19]	USA	119	open	46 (38.6%)	n.s.	n.s.	n.s.
Donepudi[20]	USA	110	open	69 (62.7%)	n.s.	n.s.	n.s.
Diehl, 2021[21]	Germany	52	fetoscopic	16/30 (53.3%)	23/42 (55%)	n.s.	n.s.
Houtrow[22]	USA	76	open	n.s.	39/76 (51.3%)	n.s.	n.s.
Parizi[23]	Brazil	81	open	n.s.	n.s.	50 (71.6%)	n.s.
Wille[24]	Switzerland	61	open	19/46 (41.3%)	n.s.	n.s.	n.s.
Lapa[25]	Brazil	170	fetoscopic	68/103 (66%)	32/59 (54.2%)	36/59 (61%)	n.s.
Worley[26]	USA	239	open	110/239 (46%)	n.s.	n.s.	n.s.
Corroenne[27]	USA	103	open and fetoscopic	n.s.	82/93 (79.6%)	n.s.	n.s.
Sanz Cortes[28]	International	300	fetoscopic	88/201 (43.8%)	n.s.	n.s.	n.s.

Abbreviation: n.s.: Not stated.

Continence disorders are vital outcomes to study in the post-MOMS era, with an estimated rate ranging between 12 to 71% in children with OSB.[31] Fortunately, only a small percentage of these children required major urological surgical intervention. However, the available data regarding urological outcomes of prenatal surgery remains deficient, and further evaluation of those children in the long term is needed.

In summary, the MOMS trial permanently reshaped neurosurgical care for OSB by establishing prenatal myelomeningocele repair as a practice-changing intervention that reduces CSF diversion and improves functional motor outcomes, while defining the foundation for modern fetal neurosurgery.

REFERENCES

1. Danzer E, Gerdes M, Bebbington MW, et al. Lower extremity neuromotor function and short-term ambulatory potential following in utero myelomeningocele surgery. Fetal Diagn Ther. 2009;25(1):47–53. doi:10.1159/000197359
2. Lee NG, Gomez P, Uberoi V, et al. In utero closure of myelomeningocele does not improve lower urinary tract function. J Urol. 2012;188(4 Suppl):1567–1571. doi: 10.1016/j.juro.2012.06.034
3. Faria TC, Cavalheiro S, Hisaba WJ, et al. Improvement of motor function and decreased need for postnatal shunting in children who had undergone intrauterine myelomeningocele repair. Arq Neuropsiquiatr. 2013;71(9a):604–608. doi:10.1590/0004-282x20130104
4. Zamlynski J, Olejek A, Koszutski T, et al. Comparison of prenatal and postnatal treatments of spina bifida in Poland–a non-randomized, single-center study. J Matern Fetal Neonatal Med. 2014;27(14):1409–1417. doi:10.3109/14767058.2013.858689
5. Macedo A, Jr., Leal M, Rondon A, et al. Urological evaluation of patients that had undergone in utero myelomeningocele closure: a prospective assessment at first presentation and early follow-up. Do their bladder benefit from it? Neurourol Urodyn. 2015;34(5):461–464. doi:10.1002/nau.22576
6. Moldenhauer JS, Soni S, Rintoul NE, et al. Fetal myelomeningocele repair: the post-MOMS experience at the Children's Hospital of Philadelphia. Fetal Diagn Ther. 2015;37(3):235–240. doi:10.1159/000365353
7. Tulipan N, Wellons JC, 3rd, Thom EA, et al. Prenatal surgery for myelomeningocele and the need for cerebrospinal fluid shunt placement. J Neurosurg Pediatr. 2015;16(6): 613–620. doi:10.3171/2015.7.Peds15336
8. Graf K, Kohl T, Neubauer BA, et al. Percutaneous minimally invasive fetoscopic surgery for spina bifida Aperta. Part III: Neurosurgical intervention in the first postnatal year. Ultrasound Obstet Gynecol. 2016;47(2):158–161. doi:10.1002/uog.14937
9. Pedreira DA, Zanon N, Nishikuni K, et al. Endoscopic surgery for the antenatal treatment of myelomeningocele: the CECAM trial. Am J Obstet Gynecol. 2016;214(1):111.e1-.e11. doi:10.1016/j.ajog.2015.09.065
10. Elbabaa SK, Gildehaus AM, Pierson MJ, et al. First 60 fetal in-utero myelomeningocele repairs at Saint Louis Fetal Care Institute in the post-MOMS trial era: hydrocephalus treatment outcomes (endoscopic third ventriculostomy versus ventriculo-peritoneal shunt). Childs Nerv Syst. 2017;33(7):1157–1168. doi:10.1007/s00381-017-3428-8
11. Farmer DL, Thom EA, Brock JW, 3rd, et al. The management of myelomeningocele study: full cohort 30-month pediatric outcomes. Am J Obstet Gynecol. 2018;218(2): 256.e1-.e13. doi:10.1016/j.ajog.2017.12.001
12. Moron AF, Barbosa MM, Milani H, et al. Perinatal outcomes after open fetal surgery for myelomeningocele repair: a retrospective cohort study. BJOG Int J Obstet Gynaecol. 2018;125(10):1280–1286. doi:10.1111/1471-0528.15312

13. Pastuszka A, Bohosiewicz J, Koszutski T. Prenatal myelomeningocele repair improves urinary continence and reduces the risk of constipation. Neurourol Urodyn. 2018;37(8):2792–2798. doi:10.1002/nau.23771
14. Vonzun L, Winder FM, Meuli M, et al. Prenatal sonographic head circumference and cerebral ventricle width measurements before and after open fetal myelomeningocele repair - prediction of shunting during the first year of life. Ultraschall Med. 2020;41(5): 544–549. doi:10.1055/a-0756-8417
15. Spoor JKH, Gadjradj PS, Eggink AJ, et al. Contemporary management and outcome of myelomeningocele: the Rotterdam experience. Neurosurg Focus. 2019;47(4):E3. doi:10.3171/2019.7.Focus19447
16. Brock JW, 3rd, Thomas JC, Baskin LS, et al. Effect of prenatal repair of myelomeningocele on urological outcomes at school age. J Urol. 2019;202(4):812–818. doi:10.1097/ju.0000000000000334
17. Carrabba G, Macchini F, Fabietti I, et al. Minimally invasive fetal surgery for myelomeningocele: preliminary report from a single center. Neurosurg Focus. 2019;47(4): E12. doi:10.3171/2019.8.Focus19438
18. Möhrlen U, Ochsenbein-Kölble N, Mazzone L, et al. Benchmarking against the MOMS trial: Zurich results of open fetal surgery for spina bifida. Fetal Diagn Ther. 2020;47(2): 91–97. doi:10.1159/000500049
19. Flanders TM, Heuer GG, Madsen PJ, et al. Detailed analysis of hydrocephalus and hindbrain herniation after prenatal and postnatal myelomeningocele closure: report from a single institution. Neurosurgery. 2020;86(5):637–645. doi:10.1093/neuros/nyz302
20. Donepudi R, Brock C, Schulte S, et al. Trend in ventricle size during pregnancy and its use for prediction of ventriculoperitoneal shunt in fetal open neural tube defect. Ultrasound Obstet Gynecol. 2020;56(5):678–683. doi:10.1002/uog.21928
21. Diehl D, Belke F, Kohl T, et al. Fully percutaneous fetoscopic repair of myelomeningocele: 30-month follow-up data. Ultrasound Obstet Gynecol. 2021;57(1):113–118. doi:10.1002/uog.22116
22. Houtrow AJ, MacPherson C, Jackson-Coty J, et al. Prenatal repair and physical functioning among children with myelomeningocele: a secondary analysis of a randomized clinical trial. JAMA Pediatr. 2021;175(4):e205674. doi:10.1001/jamapediatrics.2020.5674
23. Parizi JLG, Leal da Cruz M, Andrade MC, et al. A comparative analysis of bladder pattern of patients who underwent in utero versus postnatal myelomeningocele repair. J Urol. 2020; 203(1):194–199. doi:10.1097/ju.0000000000000521
24. Wille DA, Padden B, Moehrlen U, et al. Impact of brain malformations on neurodevelopmental outcome in children with a history of prenatal surgery for open spina bifida. Fetal Diagn Ther. 2021;48(8):588–595. doi:10.1159/000517972
25. Lapa DA, Chmait RH, Gielchinsky Y, et al. Percutaneous fetoscopic spina bifida repair: effect on ambulation and need for postnatal cerebrospinal fluid diversion and bladder catheterization. Ultrasound Obstet Gynecol. 2021;58(4):582–589. doi:10.1002/uog.23658
26. Worley G, Greenberg RG, Rocque BG, et al. Neurosurgical procedures for children with myelomeningocele after fetal or postnatal surgery: a comparative effectiveness study. Dev Med Child Neurol. 2021;63(11):1294–1301. doi:10.1111/dmcn.14792
27. Corroenne R, Sanz Cortes M, Johnson RM, et al. Impact of the cystic neural tube defects on fetal motor function in prenatal myelomeningocele repairs: a retrospective cohort study. Prenat Diagn. 2021;41(8):965–971. doi:10.1002/pd.5992
28. Sanz Cortes M, Chmait RH, Lapa DA, et al. Experience of 300 cases of prenatal fetoscopic open spina bifida repair: report of the International Fetoscopic Neural Tube Defect Repair Consortium. Am J Obstet Gynecol. 2021;225(6):678.e1–e11. doi:10.1016/j.ajog.2021.05.044
29. Mustafa HJ, Arab K, Javinani A, et al. Prenatal predictors of need for cerebrospinal fluid diversion in infants following prenatal repair of open spina bifida; systematic review and meta-analysis. Am J Obstet Gynecol MFM. 2023;5(8):100983. doi:10.1016/j.ajogmf.2023.100983

30. Mustafa HJ, Arab K, Javinani A, et al. Prenatal predictors of ambulation without assistance by 30 months of age in children following prenatal repair of open spina bifida, a systematic review and meta-analysis. Reprod Female Child Health. 2024;3(2):e85. doi: 10.1002/rfc2.85
31. Buoro RS, Nogueira MP. Quality of life and challenges of family members of children with meningomyelocele. Acta Ortop Bras. 2020;28(6):291–295. doi:10.1590/1413-785220202806237160

CHAPTER 22

Incidence and Evolution of Subependymal and Intraventricular Hemorrhage: A Study of Infants Less Than 1,500 gm

Papile LA, Burstein J, Birstein R, Koffler H. J Pediatr. 1978 Apr;92(4):529–534

Reviewed by Lu-Ann Papile

Research Objective To determine the frequency and severity of subependymal and intraventricular hemorrhage (PIVH) in a cohort of preterm infants weighing <1500 g at birth (very low birth weight [VLBW]) using computed tomography (CT) brain imaging.

Study Design CT brain scans were obtained in 46 consecutive live-born VLBW infants admitted to the University of New Mexico Newborn Intensive Care Unit. Living infants were studied at 4 to 7 days of age and weekly thereafter. If an infant died before 4 days old, a postmortem CT brain scan was performed within 6 hours of death and before brain fixation. The infants were transferred between the newborn intensive care unit and the radiology department in a heated transport isolette. The heart rate was continuously monitored and heat loss was minimized by using heat lamps and covering the infant with a plastic sheet. A neonatologist was present throughout the procedure.

Sample Size 46 consecutive live-born VLBW infants.

Follow-Up N/A

Inclusion/Exclusion Criteria N/A

Intervention or Treatment Received Because the size of the smallest commercially available head cone exceeded the head size of the infants studied, a foam rubber sheet 2.54 cm thick was placed between the plastic head cone and the rubber head bag. Water-filled latex surgical gloves were placed around the head for support when necessary.

Results The frequency of PIVH was 43% (20/46). Among the 29 infants who survived, 31% had PIVH (9/29). Four grades of PIVH were described: Grade I and II lesions resolved spontaneously. Hydrocephalus developed in infants with grade III and IV lesions. Clinical signs of PIVH were not evident in most of the surviving

DOI: 10.1201/9781003416197-22

infants with PIVH (7/9). There were no significant differences between the infants with and without PIVH in birth weight, gestational age, 1- and 5-minute Apgar scores, or the need for resuscitation at birth or for subsequent respiratory assistance.

Conclusion PIVH is not only common in surviving VLBW infants, but also clinically silent in most cases.

Author/Reviewer Commentary In 1973, during my neonatal/perinatal fellowship, I cared for a VLBW infant who manifested a rapidly increasing head circumference at 1 month of age. The infant was thought to have a subdural hemorrhage and on the recommendation of the neurosurgery team, the infant underwent daily serial taps to remove blood from the subdural space. Because the hydrocephalus did not resolve after a month of treatment, a pneumo-encephalogram was recommended. The study revealed hydrocephalus most likely posthemorrhagic and several porencephalic tracks resulting from repeated ventricular taps. This index case was the impetus for my research regarding brain injury in the VLBW infant.

Before the advent of non-invasive cranial imaging, the diagnosis of presumed PIVH was based on the presence of a constellation of clinical signs that included hypotonia, hypotension, a bulging fontanelle, and seizure-like activity accompanied by a fall in hematocrit and a metabolic acidosis. Affected infants had a high rate of death and at necropsy, a frequent finding was PIVH, a lesion that was particular to VLBW infants.

In 1973, the first report of the clinical application of CT in the United States was published. In 1974, our institution acquired a CT scanner. In collaboration with a junior colleague in radiology, Jerome Burstein, I submitted a proposal to explore the feasibility of performing CT brain imaging in VLBW infants. Because we had an active neonatal transport team that traveled throughout the Southwest to bring medically fragile and preterm infants to our Newborn Intensive Care Unit, there was an established protocol in place for monitoring babies during transport. Monitoring consisted of measuring heart rate continuously and rectal temperature intermittently. The adequacy of the infants' oxygen saturation was assessed clinically (portable pulse oximetry for VLBW infants was not available clinically until 1995). The smallest commercially available head cone for the CT scanner far exceeded the size of the VLBW infants' heads, so we devised a method to minimize the space in order to improve the quality of the image.

Enrollment of VLBW infants in our observational study began in 1975. Our first published study,[1] which included the first 17 enrolled infants, demonstrated the feasibility of utilizing a CT brain scan to diagnose PIVH. A comparison of postmortem brain sections cut in the same plane as the CT brain scan sections of the 8 infants who died demonstrated excellent correlation with no false-positive or false-negative diagnoses.

The clinical observational study outlined in this chapter,[2] was a continuation of our initial study. It was the first published study to demonstrate that PIVH occurred in approximately a third of surviving VLBW infants, a much higher incidence than was clinically suspected. More important was the finding that most of the affected infants who survived the onset of hemorrhage did not have any of the clinical signs associated with PIVH, indicating that the onset was clinically silent. The report also described four separate grades of PIVH:

- Grade I – subependymal hemorrhage
- Grade II – intraventricular hemorrhage without ventricular dilatation
- Grade III – intraventricular hemorrhage with ventricular dilatation
- Grade IV – intraventricular hemorrhage with parenchymal hemorrhage

We subsequently enrolled an additional 54 infants into the study.[3] In this cohort of 100 consecutive VLBW infants, the frequency of PIVH among surviving infants was 34% (32/57), essentially the same as in our smaller study (31%). In addition, the rate of "silent" PIVH was also similar (68% vs 77%). Grade I and II PIVH resolved spontaneously; however, 8/9 infants with grade III and IV PIVH developed posthemorrhagic hydrocephalus (PHH). Posthemorrhagic hydrocephalus and its subsequent progression were detected weeks before the clinical diagnosis of hydrocephalus.

We also conducted the earliest outcome study of surviving infants with PIVH,[4] in which we described the relationship of PIVH and early childhood developmental and neuromotor disabilities. Overall, major handicaps were three times more likely among infants with PIVH than among infants without PIVH. Infants with grade I and II PIVH had the same rate of handicap as those without PIVH. Among infants with grade III and IV PIVH, the rate was 36% and 76%, respectively.

The results of our studies and several later studies established that PIVH was common in surviving VLBW infants. Additionally, screening VLBW infants for PIVH was feasible and serial evaluation was helpful in identifying the presence and progression of PHH. However, the necessity of transporting VLBW infants to the CT suite was an obstacle to the widespread adoption of screening. It was not until the 1980s, when portable bedside ultrasonography suitable for visualizing the brain of VLBW infants became available, that screening for PIVH became routine. Since then, there have been over 100 published manuscripts related to the use of head ultrasound (HUS) for the detection of PIVH.

In 2002, the American Academy of Neurology, in conjunction with the Child Neurology Society, issued a practice parameter recommending that all infants born at less than 30 weeks' gestation undergo screening with HUS for PIVH.[5] In 2020, the American Academy of Pediatrics published detailed recommendations for routine neuroimaging in the preterm brain, noting that CT and magnetic resonance imaging are not recommended.[6]

Despite the remarkable advances made in the care of VLBW infants that have occurred since our 1978 study, PIVH remains a major morbidity and is the most common hemorrhagic lesion encountered in this population. Currently, the rate of PIVH is approximately 20–25% overall for VLBW infants, with rates as high as 45% in infants with birthweights less than 750 g. Unresolved treatment issues include the optimal timing for intervention in VLBW infants who develop PHH, as well as what is the most efficacious method.

REFERENCES

1. Burstein J, Papile LA, Burstein R. Subependymal germinal matrix and intraventricular hemorrhage in preterm infants: diagnosis by CT. Am J Roentgenol. 1977;128:971–978.
2. Papile LA, Burstein J, Burstein R, Koffler H. Incidence and evolution of subependymal and intraventricular hemorrhage: a study of infants less than 1,500 gm. J Pediatr. 1978; 92:529–532.
3. Burstein J, Papile LA, Burstein R. Intraventricular hemorrhage and hydrocephalus in premature newborns: a prospective study with CT. AJR. 1979;132:631–635.
4. Papile LA, Munsick-Bruno G, Schaefer A. Relationship of cerebral intraventricular hemorrhage and earl childhood neurologic handicaps. J Pediatr. 1983;103:273–277. doi:10.1016/s0022-3476(83)80366-7
5. Ment L, Sada HS, Barnes P, et al. Practice parameter: neuroimaging of the neonate: report of the Quality Standards Subcommittee of the American Academy of Neurology and the Practice Committee of the Child Neurology Society. Neurology. 2002;58:1726–1738. doi:10.1212/wnl.58.12.1726
6. Hand IL, Shellhaas RA, Milla SS, et al. Routine neuroimaging of the preterm brain. Pediatrics. 2020;146(1–3):e2020029082.

CHAPTER 23

Intrinsic Brain-Stem Tumors of Childhood: Surgical Indications

Epstein F, McCleary EL, J Neurosurg. 1986;64:11–15

Reviewed by Alan R Cohen

Research Question/Objective This was a single-institution analysis of the indications for surgery for the management of intrinsic non-exophytic brainstem tumors in children.

Study Design Retrospective review.

Sample Size 34 pediatric patients.

Follow-Up 24 months.

Inclusion Criteria

- All patients were children.
- Age was not specified.
- Tumors were divided into three subgroups: focal (circumscribed mass with diameter <2 cm, no edema), diffuse (size >2 cm, with edema), and cervicomedullary (occurring at the junction of the medulla and cervical spinal cord).

Intervention or Treatment Received All patients underwent radical microsurgical tumor resection. The operative approach was chosen to enter the portion of the tumor that was closest to the surface of the brainstem. For the first 15 patients in the series, the resection was carried out using a Cavitron ultrasonic surgical aspirator. For the last 19 patients, the resection was performed using a laser. Brainstem evoked potential monitoring was carried out in the last 10 patients.

Results There were 4 focal tumors (3 benign Word Health Organization [WHO] grades I–II, 1 malignant WHO grades III–IV), 22 diffuse tumors (all malignant WHO grades III–IV), and 8 cervicomedullary tumors (all benign WHO grades III–IV). Two of the 4 focal astrocytomas and all of the 8 cervicomedullary astrocytomas either stabilized or improved after surgery. The one patient with a

DOI: 10.1201/9781003416197-23

malignant focal astrocytoma died of tumor progression 6 months after surgery. None of the 22 patients with diffuse astrocytomas benefited from surgery. Three patients with diffuse astrocytomas died within a month of surgery and four were more impaired postoperatively from cranial nerve palsies. All patients with diffuse astrocytomas died from tumor progression within 6 to 12 months of surgery.

Study Limitations This was a preliminary investigation with a small patient cohort and a retrospective analysis with a relatively short duration of follow-up. Its strength was that it provided a basis of structure to a poorly understood field and offered hope for future novel therapies.

Conclusion Radical surgery is recommended for cervicomedullary tumors, which are often benign. Radical surgery is not indicated for diffuse tumors, which are usually malignant and for which radiation therapy is the treatment of choice.

Reviewer Commentary This report from Epstein and McCleary, published almost four decades ago, was a landmark study. Surgery of the brainstem was once considered a fool's errand, too dangerous to even consider, with high rates of morbidity and mortality. I have a very personal memory of this work, as I was Epstein's resident at the time of publication and had a role assisting him in surgery on several of the cases. And McCleary, who collected the data and performed the analysis, was my co-resident, a brilliant physician and a close friend.

Epstein was a bold thinker who had already shaken up the field of pediatric neurosurgery by realizing that many intramedullary spinal cord tumors in children were low grade and could often be debulked safely, similar to the way cerebellar astrocytomas of childhood could be managed. He was also an innovative thinker and began to classify brainstem tumors according to their location. Epstein recognized early that intrinsic cervicomedullary tumors were usually low grade and could be approached safely using meticulous operative technique. He recognized that tumors rostral to the medulla were more likely to be malignant and less likely to be amenable to radical resection.

It is important to remember the era in which Epstein worked. Magnetic resonance imaging was a relatively new tool and many of the patients in his series were imaged with computerized tomography alone. Intraoperative neurophysiologic monitoring was new on the horizon, as was intraoperative image guidance. Epstein was a courageous, forward-thinking surgeon whose efforts set the stage to advance surgery of the brainstem as we practice it today.

Looking back, the pathological identification of brainstem tumors was also relatively primitive at the time of this publication. The WHO had used a conventional classification system based on histology, ultrastructure, and immunohistochemistry. The modern WHO classification system is a hybrid taxonomy that has added molecular diagnostic features, including mutations and fusions that can potentially be targeted.

We now know, for example, that selected tumors of the midbrain tectum are often low grade. Diffuse tumors of the pons, formerly called diffuse intrinsic pontine gliomas, are lethal. These tumors have now been renamed diffuse midline gliomas (DMGs). We now know that there are driver mutations in the histone remodeling gene family *histone H3* that are usually present in DMGs that promote tumorigenesis.[1] And the presence of these histone alterations supersedes histology in determining the prognosis of these tumors. Modern hybrid WHO classification schemes should lead to more opportunities to selectively target brainstem tumors with designer drugs for personalized medicine.[2]

None of this information was available to Epstein and McCleary when they created their initial classification of brainstem neoplasms. But their early work set a foundation for what was to come. Their use of meticulous microsurgery with surgical adjuncts available at the time, including primitive neuro-monitoring, predated the high-tech neuro-monitoring we use routinely today. They also had the wisdom to approach these intrinsic brainstem tumors using a pathway that minimized the distance they would have to use to traverse normal tissue. Modern microsurgery employs Spetzler's refinement of the "two-point technique,"[3] and advances in the understanding of brainstem microanatomy have led to the finding of "safe zones" in which to enter the brainstem.[4]

Epstein and McCleary were among the first to recognize that intramedullary tumors at the cervicomedullary junction were usually low grade and could be approached surgically, though with considerable attention to technique. These lesions were often low-grade astrocytomas that were not encapsulated but had an identifiable interface with the normal brainstem. They were among the first to recognize that the prognosis for tumors of the brainstem was different depending on their geographic location, among other factors.

Epstein and McCleary also discussed the option of biopsy for intrinsic brainstem tumors. This is a topic that has been debated by pediatric neurosurgeons for decades. In their 1986 article, they recommended against biopsy, noting that the benefit was not worth the risk. At the time, that made sense, as there were limited therapeutic options available. But now that we live in a molecular world, biopsy may offer new insights for targeted therapy and the pendulum has swung back in favor of biopsy.

Fred Epstein used to have a sign on his desk that read, "The Brainstem Is an Over-Rated Structure." It was meant to be a tongue-in-cheek statement, as no one had more respect for the intricacies of the brainstem than Epstein. But it was also a reflection of his eternal optimism, which led to his pioneering work in unraveling some of the mysteries of brainstem surgery.

REFERENCES

1. Cohen AR. Brain tumors in children. N Engl J Med. 2022;386:1922–1931. doi:10.1056/NEJMra2116344
2. Rehder R, Cohen AR. Comprehensive Management of Pediatric Brainstem Tumors. In Spetzler R, Yashar M, Kalani S, Lawton MT, eds. Chapter 14. Surgery of the Brainstem. New York, Thieme; 2020.
3. Cavalcanti DD, Preul, MC, Yashar M, Kalani S, Spetzler RF. Microsurgical anatomy of safe entry zones to the brainstem. J Neurosurg. 2015;24:1359–1376. doi:10.3171/2015.4.JNS141945
4. Yashar M, Kalani S, Yagmurlu K, Martirosyan NL, Cavalcanti DD, Spetzler RF. Approach selection for intrinsic brainstem. J Neurosurg. 2016;125:1596–1607. doi:10.3171/2016.6.JNS161043

CHAPTER 24

Molecular Subgroups of Medulloblastoma: The Current Consensus

Taylor MD, Northcott PA, Korshunov A, Remke M, Cho YJ, Clifford SC, Eberhart CG, Parsons DW, Rutkowski S, Gajjar A, Ellison DW, Lichter P, Gilbertson RJ, Pomeroy SL, Kool M, Pfister SM, Acta Neuropathol. 2012 Apr;123(4):465–472

Reviewed by Trenton A Line and Jignesh Tailor

Objective/Research Question The objective was to develop a unified system for classifying medulloblastoma based on molecular genomics.

Study Design Consensus statement.

Sample Size Molecular data from four major research groups (St Jude, Netherlands, Toronto, and Boston) with over 400 patients.

Inclusion/Exclusion Criteria N/A

Intervention or Treatment Received N/A

Results and Conclusion A consensus on four molecular subgroups of medulloblastoma was achieved: SHH (Sonic Hedgehog-activated), WNT (Wingless-activated), group 3, and group 4. The demographics, clinical features, molecular alterations, gene expression, and prognosis were described (Figure 24.1).

Reviewer Commentary For many years, medulloblastoma was approached clinically as a single disease, with treatment strategies guided largely by age, metastatic status, histopathology, and extent of surgical resection. While these variables provided a practical framework for risk stratification, they offered limited insight into the underlying biology of the tumor and could not fully account for the striking heterogeneity in clinical behavior and outcomes observed across patients. By the late 2000s, it had become increasingly clear that medulloblastoma represented not one disease, but several biologically distinct entities.[1–4]

This publication represents a pivotal moment in this transition. Rather than introducing a new dataset, this paper synthesized a rapidly expanding body of

DOI: 10.1201/9781003416197-24

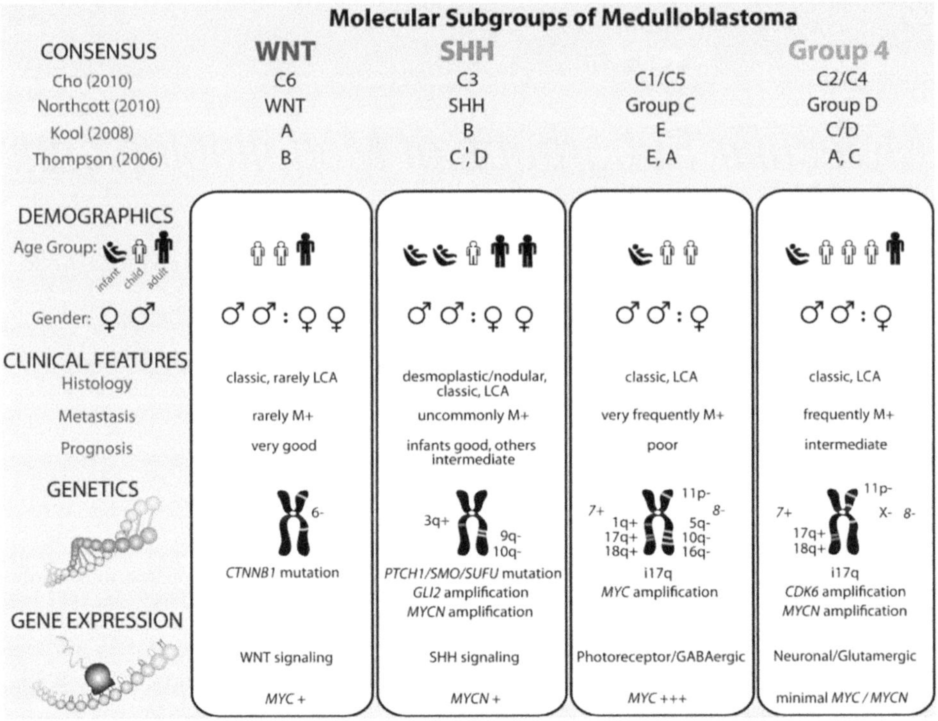

Figure 24.1 Molecular subgroups of medulloblastoma. (From Taylor et al., Acta Neuropathol. 123(4), 465–472, 2012.)

genomic evidence into a unified and clinically meaningful classification. By establishing four core molecular subgroups, WNT, SHH, group 3, and group 4, the authors provided a common biological language that has since underpinned nearly all advances in medulloblastoma research and clinical care. In doing so, this work marked the true beginning of the molecular era in pediatric neuro-oncology.

The impact of this paper is reflected in its extraordinary reach. It has been cited well over 3,000 times, placing it among the most highly cited articles in the field. The summary figure from this manuscript (Figure 24.1) has become one of the most widely used and reproduced figures in medulloblastoma worldwide. By integrating molecular subgroups with genetics, demographics, histology, and clinical outcome, this schematic provided a clear and intuitive framework that could be readily understood by clinicians, researchers, and trainees alike.

Historical Context The years preceding this consensus were marked by rapid progress in transcriptomic profiling of medulloblastoma. Independent groups using gene-expression arrays consistently demonstrated that medulloblastoma tumors clustered into distinct molecular groups. However, differences in cohort size, analytical methods, and subgroup naming conventions led to variability in how these findings were reported. Early studies by Thompson et al. and Kool et al. described five molecular subgroups using letter-based systems (A–E), while later large-scale analyses from Toronto (SHH, WNT, group C, group D) and Boston (C1–6) proposed four and six subgroups, respectively, with different nomenclature and degrees of substructure.[1–4]

Despite these differences, there was strong agreement on several key points. WNT-activated and SHH-activated tumors were consistently identified across all studies and were readily distinguished from other medulloblastomas based on the transcriptional profile, genetics, and clinical behavior. The principal uncertainty lay in the number and biological identity of the remaining non-WNT/non-SHH tumors. Some analyses suggested a single large group, while others proposed multiple distinct entities.[5]

Recognizing the need for clarity, leaders in the field convened to review the accumulated evidence. The result was the consensus articulated in this paper, which proposed four core subgroups supported by the greatest weight of available data. The deliberately neutral naming of groups 3 and 4 reflected both biological distinction and humility, acknowledging that their underlying biology was still incompletely understood.

Impact on Surgical Practice One of the most important downstream effects of molecular subgrouping has been its influence on neurosurgical decision-making, particularly regarding the extent of resection. Historically, aggressive surgical resection was considered a cornerstone of medulloblastoma management. Residual tumor burden, often dichotomized using a threshold of 1.5 cm^2, was incorporated into risk stratification schemes and frequently prompted second-look surgeries or the escalation of adjuvant therapy.[6,7]

The integration of molecular subgroup information fundamentally reshaped this paradigm. In 2016, Thompson et al. examined 787 medulloblastoma patients with known molecular subgroup affiliation.[8] This study, published in *Lancet Oncology*, demonstrated that the apparent prognostic benefit of gross total resection was substantially attenuated once the molecular subgroup was accounted for. Across WNT, SHH, and group 3 tumors, there was no significant progression-free or overall survival advantage for gross total resection compared with near-total resection.

A modest benefit of more extensive resection was observed primarily in group 4 tumors, particularly in patients with metastatic disease. Even in this setting, however, the magnitude of benefit was small relative to the prognostic impact of molecular subgroup, metastatic status, and adjuvant therapy. Importantly, near-total resection was consistently equivalent to gross total resection across all subgroups.[8]

These findings have had direct implications for operative strategy. They support a shift away from a dogmatic pursuit of gross total resection at all costs and toward a philosophy of maximal safe resection. When a residual tumor is adherent to critical structures such as the brainstem or floor of the fourth ventricle, leaving a small residual, particularly less than 1.5 cm^2, may avoid significant neurological morbidity without compromising oncologic outcome for most patients.

This molecularly informed perspective has also influenced decisions regarding second-look surgery. In the absence of a clear survival benefit for converting a near-total resection to a gross total resection, the risks of additional surgery, delayed adjuvant therapy, neurological injury, and posterior fossa syndrome must be weighed carefully against modest or uncertain gains.[8–11]

Relevant Studies Following the establishment of the four-subgroup framework, numerous studies validated its clinical relevance and extended its implications. Significant international efforts have confirmed the reproducibility of these subgroups across institutions and analytic platforms and have helped clarify subgroup-enriched patterns of clinical behavior.[12,13]

Subsequent work demonstrated subgroup-specific patterns of recurrence, with group 3 and group 4 tumors more likely to recur at metastatic sites rather than at the primary tumor bed, further diminishing the presumed importance of aggressive local resection as a universal determinant of outcome.[14]

Advances in molecular diagnostics, including rapid subgroup assays, have enabled increasingly precise classification in routine clinical settings and have accelerated the clinical translation of subgroup-aware risk stratification.[15] While additional subtypes within each subgroup have since been described through methylation profiling and multiomic approaches, these refinements build directly upon the foundation laid by the consensus classification rather than replacing it.[16–19]

Study Limitations The generic naming of group 3 and group 4 reflects an intentional acknowledgment of incomplete biological understanding at the time. With hindsight, we now recognize substantial heterogeneity within these groups.[16–20]

Conclusion This publication represents a defining inflection point in pediatric neuro-oncology. By establishing a unified molecular classification, it transformed medulloblastoma from a histologically defined tumor into a biologically stratified disease. The framework introduced in this paper has reshaped clinical trials, refined surgical decision-making, and laid the groundwork for risk-adapted and biologically informed therapy. Its influence continues to be felt across disciplines, and it remains central to how medulloblastoma is understood and treated in the "molecular era."

REFERENCES

1. Thompson MC, Fuller C, Hogg TL, et al. Genomics identifies medulloblastoma subgroups that are enriched for specific genetic alterations. J Clin Oncol. 2006;24(12):1924–1931.
2. Kool M, Koster J, Bunt J, et al. Integrated genomics identifies five medulloblastoma subtypes with distinct genetic profiles, pathway signatures and clinicopathological features. PLoS One. 2008;3(8):e3088.

3. Northcott PA, Korshunov A, Witt H, et al. Medulloblastoma comprises four distinct molecular variants. J Clin Oncol. 2011;29(11):1408–1414.
4. Cho YJ, Tsherniak A, Tamayo P, et al. Integrative genomic analysis of medulloblastoma identifies a molecular subgroup that drives poor clinical outcome. J Clin Oncol. 2011; 29(11):1424–1430.
5. Northcott PA, Dubuc AM, Pfister S, Taylor MD. Molecular subgroups of medulloblastoma. Expert Rev Neurother. 2012;12(7):871–884.
6. Albright AL, Wisoff JH, Zeltzer PM, Boyett JM, Rorke LB, Stanley P. Effects of medulloblastoma resections on outcome in children: a report from the Children's Cancer Group. Neurosurgery. 1996;38(2):265–271.
7. Zeltzer PM, Boyett JM, Finlay JL, et al. Metastasis stage, adjuvant treatment, and residual tumor are prognostic factors for medulloblastoma in children: conclusions from the Children's Cancer Group 921 randomized phase III study. J Clin Oncol. 1999;17(3):832–845.
8. Thompson EM, Hielscher T, Bouffet E, et al. Prognostic value of medulloblastoma extent of resection after accounting for molecular subgroup: an integrated clinical and molecular analysis. Lancet Oncol. 2016;17(4):484–495.
9. Korah MP, Esiashvili N, Mazewski CM, et al. Incidence, risks, and sequelae of posterior fossa syndrome in pediatric medulloblastoma. Int J Radiat Oncol Biol Phys. 2010;77(1): 106–112.
10. Robertson PL, Muraszko KM, Holmes EJ, et al. Incidence and severity of postoperative cerebellar mutism syndrome in children with medulloblastoma: a prospective study by the Children's Oncology Group. J Neurosurg. 2006;105(6 Suppl):444–451.
11. Levisohn L, Cronin-Golomb A, Schmahmann JD. Neuropsychological consequences of cerebellar tumour resection in children: cerebellar cognitive affective syndrome in a paediatric population. Brain. 2000;123(Pt 5):1041–1050.
12. Northcott PA, Jones DTW, Kool M, et al. Medulloblastomics: the end of the beginning. Nat Rev Cancer. 2012;12(12):818–834.
13. Northcott PA, Korshunov A, Pfister SM, Taylor MD. The clinical implications of medulloblastoma subgroups. Nat Rev Neurol. 2012;8(6):340–351.
14. Ramaswamy V, Remke M, Bouffet E, et al. Recurrence patterns across medulloblastoma subgroups: an integrated clinical and molecular analysis. Lancet Oncol. 2013;14(12):1200.
15. Northcott PA, Shih DJH, Remke M, et al. Rapid, reliable, and reproducible molecular subgrouping of clinical medulloblastoma samples. Acta Neuropathol. 2012;123(4): 615–626.
16. Hovestadt V, Ayrault O, Swartling FJ, Robinson GW, Pfister SM, Northcott PA. Medulloblastomics revisited: biological and clinical insights from thousands of patients. Nature Reviews Cancer. 2020;20(1):42–56.
17. Juraschka K, Taylor MD. Medulloblastoma in the age of molecular subgroups: a review. J Neurosurg Pediatr. 2019;24(4):353–363.
18. Schwalbe EC, Lindsey JC, Nakjang S, et al. Novel molecular subgroups for clinical classification and outcome prediction in childhood medulloblastoma: a cohort study. Lancet Oncol. 2017;18(7):958–971.
19. Sharma T, Schwalbe EC, Williamson D, et al. Second-generation molecular subgrouping of medulloblastoma: an international meta-analysis of group 3 and group 4 subtypes. Acta Neuropathologica. 2019;138(2):309–326.
20. Cavalli FMG, Remke M, Rampasek L, Peacock J, Shih DJH, Luu B, et al. Intertumoral heterogeneity within medulloblastoma subgroups. Cancer Cell. 2017;31(6):737–754.e6.

Chapter 25

Pial Synangiosis for Moyamoya Syndrome in Children

Adelson PD, Scott RM, Pediatr Neurosurg. 1995;23(1):26–33

Reviewed by Edward R Smith

Research Question/Objective The authors describe a modification of the encephalo-duro-arterio-synangiosis (EDAS) surgical technique for patients with moyamoya syndrome. The two key differences of the new approach included widely opening the arachnoid and suturing the donor graft of the superficial temporal artery (STA) directly to the brain.

Study Design Retrospective single-center case series review.

Sample Size A total of 34 pediatric patients (age 1–19 years, 22 female, 12 male) were studied covering a period of 9 years (1985–1994). Within this group, 68 pial synangioses were performed in 50 procedures (18 patients had bilateral operations under a single anesthetic for 36 synangioses and 16 patients had staged operations for the remaining 32 synangioses).

Follow-Up Follow-up ranged from 1 month to 9.5 years, with 19/34 patients (56%) having at least 1 year of postoperative data. Clinical data for outcomes was determined solely from the patients with at least 1 year of data to ensure that the results were durable. Postoperative angiography was performed in 34/36 (94%) of the patients at 10–12 months after surgery.

Inclusion/Exclusion Criteria

- Inclusion Criteria
  - Pediatric patients with radiographic evidence of moyamoya and cerebral ischemia (either radiographic or clinical).
  - All patients had imaging, including catheter angiography, to confirm the presence of moyamoya arteriopathy.
  - "Most" were symptomatic (numbers not reported) with recurrent strokes or transient ischemic attacks (TIAs).

DOI: 10.1201/9781003416197-25

- Exclusion Criteria
  - While exclusion criteria are not defined in this paper, subsequent publications on this topic by the senior author and colleagues have noted that recent major stroke, infection, or hemorrhage may be contraindications, with patients' neurologic status at the time of presentation one of the major predictors of long-term outcome.[1,2]

Intervention or Treatment Received The patients in this study underwent surgical revascularization of the cerebral hemispheres in the middle cerebral artery territories, using a novel modification of an indirect bypass, which the authors termed "pial synangiosis." This approach mimics EDAS, with the use of the parietal branch of the STA as the primary donor (along with the dura), using a wide opening over the affected hemisphere. There are two key changes that differentiate pial synangiosis as a distinct procedure. First, the STA is affixed directly to the surface of the brain with 10–0 nylon sutures, in contrast to the EDAS method of suturing the STA to the dura. In addition, dura is left open without closure to increase the availability of the open edges of vascularized dural leaflets as an adjunct to collateralization from middle meningeal branches within the dura. Second, in pial synangiosis, the arachnoid is opened, with efforts made to better expose the donor tissue to the underlying brain by removing the barrier of the arachnoid. In combination, these changes were designed to increase the access of the donor tissue to form collaterals with the ischemic cortex.

In addition to these technical changes, the authors also reported the use of intraoperative electroencephalography (EEG) in the last six patients of the series, foreshadowing the subsequent adoption of this monitoring tool as routine for moyamoya revascularization cases. The precedent for EEG use came from its role in carotid endarterectomy operations in adults, with the premise that real-time awareness of altered cerebral perfusion (with ischemia manifest as slowing of EEG recordings in the affected territories) could empower the operative team to perform immediate interventions to mitigate stroke risk, such as changes in blood pressure or anesthetic agents.[3,4]

Finally, while the primary focus of the article centered on the technical aspects of the operation, the authors also pioneered the practice of bilateral revascularization under a single anesthetic. The ease and safety of pial synangiosis meant that both sides of patients with bilateral disease could be treated quick enough and with low enough risk to justify this two-sided surgery.

Results The authors performed 68 synangioses in 34 patients with a total of 50 operations, with 18 of the 34 patients undergoing bilateral operations under a single anesthetic. They had follow-up ranging from 1 month to 9.5 years, with 19/34 patients having at least 1 year of follow-up. Clinical outcomes were determined from these 19 patients with at least 1 year of follow-up to ensure that results were durable.

Of the 19 patients with longer follow-up, 15 (79%) had "excellent" outcomes, defined as no further TIAs or seizures and 2 (11%) patients had "good" outcomes, defined as a significant reduction in TIAs. The remaining 2 patients had "fair" outcomes, although 1 of these 2 patients stopped having ischemic events at the 1-year mark. In total, 2/34 patients (6%) had perioperative strokes, one of whom had moyamoya related to prior cranial radiation therapy and the other was a very young child, at 2.5 years of age. This is relevant, as these findings foreshadowed two of the highest risk cohorts of pediatric moyamoya operative candidates, the very young and those who had radiation-associated moyamoya.[5–9]

Radiographically, 28 hemispheres had follow-up imaging available for analysis. Of these, 24 (85%) had "excellent" (Matsushima A) collaterals, and the authors noted that the remaining four hemispheres with less robust surgical vascularization had less disease than the contralateral hemisphere of the same patient, implying that the degree of ischemia serves as a driver for collateral formation.[10] Again, this observation set the foundation for subsequent work that revealed that a "hungry" brain with evidence of ischemia not only had a propensity for developing spontaneous transdural collaterals preoperatively, but that these patients tended to have better responses to surgery, likely due to elevated levels of pro-angiogenic molecules that augmented revascularization.[11–15]

Conclusion Pial synangiosis, as a modification of EDAS distinguished by suturing the STA directly to the brain and widely opening the arachnoid, provides robust revascularization in pediatric moyamoya patients with clinical and radiographic outcomes comparable or better than contemporary approaches.

Reviewer Commentary The initial description of pial synangiosis as a method to revascularize the brain in pediatric moyamoya patients was a significant advance, facilitating improved angiogenesis through relatively simple technical modifications to an existing approach. It serves as an example of the importance of surgeons looking critically at their methods and exercising a willingness to test new hypotheses. In this case, the idea of putting the donor graft in closer approximation to the recipient tissue seems simple in hindsight, but was novel at the time, and has led to investigation into the molecular drivers of this phenomenon.[11,13,16–18] Subsequent analyses with thousands of cases have repeatedly validated the robustness of this technique, ultimately leading to its incorporation into the current national guidelines for pediatric stroke management as a preferred operation.[19,20]

While the focus of the authors was centered on the technical advances, sewing the STA to the pia and opening the arachnoid, there are several other advances reported here that are arguably as important (if not more so) than the operative technique. The use of intraoperative EEG, the advent of bilateral revascularization under a single anesthetic, and the importance of long-term follow-up are all innovations that have fundamentally changed the practice of pediatric moyamoya treatment.[4,7,8,14,21–24] All of these practices are now routine in major centers and have been shown to reduce risk and improve outcomes.[19] Finally, this paper was also impactful for the careful attention paid to studying why individual patients did better or worse after surgery. This meticulous analysis was a key characteristic of the senior author, Michael Scott, and led to decades of research that advanced the understanding and treatment of moyamoya around the world.

Study Limitations As a single-center, retrospective study, the work is limited by possible selection bias, small numbers, and potential heterogeneity with individual operative approaches. In addition, the average follow-up was limited and not directly compared to a natural history cohort or alternative operative approach.

Relevant Studies The importance of this pioneering work is highlighted by the abundance of subsequent related studies. While many are noted in the prior review of the results, there are several that merit specific attention. The first is the far larger series following up on this initial paper, published by Scott in 2004, involving 143 patients, which supported the utility of this approach.[25] The identification of multiple moyamoya subtypes, each associated with distinct risks and responses to surgical treatment, led to the hypothesis that moyamoya is not a single disease entity. Rather, it is an umbrella term describing a common end-stage arteriopathy that arises from a diverse range of underlying pathophysiologies, including RNF213 mutations, Down syndrome, and prior cranial irradiation. This paradigm is now widely accepted and has been reported in numerous studies, including those published in the *New England Journal of Medicine*.[18,19,26,27] Finally, the critical importance of long-term follow-up for these patients was evidenced in one of Scott's final papers, a decades-long review of his operative series, which offers tremendous insight into the durability of pial synangiosis and its ability to provide meaningful lives for countless children.[7]

REFERENCES

1. Smith ER, Scott RM. Spontaneous occlusion of the circle of Willis in children: pediatric moyamoya summary with proposed evidence-based practice guidelines. A review. J Neurosurg Pediatr. 2012;9:353–360.
2. Roach ES et al. Management of stroke in infants and children: a scientific statement from a Special Writing Group of the American Heart Association Stroke Council and the Council on Cardiovascular Disease in the Young. Stroke. 2008;39, 2644–2691.
3. Vendrame M et al. Electroencephalogram monitoring during intracranial surgery for moyamoya disease. Pediatr Neurol. 2011;44, 427–432.
4. Scott RM et al. Long-term outcome in children with moyamoya syndrome after cranial revascularization by pial synangiosis. J Neurosurg. 2004;100:142–149.
5. Koss M, Scott RM, Irons MB, Smith ER, Ullrich NJ. Moyamoya syndrome associated with neurofibromatosis type 1: perioperative and long-term outcome after surgical revascularization. J Neurosurg Pediatr. 2013;11:417–425.
6. Smith ER, Scott RM. Progression of disease in unilateral moyamoya syndrome. Neurosurg Focus. 2008;24:E17.
7. Riordan CP, Storey A, Cote DJ, Smith ER, Scott RM. Results of more than 20 years of follow-up in pediatric patients with moyamoya disease undergoing pial synangiosis. J Neurosurg Pediatr. 2019;23:1–7. doi:10.3171/2019.1.PEDS18457

8. Jackson EM, Lin N, Manjila S, Scott RM, Smith ER. Pial synangiosis in patients with moyamoya younger than 2 years of age. J Neurosurg Pediatr. 2014;13:420–425.
9. Lee JS, Storey A, Lanpher A, Smith ER. Development of moyamoya arteriopathy following treatment of intracranial tumors: clinical and radiographic characterization. J Neurosurg Pediatr. 2024;34:1–6. doi:10.3171/2024.3.PEDS23479
10. Yamada I, Matsushima Y, Suzuki S. Childhood moyamoya disease before and after encephalo-duro-arterio-synangiosis: an angiographic study. Neuroradiology. 1992; 34:318–322.
11. Soriano SG, Cowan DB, Proctor MR, Scott RM. Levels of soluble adhesion molecules are elevated in the cerebrospinal fluid of children with moyamoya syndrome. Neurosurgery. 2002;50:544–549.
12. Pricola Fehnel K et al. Using urinary bFGF and TIMP3 levels to predict the presence of juvenile pilocytic astrocytoma and establish a distinct biomarker signature. J Neurosurg Pediatr. 2016;18:396–407.
13. Sesen J et al. Non-invasive urinary biomarkers in moyamoya disease. Front Neurol. 2021;12:661952.
14. Storey A, Michael Scott R, Robertson R, Smith E. Preoperative transdural collateral vessels in moyamoya as radiographic biomarkers of disease. J Neurosurg Pediatr. 2017;19:289–295.
15. Montaser AS et al. Ivy sign: a diagnostic and prognostic biomarker for pediatric moyamoya. J Neurosurg Pediatr. 2021;1–9. doi:10.3171/2021.11.PEDS21384
16. Duggins-Warf M et al. Disease specific urinary biomarkers in the central nervous system. Sci Rep. 2023;13, 19244.
17. Fehnel KP et al. Dysregulation of the EphrinB2-EphB4 ratio in pediatric cerebral arteriovenous malformations is associated with endothelial cell dysfunction in vitro and functions as a novel noninvasive biomarker in patients. Exp Mol Med. 2020;52:658–671.
18. Kahle KT, Duran D, Smith ER. Increasing precision in the management of pediatric neurosurgical cerebrovascular diseases with molecular genetics. J Neurosurg Pediatr. 2023;31:228–237.
19. Ferriero DM et al. Management of stroke in neonates and children: a scientific statement from the American Heart Association/American Stroke Association. Stroke. 2019;50:e51–e96.
20. Macyszyn L et al. Direct versus indirect revascularization procedures for moyamoya disease: a comparative effectiveness study. J Neurosurg. 2017;126:1523–1529.
21. Vendrame M et al. Electroencephalogram monitoring during intracranial surgery for moyamoya disease. Pediatr Neurol. 2011;44:427–432.
22. Penn DL et al. General principles for pial synangiosis in pediatric moyamoya patients: 2-dimensional operative video. Oper Neurosurg (Hagerstown). 2019;16:E14–E15.
23. Rosi A, Riordan CP, Smith ER, Scott RM, Orbach DB. Clinical status and evolution in moyamoya: Which angiographic findings correlate? Brain Commun. 2019;1:fcz029.
24. Titsworth WL, Scott RM, Smith ER. National analysis of 2454 pediatric Moyamoya admissions and the effect of hospital volume on outcomes. Stroke. 2016;47:1303–1311.
25. Scott RM et al. Long-term outcome in children with moyamoya syndrome after cranial revascularization by pial synangiosis. J Neurosurg Spine. 2004;100:142–149.
26. Scott RM, Smith ER. Moyamoya disease and moyamoya syndrome. N Engl J Med. 2009;360:1226–1237.
27. Ganesan V, Smith ER. Moyamoya: defining current knowledge gaps. Dev Med Child Neurol. 2015;57:786–787.

Chapter 26

Hypothermia Therapy after Traumatic Brain Injury in Children

Hutchison JS, Ward RE, Lacroix J, Hébert PC, Barnes MA, Bohn DJ, Dirks PB, Doucette S, Fergusson D, Gottesman R, Joffe AR, Kirpalani HM, Meyer PG, Morris KP, Moher D, Singh RN, Skippen PW; for the Hypothermia Pediatric Head Injury Trial Investigators and the Canadian Critical Care Trials Group,
N Engl J Med. 2008 Jun 5;358(23):2447–2456

Reviewed by Anoop Chinthala and Gordan Mao

Study Design Multicenter randomized, controlled trial.

Randomization and Stratification Patients were randomized by a central telephone system with stratification by center and age (<7 years vs ≥7 years).

Class of Evidence I

Research Question/Objective To determine whether moderate hypothermia therapy (32–33°C for 24 hours, initiated within 8 hours after injury) improves neurologic outcomes and survival compared to normothermia in children with severe traumatic brain injury (TBI).

Study Design Multicenter, international randomized controlled trial conducted at 17 centers in 3 countries. Patients were randomized to either hypothermia therapy or normothermia. Temperature management protocols and guidelines for intracranial pressure (ICP) and cerebral perfusion pressure (CPP) were standardized across centers.

Inclusion/Exclusion Criteria

- Inclusion Criteria
  - Children less than 18 years of age with severe TBI (Glasgow Coma Scale ≤ 8)
  - Acute brain injury on computerized tomography, requiring mechanical ventilation

- Exclusion Criteria
  - Screened >8 hours after injury
  - Refractory shock

DOI: 10.1201/9781003416197-26

- Suspected brain death
- Nonaccidental injury
- Prolonged cardiac arrest
- High cervical cord injury
- Severe pre-injury neurodevelopmental disability
- Gunshot wounds
- Isolated epidural hematoma
- Pregnancy

Intervention or Treatment Received

- **Hypothermia group** Target 32.5 ± 0.5°C maintained for 24 hours via surface cooling; rewarming at 0.5°C every 2 hours.
- **Normothermia group** Target 37.0 ± 0.5°C maintained until intracranial hypertension resolved.

Outcome Measures

- **Primary endpoint** Proportion of patients with unfavorable outcomes (severe disability, persistent vegetative state, or death) at 6 months, assessed using the Pediatric Cerebral Performance Category scale.
- **Secondary endpoints** Mortality, intensive care unit/hospital stay, ICP, CPP, hypotension, infection, bleeding, arrhythmias, cointerventions, and neuropsychological testing (measures of intelligence, memory functioning, and speed of information processing) at 3 and 12 months.

Statistical Analysis Sample size powered for a 20% absolute reduction in unfavorable outcomes. Analyses were intention-to-treat. Subgroup and sensitivity analyses were conducted, with logistic regression used to adjust for confounders.

Results

- **Enrollment** 225 patients (108 hypothermia, 117 normothermia).
- **Primary outcome** 31% in hypothermia vs 22% in normothermia had unfavorable outcomes (RR 1.41; 95% CI, 0.89–2.22; $p = 0.14$).
- **Mortality** 21% in hypothermia vs 12% in normothermia (RR 1.40; 95% CI, 0.90–2.27; $p = 0.06$).
- **Adverse events** Hypotension and vasoactive drug use were more common during rewarming in hypothermia patients. No significant differences in infection, bleeding, or arrhythmias. Neuropsychological follow-up showed worse visual memory at 12 months in the hypothermia group ($p = 0.05$).

Conclusion Hypothermia therapy initiated within 8 hours of severe pediatric TBI and maintained for 24 hours did not improve neurologic outcomes and was associated with a trend toward increased mortality. These results suggest that this hypothermia protocol should not be routinely used in children with severe TBI.

Author/Reviewer Commentary This trial is widely regarded as a landmark in pediatric neurocritical care because it provided the first adequately powered, multicenter, randomized evidence that directly tested the long-standing hypothesis that induced hypothermia improves outcomes after TBI in children. Before this study, enthusiasm for hypothermia stemmed from compelling preclinical data in rodents and small single-center or phase II pediatric studies suggesting physiologic benefits and possible safety.[1–4] However, the field lacked convincing outcome data in children. By moving beyond surrogate markers (e.g. intracranial pressure control) to a patient-centered primary endpoint (6-month Pediatric Cerebral Performance Category) and enrolling across 17 international centers with standardized temperature, intracranial pressure (ICP), and cerebral perfusion pressure (CPP) protocols, the investigators were able to not only analyze short term outcome but long-term effects.

The study demonstrated no improvement in unfavorable neurological outcomes with 24 hours of moderate hypothermia initiated within 8 hours of injury and, importantly, identified concerning safety signals, greater hypotension, and vasoactive requirements during rewarming and a trend toward higher mortality in the hypothermia arm. It suggested that any neuroprotective benefits of hypothermia seen in preclinical TBI models may be offset clinically by systemic side-effects, especially during rewarming (e.g. hypotension and reduced CPP), or that the therapeutic window and dose–duration used here (32–33°C for 24 hours) were suboptimal for pediatric TBI. By partnering with psychiatrists and utilizing neuropsychiatric testing, this trial provided insight into the long-term cognitive effects of hypothermia treatment. They found long-term visual memory scores were significantly worse in the hypothermia group than in the normothermia group 12 months after injury.

Not only did this trial demonstrate no functional benefit, but it also showed that the use of hypothermia may cause harm and adverse long-term effects, forcing clinicians and guideline panels to reconsider the routine adoption of hypothermia protocols. A subsequent pediatric phase III trial (Cool Kids) that tested earlier initiation (≤6 hours), longer duration (48–72 hours), and slow rewarming was stopped early for futility, reinforcing the lack of outcome benefit despite protocol refinements.[5] Parallel pediatric work in Australia/New Zealand demonstrated the feasibility and safety of prolonged hypothermia but again showed no improvement in 12-month outcomes, further tempering expectations.[6] In practice, the study redirected standard care from prophylactic hypothermia toward strict fever avoidance, sustained normothermia, hemodynamic stability, and preservation of CPP targets. The 2019 *Guidelines for the Management of Pediatric Severe TBI* (Brain Trauma Foundation) recommend against prophylactic moderate hypothermia to improve overall outcomes and advise very slow rewarming if hypothermia is used for ICP control.[7] Contemporary reviews likewise emphasize normothermia as standard care and reserve hypothermia, if at all, for refractory ICP with careful hemodynamic management.

This trial contextualized pediatric findings within the broader literature of adult randomized evidence and meta-analyses that similarly failed to show a meaningful benefit of post-traumatic hypothermia. In doing so, it tempered a decade of optimism and redirected care to focus on normothermia maintenance in children.

REFERENCES

1. Clifton GL, Jiang JY, Lyeth BG, Jenkins LW, Hamm RJ, Hayes RL. Marked protection by moderate hypothermia after experimental traumatic brain injury. J Cereb Blood Flow Metab. 1991;11:114–121.
2. Clark RS, Kochanek PM, Marion DW, et al. Mild posttraumatic hypothermia reduces mortality after severe controlled cortical impact in rats. J Cereb Blood Flow Metab. 1996;16:253–261.
3. Biswas AK, Bruce DA, Sklar FH, Bokovoy JL, Sommerauer JF. Treatment of acute traumatic brain injury in children with moderate hypothermia improves intracranial hypertension. Crit Care Med. 2002;30:2742–2751.
4. Adelson PD, Ragheb J, Kanev P, et al. Phase II clinical trial of moderate hypothermia after severe traumatic brain injury in children. Neurosurgery. 2005;56:740–754.
5. Adelson PD, Wisniewski SR, Beca J, et al. Comparison of hypothermia and normothermia after severe traumatic brain injury in children (cool kids): a phase 3, randomised controlled trial. Lancet Neurol. 2013;12(6):546–553. doi:10.1016/S1474-4422(13)70077-2
6. Beca J, McSharry B, Erickson S, et al. Hypothermia for traumatic brain injury in children: a phase II randomized controlled trial. Crit Care Med. 2015;43(7):1458–1466. doi:10.1097/CCM.0000000000000947
7. Kochanek PM, Tasker RC, Carney N, et al. Guidelines for the Management of Pediatric Severe Traumatic Brain Injury, Third Edition: update of the Brain Trauma Foundation guidelines, executive summary. Neurosurgery. 2019;84(6):1169–1178. doi:10.1093/neuros/nyz051

CHAPTER 27

The First Clinical Trial to Establish Deep Brain Stimulation of the Subthalamic Nucleus as an Evidence-Based Treatment for Parkinson's Disease

Deuschl G, et al.; for the German Parkinson Study Group, Neurostimulation Section, N Engl J Med. 2006 Aug 3;355(9):896–908

Reviewed by Günther Deuschl

Research Question/Objective Subthalamic nucleus deep brain stimulation (STN-DBS) was found in uncontrolled studies to reduce levodopa-related motor complications in advanced Parkinson's disease. We compared STN-DBS plus medication with the best medical treatment alone.[1]

Study Design 156 patients with advanced disease and fluctuations of mobility were randomized to STN-DBS or BMT. Both life quality (measured with the Parkinson's Disease Questionnaire [PDQ]-39) and severity of motor symptoms (measured with the Unified Parkinson's Disease Rating Scale [UPDRS-III, OFF-state]) were used as primary outcomes to compare these treatments after 6 months.

Inclusion/Exclusion Criteria

- Inclusion Criteria
  - Patients under 75 years of age had to have fluctuations in their mobility and/or dyskinesia and/or tremor.
  - A positive response to Levodopa of more than 30%.

- Exclusion Criteria N/A

Results STN-DBS caused greater improvements in the quality of life of 27% and a 41% improvement of the motor score (UPDRS-III) in the OFF-condition compared to medical treatment. Dyskinesia, activities of daily living, and levodopa dosage were all clinically relevantly and significantly improved. There was no worsening of depression, cognition, and psychiatric rating scales. Serious adverse events were more common for STN-DBS, including three deaths in the STN and one in the BMT group, but the overall frequency of adverse events was higher for the BMT group.

DOI: 10.1201/9781003416197-27

Conclusion In this 6-month study of patients under 75 years of age with severe motor complications of Parkinson's disease, neurostimulation of the subthalamic nucleus was more effective than medical management alone. Serious adverse events were more common in the DBS group.

Author/Reviewer Commentary Although deep brain stimulation (DBS) was introduced in 1987 for the treatment of the target symptom "tremor" by stimulating the ventral intermediate nucleus of the thalamus,[2] this intervention did not improve akinesia and rigidity, the two cardinal symptoms that most profoundly lead to a deterioration in the quality of life in patients with Parkinson's disease. The observation that the subthalamic nucleus is a key regulatory structure of the basal ganglia, and that its destruction in a monkey model of Parkinson's disease could lead to an improvement of parkinsonian symptoms,[3] paved the way for the next step in this sequence of exciting discoveries. This work ultimately led to the first implantation of an electrode into this nucleus by Alim Benabid and Pierre Pollak in 1993.[4] This was a groundbreaking development, as the subthalamic nucleus had been considered a no-go area for neurosurgeons since 1927, when Martin et al.[5] demonstrated that lesioning of this nucleus could result in untreatable ballism. Information about this advance spread rapidly within the scientific community, and other groups soon began operating on the first patients; nevertheless, the first large case series was published by the Grenoble group only in 1998.[6]

At that time, the state of clinical research in this border area between neurology and neurosurgery was still in its infancy. German neurosurgeons, in particular, were still deeply affected by the public condemnation of lesional stereotactic surgery in the 1970s,[7] which followed functional neurosurgical interventions for psychiatric conditions which, at the time, lacked a solid scientific basis. As a consequence, functional stereotaxis became largely restricted to neurological indications, where it indeed had the potential for major clinical success. Neurologists were rarely involved in these procedures, and the two disciplines, whose combined expertise was essential for successful treatment, remained largely separated.

In 1998, an initiative emerged within the German movement disorder community to apply to the German Ministry of Research for an overarching research funding structure for Parkinson's disease under the leadership of Wolfgang Oertel; this application was successful in 1999. The German implantation centers, which were then just emerging, were open to joining a DBS study group, which I had the pleasure of leading.

This new beginning offered the opportunity to rethink the study concepts for DBS trials. Whereas most earlier investigations of functional neurosurgical procedures had been uncontrolled, we aimed to include a meaningful control group and therefore chose a waiting-group design. At that time, the main outcome measure traditionally used was the reduction of off-time, reflecting the legacy of medication studies. However, we chose quality of life, measured by the PDQ-39, as the primary outcome parameter of a clinical trial for the first time in Parkinson's disease interventions. We felt that a surgical intervention carrying specific risks should be associated with an improvement in this integral parameter for the assessment of a health intervention. The results turned out to be clearly positive. Naturally, all other outcomes standard for clinical trials in advanced Parkinson's disease were also included, in particular, the UPDRS motor score, as well as measures of immobility, dyskinesia, off-time, and questionnaires assessing depression, cognition, and neuropsychiatric symptoms.

Since this first publication in 2006, several high-quality controlled studies have been published. These compared DBS of the subthalamic nucleus or the globus pallidus internus with best medical treatment alone in 2009[8] and 2010,[9] compared DBS of the subthalamic nucleus with DBS of the globus pallidus internus in 2010[10] and 2012,[11] and explored the effects of stimulation ON versus stimulation OFF in patients with implanted DBS electrodes in studies published in 2012[12] and 2020.[13] Overall, all studies comparing STN-DBS with medical treatment alone confirmed the superior efficacy of STN-DBS in eligible patients.

A special role was played by the so-called Earlystim trial, a German–French multicenter study that I had the pleasure of leading together with close colleagues.[14] This trial recruited patients with motor fluctuations of no more than 3 years' duration and compared STN-DBS with best medical treatment. At this disease stage, patients with Parkinson's disease can usually still be treated adequately with medication alone; nevertheless, the study demonstrated that STN-DBS resulted in superior quality of life and better outcomes across almost all motor parameters compared with standardized best medical treatment. Earlier stimulation can therefore improve life in eligible patients with Parkinson's disease. This study represents the most important reason why the mean age of patients undergoing STN stimulation has continuously decreased since 2013.

The pivotal studies provided convincing evidence of improvements in both quality of life and motor outcomes. It also became clear that quality of life is not merely a reflection of motor symptoms; rather, it is strongly influenced by non-motor symptoms, as we now know.[15] Several open-label and registry studies have demonstrated beneficial effects of STN-DBS on a variety of non-motor symptoms, including sleep, urinary, emotional, and cognitive symptoms.[16,17]

STN-DBS remains a surgical procedure and, accordingly, neurosurgical complications can occur. Surgically related serious adverse events (SAEs), such as hemorrhage or infection, device-related SAEs such as lead breakage, and stimulation-induced SAEs such as dyskinesia have all been reported. In our first trial,[1] we observed more such complications than are seen today,[13] largely due to subsequent improvements in hardware and surgical techniques. The later Earlystim trial also reported more than 20 neurosurgical SAEs among 256 patients; however, all of these complications had resolved after 2 years.[14]

Meanwhile, DBS has also received favorable evaluations from the perspective of evidence-based medicine, as reflected in several reviews of treatment options for Parkinson's disease[18–20] and in a recent guideline on the use of "invasive therapies" for Parkinson's disease.[21] Although controlled studies have assessed treatment effects for periods of up to 2 years, longer-term studies cannot be conducted under controlled conditions. Nevertheless, many monocentric and, in part, multicentric studies have demonstrated sustained improvements in core symptoms such as rigidity and tremor over periods of up to 15 or even 20 years, as summarized in several reviews.[22–24] A slight prolongation of life expectancy, of approximately 1 year, has also been reported.[22] Importantly for patients and their families, however, the treatment cannot halt disease progression with respect to dementia, gait disturbance, and later speech and voice changes. In this sense, STN-DBS can create "A Second Honeymoon for Parkinson's Disease," as one editorial accompanying the Earlystim study aptly phrased it.[25]

Given the wealth of high-quality clinical trials, DBS has become one of the most extensively studied treatments for Parkinson's disease. The study reported here was the first to demonstrate the efficacy of DBS of the subthalamic nucleus in a large cohort of patients and has served as a template for subsequent high-quality studies, which have expanded the field to encompass many additional aspects and facets of this treatment.

REFERENCES

1. Deuschl G, Schade-Brittinger C, Krack P, et al. A randomized trial of deep-brain stimulation for Parkinson's disease. N Engl J Med. 2006;355:896–908.
2. Benabid AL, Pollak P, Gervason C, et al. Long-term suppression of tremor by chronic stimulation of the ventral intermediate thalamic nucleus. Lancet. 1991;337:403–406.
3. Bergman H, Wichmann T, DeLong MR. Reversal of experimental parkinsonism by lesions of the subthalamic nucleus. Science. 1990;249:1436–1438.
4. Limousin P, Pollak P, Benazzouz A, et al. Bilateral subthalamic nucleus stimulation for severe Parkinson's disease. Mov Disord. 1995;10:672–674.
5. Martin JP. Hemichorea resulting from a local lesion of the brain (syndrome of the body of Luys). Brain. 1927;50:637–651.
6. Limousin P, Krack P, Pollak P, et al. Electrical stimulation of the subthalamic nucleus in advanced Parkinson's disease. N Engl J Med. 1998;339:1105–1111.
7. Authorgroup. Seele unterm Messer. Der Spiegel. 1975;29:32–45.
8. Weaver FM, Follett K, Stern M, et al. Bilateral deep brain stimulation vs best medical therapy for patients with advanced Parkinson disease: a randomized controlled trial. JAMA. 2009;301:63–73.
9. Williams A, Gill S, Varma T, et al. Deep brain stimulation plus best medical therapy versus best medical therapy alone for advanced Parkinson's disease (PD SURG trial): a randomised, open-label trial. Lancet Neurol. 2010;9:581–591.
10. Follett KA, Weaver FM, Stern M, et al. Pallidal versus subthalamic deep-brain stimulation for Parkinson's disease. N Engl J Med. 2010;362:2077–2091.
11. Odekerken VJ, van Laar T, Staal MJ, et al. Subthalamic nucleus versus globus pallidus bilateral deep brain stimulation for advanced Parkinson's disease (NSTAPS study): a randomised controlled trial. Lancet Neurol. 2013;12:37–44.

12. Okun MS, Gallo BV, Mandybur G, et al. Subthalamic deep brain stimulation with a constant-current device in Parkinson's disease: an open-label randomised controlled trial. Lancet Neurol. 2012;11:140–149.
13. Vitek JL, Jain R, Chen L, et al. Subthalamic nucleus deep brain stimulation with a multiple independent constant current-controlled device in Parkinson's disease (INTREPID): a multicentre, double-blind, randomised, sham-controlled study. Lancet Neurol. 2020;19:491–501.
14. Schuepbach WM, Rau J, Knudsen K, et al. Neurostimulation for Parkinson's disease with early motor complications. N Engl J Med. 2013;368:610–622.
15. Martinez-Martin P, Rodriguez-Blazquez C, Kurtis MM, Chaudhuri KR. The impact of non-motor symptoms on health-related quality of life of patients with Parkinson's disease. Mov Disord. 2011;26:399–406.
16. Petry-Schmelzer JN, Krause M, Dembek TA, et al. Non-motor outcomes depend on location of neurostimulation in Parkinson's disease. Brain. 2019;142:3592–3604.
17. Dafsari HS, Reddy P, Herchenbach C, et al. Beneficial effects of bilateral subthalamic stimulation on non-motor symptoms in Parkinson's disease. Brain Stimul. 2016;9:78–85.
18. Fox SH, Katzenschlager R, Lim SY, et al. International Parkinson and movement disorder society evidence-based medicine review: update on treatments for the motor symptoms of Parkinson's disease. Mov Disord. 2018;33:1248–1266.
19. Seppi K, Weintraub D, Coelho M, et al. the movement disorder society evidence-based medicine review update: treatments for the non-motor symptoms of Parkinson's disease. Mov Disord. 2011;26(Suppl 3):S42–S80.
20. Fox SH, Katzenschlager R, Lim SY, et al. The movement disorder society evidence-based medicine review update: treatments for the motor symptoms of Parkinson's disease. Mov Disord. 2011;26(Suppl 3):S2–S41.
21. Deuschl G, Antonini A, Costa J, et al. European Academy of Neurology/Movement Disorder Society–European Section guideline on the treatment of Parkinson's disease: I. Invasive therapies. Mov Disord. 2022;37:1360–1374.
22. Mahlknecht P, Foltynie T, Limousin P, Poewe W. How does deep brain stimulation change the course of Parkinson's disease? Mov Disord. 2022;37:1581–1592.
23. Limousin P, Foltynie T. Long-term outcomes of deep brain stimulation in Parkinson disease. Nat Rev Neurol. 2019;15:234–242.
24. Shalash A, Alexoudi A, Knudsen K, Volkmann J, Mehdorn M, Deuschl G. The impact of age and disease duration on the long term outcome of neurostimulation of the subthalamic nucleus. Parkinsonism Relat Disord. 2014;20:47–52.
25. Tanner CM. A second honeymoon for Parkinson's disease? N Engl J Med. 2013;368: 675–676.

CHAPTER 28

The Long-Term Outcome of Microvascular Decompression for Trigeminal Neuralgia

Barker FG 2nd, Jannetta PJ, Bissonette DJ, Larkins MV, Jho HD, N Engl J Med. 1996 Apr 25;334(17):1077–1083

Reviewed by Josue Ordaz, Joao Paulo Almeida, and Mitesh Shah

Research Question/Objective The study's main objective was to describe the long-term results of microvascular decompression (MVD) for trigeminal neuralgia (TN). The authors aimed to assess the safety and efficacy of MVD, specifically evaluating pain relief and recurrence rates over an extended follow-up period.

Study Design Prospective single-center cohort study of 1,185 consecutive patients undergoing microvascular decompression for trigeminal neuralgia.

Inclusion/Exclusion Criteria

- Inclusion Criteria
  - All patients who underwent microvascular decompression of the trigeminal nerve for medically intractable trigeminal neuralgia at a single institution between 1972 and 1991 (20 years).
- Exclusion Criteria
  - Patients with trigeminal neuralgia due to multiple sclerosis or tumors were excluded.

Intervention or Treatment Received MVD was performed for the management of trigeminal neuralgia. The surgical procedure involved a microsurgical examination of the trigeminal nerve for vascular compression at or near its entry site into the brainstem, with any compressive arteries or veins repositioned or divided.

Outcome Assessment Outcomes were prospectively assessed using annual questionnaires sent to patients. The study tracked individual symptoms, operative findings, and complications, with the degree of immediate postoperative relief graded as complete, partial, or poor.

Follow-Up The median follow-up duration was 6.2 years, with all patients followed for at least 1 year.

DOI: 10.1201/9781003416197-28

Results

- *Effectiveness of MVD*: The study found that microvascular decompression is a safe and effective treatment for trigeminal neuralgia, with a high long-term success rate.
- *Long-term pain relief*: Ten years after surgery, 70% of patients were free of pain without the need for medication, while an additional 4% experienced only occasional pain that did not require long-term medication.
- *Recurrence rates*: The annual rate of recurrence of trigeminal neuralgia was less than 1% 10 years after the procedure, indicating sustained efficacy over the long term.
- *Offending vessel*: The trigeminal nerve was compressed by the superior cerebellar artery in 75% and anterior inferior cerebellar artery in 10% of patients. A vein contributed to compression in 68% and was the only compressing vessel in 12% of patients.
- *Operative risks*: Severe facial numbness occurred in 0.9% of cases after the initial procedure but it was more common in re-do procedures (8%). Likewise, facial paresis was more frequent in reoperations (0.5% vs 3%). 1.1% of patients suffered severe hearing loss after initial surgery and even less after repeat surgery. Rates of extraocular muscle palsy were about 0.9%, mostly transient and affecting the trochlear nerve. Cerebrospinal fluid leaks and chemical meningitis were observed in 1.4% and 16% of patients, respectively, and such complications were slightly more frequent after repeat surgery (2.2%, 20%).

Conclusion The authors concluded that microvascular decompression (MVD) is a safe and effective treatment for TN, with a high rate of long-term success.

Reviewer Commentary

Paper Significance and Impact The study by Barker et al. remains a landmark paper in demonstrating the safety and long-term efficacy of MVD as a treatment for TN. Since its publication, this paper has been cited more than in 1,700 publications, reflecting its profound impact on the field of neurosurgery and TN treatment. Over a 20-year period, the authors prospectively followed 1,185 patients who underwent MVD for medically intractable TN, with a median follow-up of 6.2 years. They reported that 70% of patients achieved complete relief of pain without medication 10 years post-surgery. These findings are highly significant, considering the often-debilitating nature of TN and the limitations of other treatment modalities.

Study Limitations Despite its strengths, the study by Barker et al. has several limitations. The study population was highly selective, with surgeries performed by experienced surgeons at specialized centers, which may limit the generalizability of the findings to less specialized settings or community hospitals. Additionally, the surgical techniques and equipment used during the study period (1972–1991) have since evolved, and the results may not fully reflect outcomes with current practices.

Another limitation is the lack of incorporation of modern imaging techniques, which could have improved patient selection and the identification of neurovascular compression severity. This omission may have affected the study's ability to evaluate how imaging-guided refinements in surgical planning could influence long-term outcomes. Furthermore, the study did not systematically assess postoperative quality of life or include patient-reported outcomes, missing an important aspect of treatment effectiveness.

Lastly, while the study reported long-term follow-up, it did not explore other relevant factors such as the impact of varying surgical approaches, the patient's preoperative pain characteristics, or the presence of comorbid conditions, which could have influenced the outcomes.

Overall, the Barker et al. study underscores the value of MVD as a primary treatment for TN, with enduring benefits for most patients. However, ongoing advancements in surgical techniques, imaging, and our understanding of TN's pathophysiology indicate that further studies are necessary to continue refining this approach and improving patient outcomes.

Relevant Studies More recent studies have also demonstrated the excellent efficacy of MVD for TN, showing similar long-term outcomes.[1–3] A study by Chang and colleagues reported pain-free rates of 83%, 61%, and 44% at 1, 5, and 10 years, respectively, with a median time to pain recurrence of 94 months (7.8 years).[4] Another long-term retrospective study found that 63% of patients who underwent MVD were pain-free after 20 years.[5] A meta-analysis involving 3,897 patients also showed excellent results, with a 75% pain-free rate; however, the follow-up period in this analysis was limited to a mean of 1.7 years.[6]

Alternative Treatments Medical therapy is the first-line treatment for TN with commonly used agents including carbamazepine, pregabalin, gabapentin and oxcarbamazepine. Studies have reported that up to 90 of patients experience a reduction in pain episodes with these medications.[7] However, the therapeutic window for these drugs is narrow, and side effects, such as vertigo, fatigue, diplopia, and nausea, are common.[8] Patients who become medically refractory or cannot tolerate these side effects are then referred for surgical intervention.

Alternative treatments, such as GammaKnife radiosurgery and percutaneous techniques like radiofrequency and balloon rhizotomy, have shown some effectiveness, though MVD provides longer pain-free intervals and lower recurrence rates.[9–11]

Moreover, in a retrospective study by Tronnier et al., patients undergoing radiofrequency ablation had a 50% risk of pain recurrence after 2 years.[5] In another study comparing stereotactic radiosurgery (SRS) to MVD, patients who underwent SRS had a median time to pain recurrence of 53 months (4.4 years), with pain-free rates of 71%, 47%, and 27% at 1, 5, and 10 years, respectively.[4] Percutaneous balloon rhizotomy is also an effective option, with studies showing an 8-year pain-free survival rate of 60%.[12] A more recent study reported a 94% success rate but with a median pain-free interval of only 28 months (about 2.5 years).[13] Despite the shorter pain-free durations, these procedures remain viable for patients who are unsuitable for surgery due to age, comorbidities, or personal preference.[14,15] Ongoing research into the pathophysiology of TN, particularly the role of vascular compression, continues to refine the indications and techniques for these treatments.[16,17]

Impact of Modern Imaging Techniques Advancements in neuroimaging, such as high-resolution magnetic resonance imaging (MRI) (3.0 and 7.0 Tesla), have significantly enhanced patient selection and surgical planning for MVD. Modern imaging enables more accurate identification of neurovascular compression (NVC) and other structural abnormalities contributing to TN.[18,19] This progress helps predict which patients are most likely to benefit from MVD, as those with a greater degree of NVC tend to have higher success rates. Additionally, more precise decompression, guided by improved imaging, potentially reduces the risk of recurrence.[1,4,20]

Advancements in Surgical Techniques Since 1996 Since the original Barker et al. study, surgical techniques for MVD have evolved. New approaches, such as internal neurolysis and partial neurectomy, have been introduced to address cases without clear neurovascular compression. These newer methods aim to reduce complications and improve patient outcomes.[21,22] A retrospective study by Ko et al. demonstrated pain-free survival rates of 58% at 1 year and 47% at 5 years in patients without NVC who underwent internal neurolysis.[23] These advancements reflect a trend toward more tailored surgical interventions, considering the individual patient's anatomical and pathological characteristics.

Research on the Pathophysiology of Trigeminal Neuralgia Recent studies have deepened our understanding of the underlying mechanisms of TN, highlighting the roles of vascular compression, neuroinflammation, and changes within the central nervous system. These insights emphasize the complexity of TN and suggest that a multifaceted treatment approach, combining both surgical and medical therapies, may be necessary for optimal management.[24,25] A better understanding of these mechanisms can also aid in predicting which patients are most likely to benefit from MVD or alternative treatments.

Quality-of-Life Outcomes Studies have reported significant improvements in quality-of-life metrics following MVD, including reductions in headaches, body pain, and depression.[26,27] More comprehensive evaluations of these outcomes are needed to fully understand the broader impact of MVD on patients' daily lives and overall well-being.

Summary Barker et al. established microvascular decompression as the gold-standard surgical treatment for medically refractory trigeminal neuralgia. Their landmark study demonstrated durable long-term pain relief with low morbidity and continues to serve as the benchmark against which contemporary surgical outcomes are measured.

REFERENCES

1. Sindou M, Leston J, Decullier E, Chapuis F. Microvascular decompression for primary trigeminal neuralgia: long-term effectiveness and prognostic factors in a series of 362 consecutive patients with clear-cut neurovascular conflicts who underwent pure decompression. J Neurosurg. 2007;107(6):1144–1153.
2. Sarsam Z, Garcia-Fiñana M, Nurmikko TJ, Varma TR, Eldridge P. The long-term outcome of microvascular decompression for trigeminal neuralgia. Br J Neurosurg. 2010;24(1):18–25.
3. Wei Y, Pu C, Li N, Cai Y, Shang H, Zhao W. Long-term therapeutic effect of microvascular decompression for trigeminal neuralgia: Kaplan-Meier analysis in a consecutive series of 425 patients. Turk Neurosurg. 2018;28(1):88–93.
4. Wang DD, Raygor KP, Cage TA, Ward MM, Westcott S, Barbaro NM, Chang EF. Prospective comparison of long-term pain relief rates after first-time microvascular decompression and stereotactic radiosurgery for trigeminal neuralgia. J Neurosurg. 2018;128(1):68–77.
5. Tronnier VM, Rasche D, Hamer J, Kienle A-L, Kunze S. Treatment of idiopathic trigeminal neuralgia: comparison of long-term outcome after radiofrequency rhizotomy and microvascular decompression. Neurosurgery. 2001;48:1261–1267.
6. Holste K, Chan AY, Rolston JD, Englot DJ. Pain outcomes following microvascular decompression for drug-resistant trigeminal neuralgia: a systematic review and meta-analysis. Neurosurgery. 2020;86(2):182–190.
7. Yuan M, Zhou H-Y, Xiao Z-L, Wang W, Li X-L, Chen S-J, Yin X-P, Xu L-J. Efficacy and safety of gabapentin vs. carbamazepine in the treatment of trigeminal neuralgia: a meta-analysis. Pain Practice. 2016;16(8):1083–1091.
8. Al-Quliti KW. Update on neuropathic pain treatment for trigeminal neuralgia. Neurosciences (Riyadh). 2015;20(2):107–114.
9. Little AS, Shetter AG, Shetter ME, Bay C, Rogers CL. Long-term pain response and quality of life in patients with typical trigeminal neuralgia treated with GammaKnife stereotactic radiosurgery. Neurosurgery. 2008;63(5):915–924.
10. Régis J, Tuleasca C, Resseguier N, Carron R, Donnet A, Gaudart J, Levivier M. Long-term safety and efficacy of GammaKnife surgery in classical trigeminal neuralgia: a 497-patient historical cohort study. J Neurosurg. 2016;124(4):1079–1087.
11. Sheehan J, Pan H-C, Stroila M, Steiner L. GammaKnife surgery for trigeminal neuralgia: outcomes and prognostic factors. J Neurosurg. 2005;102(3):434–441.
12. Brown JA, Chittum CJ, Sabol D, Gouda JJ. Percutaneous balloon compression of the trigeminal nerve for treatment of trigeminal neuralgia. Neurosurg Focus. 1996;1(2):e4; discussion 1 p following e4.
13. Asplund P, Linderoth B, Bergenheim AT. The predictive power of balloon shape and change of sensory functions on outcome of percutaneous balloon compression for trigeminal neuralgia. J Neurosurg. 2010;113(3):498–507.
14. Martínez Moreno NE, Gutiérrez-Sárraga J, Rey-Portolés G, Jiménez-Huete A, Martínez Álvarez R. Long-term outcomes in the treatment of classical trigeminal neuralgia by GammaKnife radiosurgery. Neurosurgery. 2016;79(6):879–888.
15. Ozturk G, Samanci Y, Peker S. Long-term efficacy of GammaKnife radiosurgery on pain control in trigeminal neuralgia. Turk Neurosurg. 2023;33:691–696.

16. Cong L, Zhihua C, Zhilin G, Huoniu OY. Effects of microvascular decompression plus longitudinal nerve sectioning on recurrent trigeminal neuralgia and investigations of postoperative recurrence causes. Turkish Neurosurg. 2019;29:369–376.
17. DeSouza DD, Hodaie M, Davis KD. Abnormal trigeminal nerve microstructure and brain white matter in idiopathic trigeminal neuralgia. Pain. 2014;155(1):37–44.
18. Bachmann R, Nassenstein I, Kooijman H, Dittrich R, Stehling C, Kugel H, Niederstadt T, Kuhlenbäumer G, Ringelstein EB, Krämer S, Heindel W. High-resolution magnetic resonance imaging (MRI) at 3.0 Tesla in the short-term follow-up of patients with proven cervical artery dissection. Invest Radiol. 2007;42(6):460–466.
19. Patel B, Markus HS. Magnetic resonance imaging in cerebral small vessel disease and its use as a surrogate disease marker. Int J Stroke. 2011;6(1):47–59.
20. Loayza R, Wikström J, Grabowska A, Semnic R, Ericson H, Abu Hamdeh S. Outcome after microvascular decompression for trigeminal neuralgia in a single center-relation to sex and severity of neurovascular conflict. Acta Neurochir (Wien). 2023;165(7): 1955–1962.
21. Carpenter A, Liu JK. Surgical outcomes after MVD with internal neurolysis and partial neurectomy for patients with trigeminal neuralgia and negative neurovascular compression. Neurosurgery. 2019;66(Supplement 1):310–450.
22. Hitotsumatsu T, Matsushima T, Inoue T. Microvascular decompression for treatment of trigeminal neuralgia, hemifacial spasm, and glossopharyngeal neuralgia: three surgical approach variations: technical note. Neurosurgery. 2003;53(6):1436–1443.
23. Ko AL, Ozpinar A, Lee A, Raslan AM, McCartney S, Burchiel KJ. Long-term efficacy and safety of internal neurolysis for trigeminal neuralgia without neurovascular compression. J Neurosurg. 2015;122(5):1048–1057.
24. Wang Y, Cao D-Y, Remeniuk B, Krimmel S, Seminowicz DA, Zhang M. Altered brain structure and function associated with sensory and affective components of classic trigeminal neuralgia. Pain. 2017;158(8):1561–1570.
25. Zhang Y, Mao Z, Pan L, Ling Z, Liu X, Zhang J, Yu X. Dysregulation of pain- and emotion-related networks in trigeminal neuralgia. Front Hum Neurosci. 2018;12:107.
26. D'Amico D, Grazzi L, Usai S, Leonardi M, Raggi A. Disability and quality of life in headache: where we are now and where we are heading. Neurolog Sci. 2013;34(S1):1–5.
27. De Siqueira SRDT, Da NÓBrega JCM, Teixeira MJ, De Siqueira JTT. Masticatory problems after balloon compression for trigeminal neuralgia: a longitudinal study. J Oral Rehabil. 2007;34(2):88–96.

CHAPTER 29

A Randomized Controlled Trial of Surgery for Temporal Lobe Epilepsy

Wiebe S, Blume WT, Girvin JP, Eliasziw M; for the Effectiveness and Efficiency of Surgery for Temporal Lobe Epilepsy Study Group, N Engl J Med. 2001 Aug 2;345(5):311–318

Reviewed by Tom Larrew and Jason Chu

Research Question/Objective To determine the efficacy of surgical treatment of temporal lobe epilepsy compared to continued medical therapy for epilepsy at 1 year. The primary outcome measure was freedom from seizures impairing awareness (complex partial or generalized) at 1 year following enrollment.

Study Design Single-center randomized control trial (RCT).

Sample Size A total of 80 patients with temporal lobe epilepsy were enrolled: 40 were randomized to surgical treatment and 40 to medical therapy.

Follow-Up Following randomization, patients were followed every 3 months for 1 year by the Epilepsy Team. All patients were followed with a self-reported monthly seizure diary, which included a description of any seizure-like events. These diaries were also reviewed by two blinded, external epileptologists to determine post-intervention seizure frequency. Additional instruments of quality of life, seizure severity, psychopathology, and depression were also self-reported and reviewed by the study team (Liverpool Seizure Severity Scale, Quality of Life in Epilepsy Inventory-89, General Health Questionnaire, and the Depression Scale of the Center for Epidemiological Studies).

Inclusion/Exclusion Criteria

- Inclusion Criteria
  - At least 16 years of age with seizures of temporal lobe semiology for ≥1 year
  - Seizures occurring monthly for the preceding year
  - Use of ≥2 antiseizure medications, one of which was phenytoin, carbamazepine, or valproic acid

DOI: 10.1201/9781003416197-29

- Exclusion Criteria
    - Patients with brain lesions that required urgent surgery
    - Progressive central nervous system disorders
    - Active psychosis
    - Pseudoseizures
    - Full-scale IQ <70
    - Previous surgery for epilepsy
    - Focal extratemporal spikes or slowing on scalp-recorded electroencephalography
    - Evidence on magnetic resonance imaging (MRI) of extratemporal lesions capable of producing the patient's seizures
    - Bilateral and equally severe epileptogenic lesions in the temporal lobe

Intervention or Treatment Received Treatment group details are depicted in Table 29.1.

Results A total of 80 patients were enrolled with 40 in the surgical treatment group and 40 in the medical treatment group. There were no differences in the baseline demographic or clinical characteristics between the 2 groups. Within the surgical group, 4 patients (10%) did not undergo an operation. There were no patients who were lost to follow-up during the study period and there were no crossovers from the medical to surgical group. One patient in the medical therapy group died from sudden unexplained death in epilepsy and there were no deaths in the surgical group.

All patients in the medical group had increases in their antiseizure medication dosages and the majority had additional changes in their medications during the study period. In the surgical group, 22% had increases in their seizure medication doses.

At the primary outcome, the cumulative proportion of patients free of seizures impairing awareness was 58% in the surgical group and 8% in the medical group ($p < 0.001$) at 1 year. Those free of all seizures (including auras) was 38% in the surgical group and 3% in the medical group. After adjusting for baseline demographic and clinical characteristics, 64% of patients who underwent surgery were free of seizures impairing awareness and 42% of patients were free of all seizures. About 25% of patients continued to have seizures after surgery. The surgical complication rate was 10% within the surgical group (thalamic infarct, wound infection, decline in verbal memory).

Table 29.1 Treatment Details for the Surgical and Medical Therapy Groups

Surgical Treatment	Medical Treatment
• Non-dominant hemisphere: Maximum 6.0–6.5 cm of the anterior lateral temporal lobe • Dominant hemisphere: Maximum of 4.0–4.5 cm of the anterior lateral temporal lobe • Mesial resection included the amygdala and anterior 1.0–3.0 cm of the hippocampus (commonly 4.0 cm)	• Adjusting the doses and combination of antiseizure medications as dictated by clinical practice and patient's level of tolerance/individual requirements • Serum antiseizure medication levels

The authors found that 2 patients were required to undergo surgical intervention for their epilepsy to render 1 patient free of seizures impairing awareness at 1 year and 3 patients to render 1 patient free of all seizures at 1 year.

Quality-of-life measures were noted to be superior in the surgical group with improvements over time.

Conclusion In appropriately selected patients, surgery for temporal lobe epilepsy is an effective and robust treatment that is superior to medical therapy at 1 year. Patients who underwent surgery had significant improvements in seizure control and quality of life.

Author/Reviewer Commentary The landmark RCT by Wiebe et al. represents one of the few studies in neurosurgical literature to provide level I evidence demonstrating the superiority of surgical intervention over continued medical therapy for patients with medically refractory temporal lobe epilepsy.

Although the study was limited to a single center with a total enrollment of 80 patients, the investigators conducted a methodologically sound RCT with standardized inclusion and exclusion criteria, defined treatment protocols, and objective outcome measures. Importantly, postrandomization seizure frequency (the primary outcome) was independently adjudicated by blinded external epileptologists, minimizing the potential for reporting bias from the investigators.

The most impactful finding was that 58% of patients undergoing surgical resection were free of disabling seizures at 1 year, compared with only 8% of patients in the medical therapy group. The intention-to-treat analysis yielded a number needed to treat of 2 to 3 to achieve seizure freedom. Surgical complications were in the expected reported range. Finally, secondary analyses demonstrated significant improvements in quality of life, employment status, and school attendance among surgical patients, emphasizing a broader socioeconomic burden of epilepsy on patients, families, and caregivers. Wiebe et al. highlight the powerful and transformative nature of epilepsy surgery.

This data was reproduced in the pediatric population by Dwivedi et al.[1] In their randomized control trial, an astonishing 77% of patients in the surgical group reported International League Against Epilepsy (ILAE) Class I (completely seizure-free, no auras) outcomes at 1 year. Of those with temporal lobe epilepsy (n = 14), 100% achieved ILAE class I, whereas only 2% in the medical group achieved a similar outcome. Consistent with the adult data, quality of life, cognitive function, and behavioral outcomes were significantly improved following surgery.

Over the past two decades, scientific and technological advancements have enhanced our understanding of seizure propagation networks and improved preoperative localization of the epileptogenic zone. Techniques such as single-photon emission computed tomography, magnetoencephalography (MEG), 7T (Tesla) MRI, resting-state functional MRI, and MRI postprocessing now complement traditional phase-I workup modalities. Concurrently, the surgical armamentarium has expanded to include a broader use of stereoencephalography, robot-assisted stereotactic neurosurgery, laser interstitial thermal therapy, high-frequency ultrasound, and intracranial neuromodulation with deep brain stimulation (DBS) or responsive neurostimulation (RNS). Wiebe et al.'s study formed the basis for further surgically focused clinical trials in epilepsy, including (but not limited to) Early Randomized Surgery for Epilepsy Trial (ERSET), GammaKnife for mesial temporal sclerosis (MTS), Stimulation of the Anterior Nucleus of the Thalamus for Epilepsy (SANTE), Responsive Neurostimulation System (RNS) Pivotal Trial, Electrical Stimulation of Thalamus for Epilepsy of Lennox–Gastaut (ESTEL), NAUTILUS trial, and Stereotactic Laser Ablation for Temporal Lobe Epilepsy (SLATE).[2–6] There is no doubt that continued innovation will lead to further success for our patients undergoing surgical treatment of their epilepsy.

Despite the robust evidence to support safety and efficacy, epilepsy surgery remains an underutilized resource.[7,8] Familiarity with Wiebe et al.'s pioneering findings is essential for neurosurgeons, not only as a cornerstone for evidence-based practice but also to educate referring providers and counsel patients and families regarding the life-altering potential of epilepsy surgery.

Study Limitations The authors of the study also note that the optimal timing of surgery for epilepsy was not addressed in their RCT.

REFERENCES

1. Dwivedi R, Ramanujam B, Chandra PS, et al. Surgery for drug-resistant epilepsy in children. N Engl J Med. 2017;377:1639–1647. doi:10.1056/NEJMoa1615335
2. Engel J, McDermott MP, Wiebe S, et al. Early surgical therapy for drug-resistant temporal lobe epilepsy: a randomized trial. JAMA. 2012;307:922–930. doi:10.1001/jama.2012.220
3. Barbaro NM, Quigg M, Broshek DK, et al. A multicenter, prospective pilot study of GammaKnife radiosurgery for mesial temporal lobe epilepsy: seizure response, adverse events, and verbal memory. Ann Neurol. 2009;65:167–175. doi:10.1002/ana.21558
4. Salanova V, Witt T, Worth R, et al. Long-term efficacy and safety of thalamic stimulation for drug-resistant partial epilepsy. Neurology. 2015;84:1017–1025. doi:10.1212/WNL.0000000000001334
5. Heck CN, King-Stephens D, Massey AD, et al. Two-year seizure reduction in adults with medically intractable partial onset epilepsy treated with responsive neurostimulation: final results of the RNS system pivotal trial. Epilepsia. 2014;55:432–441. doi:10.1111/epi.12534
6. Dalic LJ, Warren AEL, Bulluss KJ, et al. DBS of thalamic centromedian nucleus for Lennox-Gastaut syndrome (ESTEL trial). Ann Neurol. 2022;91:253–267. doi:10.1002/ana.26280
7. Engel J. Why is there still doubt to cut it out? Epilepsy Curr. 2013;13:198–204. doi:10.5698/1535-7597-13.5.198
8. Samanta D, Ostendorf AP, Willis E, et al. Underutilization of epilepsy surgery. Part I: A scoping review of barriers. Epilepsy Behav. 2021;117:107837. doi:10.1016/j.yebeh.2021.107837

CHAPTER 30

Early Identification of Refractory Epilepsy

Kwan P, Brodie MJ, N Engl J Med. 2000 Feb 3;342(5):314–319

Reviewed by Rob Blake

Research Question/Objective In patients with newly diagnosed epilepsy, what is the prognosis for long-term seizure freedom and what factors are associated with subsequent poor seizure control?

Study Design The study followed a large group of newly diagnosed epilepsy patients from a single center in Scotland. A structured questionnaire was used at the initial visit to obtain demographic and clinical information. Additional studies, such as electroencephalography and brain imaging, were obtained at the clinical discretion of the epilepsy team. Patients were seen every 4 to 6 weeks for the first 6 months, then at least every 4 months thereafter. Each patient's clinical course was closely tracked, including antiseizure medication (ASM) administration, and whether patients were seizure-free. Patients were considered free of seizures if they had not had a seizure of any type for at least 12 months while taking the same dose of ASM or while not taking any ASM.

Sample Size 525 patients between the ages of 9 and 93 years.

Follow-Up Median follow-up was 5 years (range 2–16 years).

Inclusion/Exclusion Criteria

- Inclusion Criteria
  - All consecutive patients who had been newly diagnosed with epilepsy and started on antiseizure medication at a single center (Epilepsy Unit of the Western Infirmary in Glasgow, Scotland) between January 1, 1984, and December 31, 1997.

- Exclusion Criteria – Patients were excluded at the discretion of the neurologists if:
  - It was felt they were not compliant with the treatment regimen.
  - They died from any cause during treatment.
  - They did not return for follow-up after the first ASM was started.

DOI: 10.1201/9781003416197-30

Intervention or Treatment Received The patients were started on an ASM chosen at the discretion of the epilepsy team based on clinical history and testing results. If patients failed the first ASM due to continued seizures or if the patient had intolerable side effects, they were changed to another ASM. Patients who failed 2 to 3 single drugs were then treated with a combination of multiple ASMs. There was no control group. Patients were followed over time to determine if they became seizure-free or if they developed poor seizure control.

Results At the time of the last clinic visit, 333 out of 525 patients were free of seizures (63%). Of the 525 patients in the study, 470 of these had never tried any ASM before enrollment in the study. Of these 470, 222 (47%) responded to the first ASM used, meaning they were seizure-free at the last follow-up. An additional 61 (13%) responded to the second ASM, while only 18 (4%) responded to a third drug or multiple drugs (Figure 30.1).

The reason patients failed the first ASM influenced the likelihood of long-term seizure freedom. Only 11% of patients who failed the first ASM due to the medication being ineffective at controlling seizures subsequently became seizure-free, compared to 41% of patients who stopped the first ASM due to intolerable side effects, and 55% of patients who had an idiosyncratic reaction, such as a rash or hepatotoxicity.

There were factors found at baseline that increased the likelihood of patients continuing to have uncontrolled seizures. Patients were assigned to the now-defunct

Table 2. Success of Antiepileptic-Drug Regimens in 470 Patients with Previously Untreated Epilepsy.

Variable	No. (%)
Response to first drug	222 (47)
Seizure-free during continued therapy with first drug	207 (44)
Remained seizure-free after discontinuation of first drug	15 (3)
Response to second drug	61 (13)
Seizure-free during monotherapy with second drug	41 (9)
Remained seizure-free after discontinuation of second drug	20 (4)
Response to third drug or multiple drugs	18 (4)
Seizure-free during monotherapy with third drug	6 (1)
Seizure-free during therapy with two drugs	12 (3)
Total	301 (64)

Figure 30.1 Table 2 from the paper shows the success of antiepileptic drug regimens in 470 patients with previously untreated epilepsy.

classification system of idiopathic epilepsy (epilepsy presumed to have a genetic origin), symptomatic epilepsy (epilepsy considered to be caused by a known structural abnormality), or cryptogenic epilepsy (epilepsy presumed to be due to an underlying but unidentified focal abnormality). Patients in the symptomatic or cryptogenic epilepsy groups were more likely to continue to have seizures compared to those with idiopathic epilepsy (40% vs 26%, $p = 0.004$; relative risk 1.5, 95% confidence interval [CI], 1.1–2.1). In addition, the number of total seizures patients had before treatment was associated in a linear fashion with the likelihood of poor seizure control ($p < 0.001$). In particular, seizures were uncontrolled in 51% of patients who had experienced more than 20 seizures before starting on ASMs, compared to 29% of patients who had 20 seizures or fever before starting treatment ($p < 0.001$; relative risk 1.8; CI, 1.4–2.2).

Finally, the study compared patients treated with ASMs that at that time were considered "new" (lamotrigine, gabapentin, oxcarbazepine, tiagabine, topiramate, and vigabatrin) to those receiving medications considered "established" (carbamazepine, valproate sodium, phenytoin, and ethosuximide). There was no difference in seizure-freedom rates between these "new" and "established' ASM groups (69% vs 67%).

Conclusion Of the patients with newly diagnosed epilepsy never previously trialed on medications, nearly half (47%) became seizure-free with the first trialed ASM, while a smaller but still significant amount (13%) achieved seizure freedom with a second trialed medication. However, trials of a third ASM or combinations of multiple ASMs only led to seizure control in a small minority of patients (4%). After the failure of the first two first-line ASMs, patients were unlikely to achieve seizure freedom with medication alone, and consideration for non-medical treatments, such as epilepsy surgery, should be pursued.

Patients with known structural or presumed but unidentified focal causes of epilepsy were more likely to develop intractable epilepsy. Likewise, a high seizure burden, particularly those with over 20 seizures before treatment was started, had a higher likelihood of seizure intractability.

Reviewer Commentary Although Kwan and Brodie weren't the first authors to report the prognosis for patients with epilepsy,[1–3] this landmark paper established the best values for long-term seizure-freedom rates in the literature up to that time. By methodically tracking every new epilepsy case in a single center over a 14-year period, the authors were able to clearly show that while most patients with newly diagnosed epilepsy were able to obtain good seizure control, a significant portion (36% in this population) continued to have seizures despite medical treatment. Even more importantly, the data confirmed the now accepted fact that patients who have failed 2 adequately trialed ASMs are unlikely to achieve seizure freedom with further medical trials. This finding, along with other data[4,5] was instrumental in creating the International League Against Epilepsy's official definition of drug-resistant epilepsy as "failure of adequate trials of 2 tolerated, appropriately chosen and used antiepileptic drug schedules (whether as monotherapy or in combination) to achieve sustained seizure freedom."[6] As such, the recommendation to pursue epilepsy surgery as soon as patients have failed 2 ASMs is now the standard of care.

Study Limitations The study was performed at a single epilepsy center in Scotland, so generalizability to other patient populations may be limited. The study ran from the mid-1980s to the late 1990s, and the ASM prescription pattern was quite different from what is used in most modern epilepsy centers now.

Relevant Studies Kwan and Brodie followed up their original paper by publishing a subsequent article in 2018.[7] This study again included newly diagnosed epilepsy patients seen at the Epilepsy Unit of the Western Infirmary in Glasgow, Scotland, but expanded the enrollment period to over 30 years, from July 1, 1982 to October 31, 2012. By so doing, their sample size now included 1,795 patients, including many patients receiving ASMs more commonly used in current epilepsy centers. The results remained remarkably stable even with these additional data points, with 45.7% of newly diagnosed epilepsy patients becoming seizure-free on their first ASM, 11.6% on their second ASM, and only 4.4% on their third. At the end of the study, 63.7% of patients were seizure-free for at least 1 year.

A study looking at seizure control in the pediatric population was conducted in a Dutch population,[5] which again showed strikingly similar results. In this group, 388 children were prescribed ASMs, and 46% achieved at least 1 year of seizure freedom on their first ASM, 19% on their second ASM, and 9% on all additional ASM regimens.

Summary This paper was impactful because it definitively established realistic, evidence-based expectations for long-term seizure control in patients with newly diagnosed epilepsy and, in doing so, it fundamentally reshaped clinical decision-making. By rigorously demonstrating that seizure freedom is unlikely after the failure of 2 appropriately chosen antiseizure medications, Kwan and Brodie provided the empirical foundation for the modern definition of drug-resistant epilepsy and the timely referral for epilepsy surgery. Its clarity, methodological strength, and reproducibility across decades and populations transformed both prognostic counseling and standards of care, making it a true landmark in epilepsy management.

REFERENCES

1. Schmidt D, Gram L. Monotherapy versus polytherapy in epilepsy: a reappraisal. CNS Drugs. 1995;3:194–208.
2. Brodie MJ, Dichter MA. Antiepileptic drugs. N Engl J Med. 1996;334:168–175. [Erratum, N Engl J Med 1996;334:479.]
3. Devinsky O. Patients with refractory seizures. N Engl J Med. 1999;340:1565–1570.
4. Mohanraj R, Brodie MJ. Diagnosing refractory epilepsy: response to sequential treatment schedules. Eur J Neurol. 2006;13:277–282.

5. Arts WF, Brouwer OF, Peters AC, Stroink H, Peeters EA, Schmitz PI, vanDonselaar CA, Geerts AT. Course and prognosis of childhood epilepsy: 5-year follow-up of the Dutch study of epilepsy in childhood. Brain. 2004;127:1774–1784.
6. Kwan P, Arzimanoglou A, Berg AT, Brodie MJ, Allen Hauser W, Mathern G, Moshé SL, Perucca E, Wiebe S, French J. Definition of drug resistant epilepsy: consensus proposal by the ad hoc Task Force of the ILAE Commission on Therapeutic Strategies. Epilepsia. 2010;51(6):1069–1077. doi:10.1111/j.1528-1167.2009.02397.x. [Erratum in: Epilepsia. 2010 Sep;51(9):1922.]
7. Chen Z, Brodie MJ, Liew D, Kwan P. Treatment outcomes in patients with newly diagnosed epilepsy treated with established and new antiepileptic drugs: a 30-year longitudinal cohort study. JAMA Neurol. 2018;75(3):279–286. doi:10.1001/jamaneurol.2017.3949. [Erratum in: JAMA Neurol. 2018 Mar 1;75(3):384. doi: 10.1001/jamaneurol.2018.0018.]

CHAPTER 31

Vagus Nerve Stimulation for Treatment of Partial Seizures: 1. A Controlled Study of Effect on Seizures. First International Vagus Nerve Stimulation Study Group

Ben-Menachem E, Mañon-Espaillat R, Ristanovic R, Wilder BJ, Stefan H, Mirza W, Tarver WB, Wernicke JF; First International Vagus Nerve Stimulation Study Group, Epilepsia. 1994 May–Jun;35(3):616–626

Reviewed by Jason Chu and Tom Larrew

Research Question/Objective To determine whether high-parameter (therapeutic) vagus nerve stimulation reduces partial seizure frequency more effectively than low-parameter (control) stimulation.

Study Design A multicenter, prospectively randomized, parallel, double-blind study of patients with refractory partial seizures was conducted. Following a 12-week baseline seizure monitoring period, participants underwent vagus nerve simulation (VNS) implantation and were randomized to high- or low-parameter stimulation for 14 weeks. Seizure outcomes were then assessed, after which patients were permitted to cross over to high-parameter stimulation. Antiseizure medication levels were maintained at a stable level as far as possible throughout the study.

Sample Size A total of 67 patients with refractory partial (simple or complex) seizures were enrolled. Thirty-one patients were randomized to the high-stimulation paradigm and 36 patients were randomized to the low-stimulation paradigm.

Follow-Up Patients were evaluated every 4 weeks during the 12-week baseline phase, then underwent VNS implantation. After a 2-week recovery, stimulation was initiated and patients were followed at weeks 6, 10, and 14. Seizures, including auras (counted as simple partial seizures), were recorded in patient diaries. Antiseizure medication levels, vital signs, and adverse events were monitored. Seizure severity (mild, moderate, severe) and duration were documented when possible.

DOI: 10.1201/9781003416197-31

Inclusion/Exclusion Criteria

- Inclusion Criteria
    - Partial seizures not adequately controlled with medication
    - At least 6 seizures a month during the 12-week baseline period

- Exclusion Criteria
    - An unstable medical condition
    - Pregnancy
    - A seizure etiology more appropriately treated by other means (such as surgery)

Intervention or Treatment Received The two treatment paradigms are shown in Table 31.1.

Results 83 patients were enrolled; 16 were excluded before analysis (11 discontinued during baseline: 1 was not stimulated due to guardianship issues, and there was 1 generator malfunction and 3 protocol deviations), leaving 67 patients for analysis. No patients were lost to follow-up, and baseline characteristics were comparable between groups.

After 14 weeks, the high-stimulation group ($n = 31$) demonstrated a 30.9% mean reduction in seizure frequency vs 11.3% in the low-stimulation group ($n = 36$) ($p = 0.029$, t-test; $p = 0.036$, Wilcoxon). Seizure reduction from baseline was significant in the high-stimulation group ($p < 0.001$) but not in the low-stimulation group ($p = 0.072$). A ≥ 50% seizure reduction occurred in 38.7% of high-stimulation patients compared with 19.4% in the low-stimulation group.

Conclusion VNS at high-stimulation parameters results in significant seizure frequency reduction. This study confirmed that VNS is an effective treatment modality for patients with refractory partial seizures.

Table 31.1 Stimulation Parameters

	High		Low	
Parameter	**Typical**	**Range**	**Typical**	**Range**
Output current (mA)	1.5	0.25–3.0	1.25	0.25–3.0
Frequency (Hz)	30	20–50	1	1–2
Pulse width (microsecond)	500	500	130	130
On time (second)	30	30–90	30	30
Off time (minute)	5	5–10	90	60–180
Magnet parameters				
Output current (mA)	1.5	0.5–3.0	0	0
On time (second)	30	30–90	N/A	N/A
Pulse width (microsecond)	500	500	N/A	N/A

Author/Reviewer Commentary In the seminal paper by Ben-Menachem et al., the efficacy of vagus nerve stimulation (VNS) was demonstrated through the first multicenter prospective randomized control study on this topic. This study was one of the few reviewed by the Food and Drug Administration (FDA) as evidence for the approval of VNS in 1997 for patients 12 and older for the treatment of partial-onset seizures refractory to antiseizure medications. The investigators of this study concurrently published their expanded results, including safety, side effects, and tolerability in one paper and seizure outcomes after an extended follow-up in another.[1,2]

This study represents one of the earliest multicenter randomized trials in neurosurgery and was methodologically rigorous. Unlike many surgical studies, it incorporated a well-matched control group. VNS allowed effective blinding through low-parameter stimulation, enabling participants to perceive stimulation without therapeutic dosing and minimizing bias. Broad inclusion criteria enhanced generalizability, demonstrating efficacy across diverse seizure types, including simple and complex partial seizures with secondary generalization.

This study, along with similar studies at the time, demonstrated that high-parameter VNS leads to significant seizure reduction in patients with medically refractory epilepsy. The high-VNS group averaged 79 fewer seizures during the study period (median 16), while the low-VNS group only averaged 4 fewer seizures (median 5). All patients in the high-stimulation group achieved a statistically significant reduction from baseline, whereas none in the low-stimulation group did. Self-reported seizure intensity and duration were not significantly different between the two groups. Although some patients noted subjective improvements, variability, incomplete reporting, and a smaller sample size for these measures likely limited the detection of group-level differences.

Although the high-stimulation group demonstrated a mean seizure reduction of 30.9%, with 38.7% achieving ≥50% reduction, stimulation was limited to 14 weeks. Subsequent studies have shown that VNS efficacy improves over time. In the frequently cited meta-analysis by Englot et al., seizure reduction averaged 36% at 3 to 12 months and 51% at ≥1 year following implantation.[3] Subsequent studies have confirmed the efficacy of VNS in generalized epilepsy. Following FDA approval, its benefit in pediatric populations has also been well established. Elliot et al. reported a 58.9% seizure reduction in patients ≤18 years, with no significant difference between children younger than 12 years and those aged 12–18 years.[4,5]

Since FDA approval, several VNS models have been introduced. A notable advancement is auto-stimulation, which uses heart rate detection, as in the SenTiva system (LivaNova, London, UK), and has been associated with modest additional seizure reduction compared with earlier models lacking this feature.[6] Modern research on VNS includes the study of the interaction of VNS with other forms of neuromodulation, such as deep brain stimulation (DBS) and responsive neurostimulation (RNS).[7] There is some evidence that there may be synergistic efficacy when VNS is used concurrently with DBS or RNS. However, dual neuromodulation may increase stimulation-related adverse effects. One study reported such side effects in 30% of patients treated with both VNS and RNS, compared with 2% in those treated with RNS alone.[7]

In recent years, VNS has expanded beyond epilepsy to other disease states. It received FDA approval in 2005 for treatment-resistant depression (LivaNova system) and in 2025 for rheumatoid arthritis in adults with inadequate response or intolerance to at least one disease-modifying antirheumatic drug (SetPoint system). Emerging evidence also supports its potential role in inflammatory bowel disease, including Crohn's disease.[8] Based on animal studies and the hypothesis that vagal tone is decreased in Crohn's disease, select patients have undergone VNS implantation with some success, though this indication is not yet FDA approved.

Study Limitations Although rigorously designed, seizure frequency relied on patient or caregiver diaries, with all recorded events counted as seizures. This approach may have overestimated the true seizure burden. Subsequent epilepsy trials have incorporated more standardized and externally validated outcome assessments, such as the blinded review of seizure diaries by independent epileptologists, as in the study by Wiebe et al., to improve accuracy and reduce bias.[9]

Summary This trial was the first high-quality, multicenter, randomized, double-blind study to demonstrate the efficacy of VNS in medically refractory epilepsy. It established neuromodulation as a credible therapeutic strategy, set a methodological standard for device-based trials in neurosurgery, and laid the foundation for FDA approval and the widespread adoption of VNS in both adult and pediatric epilepsy.

REFERENCES

1. Ramsay RE, Uthman BM, Augustinsson LE, et al. Vagus nerve stimulation for treatment of partial seizures: 2. Safety, side effects, and tolerability. Epilepsia. 1994;35(3):627–636. doi:10.1111/j.1528-1157.1994.tb02483.x
2. George R, Salinsky M, Kuzniecky R, et al. Vagus nerve stimulation for treatment of partial seizures: 3. Long-term follow-up on first 67 patients exiting a controlled study. First International Vagus Nerve Stimulation Study Group. Epilepsia. 1994;35(3):637–643. doi:10.1111/j.1528-1157.1994.tb02484.x
3. Englot DJ, Chang EF, Auguste KI. Vagus nerve stimulation for epilepsy: a meta-analysis of efficacy and predictors of response: a review. J Neurosurg. 2011;115(6):1248–1255. doi:10.3171/2011.7.JNS11977
4. Elliott RE, Rodgers SD, Bassani L, et al. Vagus nerve stimulation for children with treatment-resistant epilepsy: a consecutive series of 141 cases: clinical article. J Neurosurg Pediatr. 2011;7(5):491–500. doi:10.3171/2011.2.PEDS10505
5. Helmers SL, Wheless JW, Frost M, et al. Vagus nerve stimulation therapy in pediatric patients with refractory epilepsy: retrospective study. J Child Neurol. 2001;16(11): 843–848. doi:10.1177/08830738010160111101

6. Santhumayor B, Karkare S, Kothare S, Rodgers S. Evaluating vagus nerve stimulation treatment with heart rate monitoring in pediatric patients with intractable epilepsy. Childs Nerv Syst. 2022;38(3):547–556. doi:10.1007/s00381-021-05416-0
7. Brown MG, Sillau S, McDermott D, et al. Concurrent brain-responsive and vagus nerve stimulation for treatment of drug-resistant focal epilepsy. Epilepsy Behav. 2022; 129:108653. doi:10.1016/j.yebeh.2022.108653
8. Bonaz B, Sinniger V, Hoffmann D, et al. Chronic vagus nerve stimulation in Crohn's disease: a 6-month follow-up pilot study. Neurogastroenterol Motil. 2016;28(6):948–953. doi:10.1111/nmo.12792
9. Wiebe S, Blume WT, Girvin JP, Eliasziw M. A randomized, controlled trial of surgery for temporal-lobe epilepsy. N Engl J Med. 2001;345(5):311–318. doi:10.1056/nejm 200108023450501

CHAPTER 32

Intracarotid Injection of Sodium Amytal for the Lateralization of Cerebral Speech Dominance

Wada J, Rasmussen T. 1960, J Neurosurg. 2007 Jun;106(6):1117–1133

Reviewed by Sydney McQueen and George Ibrahim

Research Question/Objective This paper details two series of experiments examining the use of intracarotid injections of sodium amytal for determining cerebral speech lateralization.

Intervention or Treatment Received Animal and human subjects received intracarotid administration of sodium amytal, a barbiturate derivative. This induced unilateral hemispheric anesthesia, or transient depression of neuronal activity and loss of function in that hemisphere. By doing so, researchers could simulate a localized lesion and determine hemispheric language lateralization.

Sample Size The first phase included eight primates, while the second phase included 20 patients.

Inclusion Criteria

- Inclusion Criteria
  - Patients included in the clinical studies were undergoing evaluation for the surgical management of epilepsy or other neurologic disorders.

Study Design During animal trials, varying concentrations of sodium amytal were injected into either the right carotid or vertebral artery of a primate subject. Dosing ranged from 7–350 mg (equivalent to 1 to 35 times the typical human dose). If multiple trials were conducted on the same subject in each experiment, at least 30 minutes was afforded between trials for vital signs and electroencephalogram (EEG) recordings to return to baseline. After the injection of sodium amytal, various physiologic parameters and behavioral indices were recorded, including vital signs, limb movements, brainstem reflexes, and EEG.

DOI: 10.1201/9781003416197-32

During clinical studies, a series of intracarotid injections were provided to patient participants. Immediately after the injection, patients underwent a series of neuropsychological assessments, including speech (counting and naming), motor function, sensation, and visual fields. Collected data were used primarily to determine lateralization of speech dominance, i.e. the ipsilateral side, where injection resulted in the termination of spontaneous speech and an inability to name objects or count.

Follow-Up N/A

Results In the first series of experiments, 16 injections of varying doses of sodium amytal were provided to primate subjects. In the second set of experiments, a total of 41 intracarotid injections of 100–200 mg 10% sodium amytal were injected across 20 participants.

Study findings demonstrated the safety of intracarotid injections of sodium amytal at standard doses. High concentrations injected into primates (210–350 mg, or approximately 20 to 35 times the comparable human dose) resulted in hypotension, bradycardia, respiratory depression, and global neurologic depression. These later effects were primarily attributed to large doses of sodium amytal mixing with the general circulation. Identified risks included microinfarctions (observed at high doses), as well as thrombosis from arterial cannulation.

Second, study data demonstrated the efficacy of the sodium amytal test in inducing transient anesthesia in the ipsilateral cerebral hemisphere, permitting the evaluation of language function. The test afforded accurate identification of the lateralization of speech; right-handed individuals were consistently found to have language localized in the left hemisphere, whereas left-handed and ambidextrous individuals demonstrated variability in language dominance.

Lastly, results demonstrated the clinical utility of the sodium amytal test. Preoperative identification of hemispheric dominance for language allowed surgeons to accurately predict which patients were at risk of transient or permanent speech deficits following a temporal lobectomy or surgical resection in the Sylvian region. The authors also report increased surgical efficiency when operating on left-handed or ambidextrous individuals, as radical excisions could be completed with confidence when language was known to be represented in the contralateral hemisphere.

Conclusion Overall, this work demonstrated the safety and efficacy of using intracarotid injections of sodium amytal in determining the lateralization of speech. Further, it demonstrated the test's clinical utility, particularly in the preoperative planning of interventions involving the Sylvian region in left-handed and ambidextrous individuals.

Reviewer Commentary Wada and Rasmussen's work was instrumental in establishing the sodium amytal test as the gold standard for assessing cerebral lateralization of language. Colloquially known as the Wada test, this technique provided researchers and clinicians with a crucial tool for understanding the functional organization of human language. It has since been employed in various fields, including cognitive neurosciences, neuropsychology, and neurosurgery for studying not only language, but also memory, emotional processing, and other cognitive abilities.[1,2]

The primary application of this work remains in epilepsy surgery. Anterior temporal lobe resection is considered in some cases of medically refractory epilepsy and results in greater than 60% of patients remaining seizure-free at least 5 years after treatment.[3] Nevertheless, operating in this region poses significant risks to language and memory when intervening in the dominant hemisphere. The Wada test allows for the accurate identification of language dominance. As such, it is particularly helpful in cases where it is more difficult to localize language, such as in left-handed and ambidextrous individuals, or in patients with epilepsy, given the higher incidence of atypical language distribution.[4] The Wada test supports preoperative planning and surgical treatment in several ways. Surgeons can accurately predict and counsel patients on the risks of postoperative language deficits and cognitive impairment.[5] The information obtained from the test is also useful in assessing the risk of amnesia, albeit with less accuracy than the risk of aphasia, given variability in memory localization.[1] Importantly, the Wada test allows surgeons to determine the area of maximal safe resection and proceed with more extensive resections when operating in the non-dominant hemisphere. This is useful beyond epilepsy surgery, such as in surgical oncology or with the resection of any lesion in the Sylvian region.

The Wada test has subsequently been validated by multiple research groups and cited in over 2,000 peer-reviewed articles. Branch et al. completed a series of 123 patients[6]; in addition to validating the technique, their work provided further clarity on the relationship between handedness and the cerebral dominance of language. Sixty-four percent of left-handed and ambidextrous individuals were found to be left-hemisphere dominant for speech. Further, left-handed individuals who had acquired left-sided brain injuries early in life were more likely to have speech localized on the right, supporting the potential for neuroplasticity with human language. Other researchers have since identified alternative agents that may be used instead of sodium amytal, including propofol, methohexital, midazolam, and perhaps, most notably, etomidate, as employed in the etomidate speech and memory test (eSAM).[7] Established alternatives allow clinicians to tailor the agent to patient tolerances and avoid delays should anesthetic shortages arise.[7]

The main limitations of this work relate to the nature of the test itself. First, test results may be inaccurate or misleading in rare situations of the bilateral representation of speech or other cognitive functions.[6] Further, the test carries inherent risks including infection, hemorrhage, thrombosis, or acute infarct, and anesthetic reactions.[8] Indeed, researchers have cited up to an 11% complication rate.[8] Modern techniques have helped reduce these risks; rather than direct carotid injection, the Wada test is now conducted as an interventional neuroradiology procedure via femoral artery access. Lastly, while the test reliably determines the lateralization of language, it does not provide additional information about distribution within the hemisphere.[4]

Although the Wada test continues to be employed in clinical practice, its use has greatly declined in favor of other noninvasive techniques for language localization, most notably with functional magnetic resonance imaging (fMRI) and magnetoencephalography (MEG). fMRI in particular has proven to be a safe and more cost-effective alternative, while also permitting assessment of the entire brain in one examination.[1] There is an increasing body of evidence demonstrating that fMRI is comparable to the Wada test for speech localization, and ongoing improvements in imaging modalities will certainly enhance accuracy.[1] Nevertheless, despite increasing reliance on fMRI in clinical practice, modern studies continue to demonstrate the value of the Wada test in predicting post-surgical changes in verbal language and memory, and it is likely to maintain its utility for the foreseeable future.[9]

Summary Wada and Rasmussen's work established the sodium amytal test as the standard tool for determining language lateralization. Clinically, this is an essential technique for preoperative language assessment, particularly in the surgical treatment of drug-resistant epilepsy.

REFERENCES

1. Qadri S, Dave H, Das R, Alick-Lindstrom S. Beyond the Wada: an updated approach to pre-surgical language and memory testing: an updated review of available evaluation techniques and recommended workflow to limit Wada test use to essential clinical cases. Epilepsy Res. 2021;174:106673. doi:10.1016/j.eplepsyres.2021.106673
2. Massot-Tarrus A, White KP, Mousavi SR, Hayman-Abello S, Hayman-Abello B, Mirsattari SM. Concordance between fMRI and Wada test for memory lateralization in temporal lobe epilepsy: a meta-analysis and systematic review. Epilepsy Behav. 2020;107:107065.
3. Téllez-Zenteno JF, Dhar R, Wiebe S. Long-term seizure outcomes following epilepsy surgery: a systematic review and meta-analysis. Brain. 2005;128(5):1188–1198.
4. Kakinuma K, Osawa SI, Hosokawa H, et al. Determination of language areas in patients with epilepsy using the super-selective Wada test. IBRO Neurosci Rep. 2022;13:156–163.
5. Htet NN, Pizarro R, Nair VA, et al. Comparison of language and memory lateralization by functional MRI and Wada test in epilepsy. Front Neurol Neurosci Res. 2021;2. Accessed October 25, 2024. https://www.ncbi.nlm.nih.gov/pmc/articles/PMC8238456/
6. Branch C, Milner B, Rasmussen T. Intracarotid sodium amytal for the lateralization of cerebral speech dominance. J Neurosurg. 1964;21:39–405. doi:10.3171/jns.1964.21.5.0399
7. Jones-Gotman M, Sziklas V, Djordjevic J, et al. Etomidate speech and memory test (e SAM): a new drug and improved intracarotid procedure. Neurology. 2005;65(11):1723–1729. doi:10.1212/01.wnl.0000187975.78433.cb
8. Loddenkemper T, Morris HH, Möddel G. Complications during the Wada test. Epilepsy Behav. 2008;13(3):551–553.
9. Conradi N, Rosenberg F, Knake S, et al. Wada test results contribute to the prediction of change in verbal learning and verbal memory function after temporal lobe epilepsy surgery. Sci Rep. 2021;11(1):10979.

Chapter 33

Assessment of Coma and Impaired Consciousness: A Practical Scale

Teasdale G, Jennett B, Lancet. 1974 Jul 13;2(7872):81–84

Reviewed by Paul Brennan

Research Question/Objective In the 1970s, clinical assessment of, and communication about, the severity of brain injury was known to be important for optimal patient care. However, the systems for describing patients with impaired consciousness were inconsistent and there was an abundance of alternative terms, often obscure (e.g. obnubilation). This created a barrier to effective care.

Teasdale and Jennett proposed that a scale was needed that was generally applicable, irrespective of the reason for impaired consciousness, and that a scale should be suitable for repeated bedside assessment. Their landmark 1974 paper describes the product of that ambition, the Glasgow Coma Scale (GCS).

Study Design N/A

Sample Size N/A

Follow-Up N/A

Inclusion/Exclusion Criteria N/A

Intervention or Treatment Received N/A

Results Teasdale and Jennett defined a scale for assessment of coma and impaired consciousness with three different aspects of behavioural response to stimulation: motor response, verbal response, and eye opening. Responses in each of these three components were to be evaluated independently of the others. Clearly defined responses were then to be accurately graded according to a rank order that indicated the degree of dysfunction. Criteria in each of the three behaviours were described, as summarized in Table 33.1.

Conclusion By plotting a patient's assessment with the GCS over time, on a chart, a patient's consciousness and how it is changing can be easily demonstrated. This has an

DOI: 10.1201/9781003416197-33

Table 33.1

Eye Opening	Best Motor Response	Best Verbal Response
• Spontaneous	• Obeying	• Orientated
• To speech	• Localizing	• Confused
• To pain	• Flexing	• Inappropriate
• None	• Extending	• Incomprehensible
	• None	• None

important role in informing clinical management decisions. The GCS can also be used for making an estimation of a patient's likely outcome. Assessment of the GCS can easily be made by the junior doctors and nurses who provide most routine care to these patients. These core attributes have contributed to the enduring popularity of the GCS.

Reviewer Commentary In 2024, the GCS marked its 50th anniversary, its status secure as the most widely used clinical tool for the assessment of consciousness in the world. Data on patient GCS and the utility of GCS in making estimations of early brain injury severity and late outcomes have become essential in reports for both clinical series and trials. A total of 37,633 articles originating from 3,924 different scientific journals were published between 1974 and 2022, with a compound annual growth rate of publications referencing the GCS of 16.7% (Figure 33.1).[1]

From the outset, Teasdale and Jennett recognized that an effective system for patient assessment had to be practical, so that it would be used in a wide range of hospitals and by staff without specialist training. The scale does not seek to define consciousness or coma in absolute terms, because these are not discrete states. Rather, the scale describes the various states of impaired consciousness encountered in clinical practice, and how they are changing. More complicated neurological examinations or investigations may offer additional insights into a patient's consciousness. However, in general, these cannot be as easily deployed at scale, repeatedly, in settings as diverse as mass casualty events and the intensive care unit, or by medical staff and allied health professionals with minimal training. The GCS is used across all these settings.

The simplicity and effectiveness of the original GCS have been central to its success, but there have been some key changes to it since 1974. For example, the original description of the scale had a "flexion" motor response, which is now subdivided into normal and abnormal flexion.[2] This subdivision positively impacts on the estimation of a patient's likely outcome and has been in use ever since. Another change is that today's users of the GCS will be familiar with communicating patient assessment using both the component parts, eye, verbal and motor, and the GCS sum score. The sum score was introduced in 1979.[3] To determine the sum score, individual scores are applied to each criterion, within each component, then summed into a single total score ranging from 3 to 15. Assessment of a patient's condition in the three component parts of the GCS carries the most clinical information, while the sum score can be utilized in tools for estimation of a patient's likely outcome or in research studies.

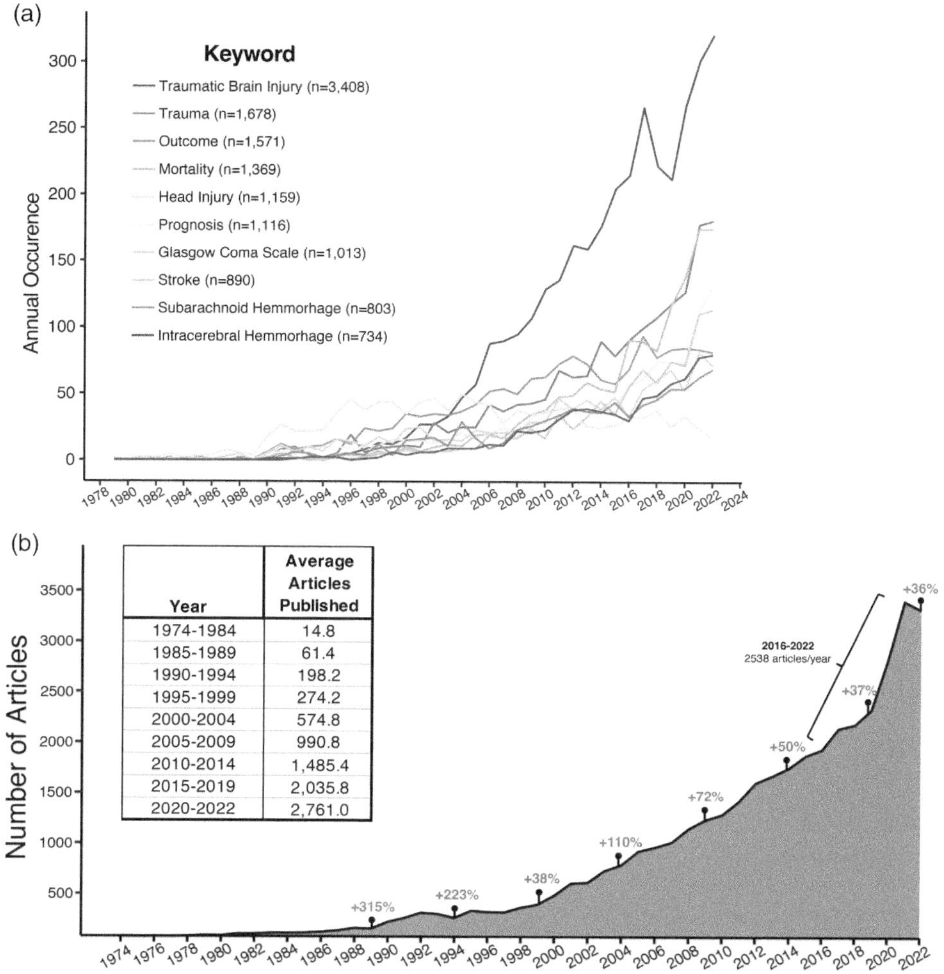

Year	Average Articles Published
1974-1984	14.8
1985-1989	61.4
1990-1994	198.2
1995-1999	274.2
2000-2004	574.8
2005-2009	990.8
2010-2014	1,485.4
2015-2019	2,035.8
2020-2022	2,761.0

Figure 33.1 Research productivity. (a) Annual incidence of author-supplied keywords in articles citing the GCS from 1974 to 2022. "Traumatic brain injury" was the most common keyword (n = 3,408). (b) Total number of published articles citing the GCS and citation rates by year from 1974 to 2022. The compounded annual growth rate was 16.67% since 1974. 2021 was the most productive year, with a total of 3,359 new publications and a 589 year-to-year marginal increase in the total number of publications employing the GCS in comparison to 2020.

Study Limitations Over the last 50 years, several new clinical scales for the assessment of consciousness have been proposed. None have supplanted GCS, but their development evidences concerns about possible limitations of the GCS.

One concern relates to consistency. Reproducibility and reliability are critical to any clinical assessment tool. Overall, the reliability of the GCS has been shown to be good to excellent. In a 2017 systematic review, Reith and colleagues[4] reviewed factors that affected the reliability of the GCS, identifying the impact of education and training, as well as the type of stimulus used. To address concerns about poor interrater reliability, in 2014, Teasdale and colleagues[5] presented GCS Aid. Its aim was to provide a standardized approach that would promote a more consistent use of the GCS, describing the findings from each response in clear terms, aimed at minimizing ambiguity. GCS Aid introduced a structured approach to assessment; check, observe, stimulate, and rate. The preliminary check is to identify factors that might interfere with assessment. Next, observe for evidence of spontaneous behaviours in each of the three components of the scale, and then, if necessary, in response to stimulation. The structured GCS Aid has been widely adopted, with translations into more than 40 languages (available free to download at glasgowcomascale.org). The GCS Aid can support education and training, so it should improve reliability, but this has yet to be confirmed.

Another potential limitation is that the GCS does not incorporate an assessment of brainstem reflexes. In their 1974 paper, Teasdale and Jennett wrote that some people may have reservations about "a system which seems to undervalue the niceties of a full neurological examination" but noted that assessment of the GCS does not prevent an additional appraisal of a patient's neurological function. Nevertheless, the Full Outline of UnResponsiveness (FOUR) Score was developed to address this putative limitation. In the FOUR score, the verbal component of the GCS is replaced with an assessment of the brainstem based on pupil and corneal reflexes and also includes an assessment of breathing. In a 2019 systematic review of the relationship of the FOUR Score to patient outcome,[6] the FOUR Score showed good to excellent prognostication of in-hospital mortality in most studies. However, there was evidence that it was the motor and eye components that had better prognostic ability, rather than the brainstem and breathing components unique to the FOUR Score. The motor and eye assessments in the FOUR Score are similar to those in the GCS.

Relevant Studies Reactivity of the pupils in response to light stimulus is a critical component of neurological assessment and is a factor other than the GCS which carries the most information about a patient's likely outcome. In 2018, Teasdale and colleagues therefore proposed the GCS-Pupils Score.[7] A Pupil Reactivity Score is derived by subtracting the number of pupils non-reactive to a light stimulus from the GCS sum score, giving a GCS-Pupils Score from 1–15. This extends the information provided about a likely patient outcome to an extent comparable to that obtained using more complex methods. Using simple prognostic charts,[8] the GCS-P can be combined with patient age and brain imaging findings to provide a rapid estimation of 6-month favorable outcome and mortality, to support clinical decision-making and communication with a patient's relatives.

For patients in whom the verbal component of the GCS cannot be assessed, for example, because they are intubated, Teasdale and colleagues[9] developed a simple, bedside verbal imputation tool. In step 1, the eye (E) and motor (M) component scores are summed. In step 2, the verbal (V) component score is identified and added to the EM sum score, giving an imputed GCS sum (EVM) score in step 3. This permits an estimation

Step 1	E + M	2	3	4	5	6	7	8	9	10
Step 2	+ V	Add 1					2	4		5
Step 3	EVM	3	4	5	6	7	9	12	13	15

Figure 33.2 Visual Aid to Imputation of a Verbal Score based on the EM Score (Sum of Eyes and Motor Component Scores).

of a patient's likely outcome to be made using tools that require a GCS sum score, when the verbal component of the GCS cannot be tested. The imputed value verbal score should not be used on clinical charts (Figure 33.2).

The success of the GCS augurs well for the next 50 years. As our understanding of the pathophysiology of brain injury evolves, there will doubtless be attempts to develop assessments that integrate additional clinical and biological data into existing models.[10] Prospective studies will be needed to determine whether any new models can outperform the stalwart of the assessment of impaired consciousness, the GCS.

REFERENCES

1. Zhang JK, Dinh TU, Teasdale G, Mercier P, Mattei TA. The message of the Glasgow Coma Scale: a comprehensive bibliometric analysis and systematic review of clinical practice guidelines spanning the past 50 years. World Neurosurg. 2024;185:93–402.e27. doi:10.1016/j.wneu.2024.02.139
2. Teasdale G, Jennett B. Assessment and prognosis of coma after head injury. Acta Neurochir. 1976;34:45–55
3. Teasdale GM, Murray G, Parker L, Jennett B. Adding up the Glasgow Coma Score. Acta Neurochir (Wien). 1979;1:13–16.
4. Reith FC, Synnot A, van den Brande R, Gruen RL, Maas AI. Factors influencing the reliability of the Glasgow Coma Scale: a systematic review. Neurosurgery. 2017;80(6):829–839. doi:10.1093/neuros/nyw178
5. Teasdale G, Allan D, Brennan P, et al. Forty years on: updating the Glasgow Coma Scale. Nurs Times. 2014;110(42):12–16.
6. Foo CC, Loan JJM, Brennan PM. The relationship of the FOUR score to patient outcome: a systematic review. J Neurotrauma. 2019;36(17):2469–2483. doi:10.1089/neu.2018.6243
7. Brennan, PM, Murray, GD, Teasdale GM. Simplifying the use of prognostic information in traumatic brain injury. Part 1: The GCS-Pupils Score: an extended index of clinical severity. J Neurosurg. 2018;128(6):1612–1620. doi:10.3171/2017.12.JNS172780
8. Murray GD, Brennan PM, Teasdale GM. Simplifying the use of prognostic information in traumatic brain injury. Part 2: Graphical presentation of probabilities. J Neurosurg. 2018;128(6):1621–1634. doi:10.3171/2017.12.JNS172782
9. Brennan PM, Murray GD, Teasdale GM. A practical method for dealing with missing Glasgow Coma Scale verbal component scores. J Neurosurg. 2020;135(1):214–219. doi:10.311/2020.6.JNS20992
10. Newcombe V, Brennan PM, Citerio G. What's new: the Glasgow Coma Scale at 50 – evolution and future directions. Intensive Care Med. 2025. doi:10.1007/s00134-024-07757-1

Chapter 34

Traumatic Acute Subdural Hematoma: Major Mortality Reduction in Comatose Patients Treated within Four Hours

Seelig JM, Becker DP, Miller JD, Greenberg RP, Ward JD, Choi SC, NEJM. 1981;25:1511–151

Reviewed by Laurie L Ackerman

Research Question/Objective To identify factors contributing to recovery after surgical decompression of patients with acute subdural hematoma (ASDH).

Study Design Retrospective case series.

Sample Size 82 patients.

Follow-Up 1 year.

Inclusion Criteria

- 82 consecutive comatose patients >2 years of age with traumatic ASDH culled from 366 consecutive patients with severe traumatic brain injury (TBI) from December 1972 to February 1980.
- Patients were breathing spontaneously, unable to speak, unresponsive to verbal commands, and had midline shift >5 mm and were operatively treated.

Intervention or Treatment Received Patients were intubated after a neurologic exam was obtained (unless in respiratory distress) and hyperventilated to a $PaCo_2$ of 25–30 mmHg. Medications included 4 mg vecuronium, 20 mg intravenous (IV) dexamethasone, 500 mg of IV phenytoin, and 60 mg of intramuscular (IM) phenobarbital. Air ventriculography was used from 1972 to mid-1975, and computed tomography thereafter. 100 g of mannitol was administered before the operating room (OR). Initial subtemporal decompression followed by a frontotemporoparietal craniotomy was performed with either a ventriculostomy

DOI: 10.1201/9781003416197-34

or a subarachnoid screw inserted opposite the craniotomy site for intracranial pressure (ICP) monitoring for at least 3 days. Elevation of ICP >20 mmHg was treated with hyperventilation, cerebrospinal fluid (CSF) drainage or mannitol alone or in combination. The last 40 patients had multimodality-evoked potentials recorded. Surviving patients went to rehabilitation. Functional recovery was defined as "good recovery or moderate disability on the Glasgow Outcome Scale."

Results

Time to Surgery The mean time to surgery in those who died was 390 +/– 38.5 vs 170 +/– 18.3 minutes in survivors ($p < 0.001$). Patients undergoing surgery within 4 hours of injury had a 30% mortality rate and a 60–70% functional recovery (as compared to those operated after 4 hours) ($p < 0.0001$). 75% of patients with ASDH were male and had a 65% mortality rate compared to females who were operated on 2 hours earlier than men ($p < 0.02$) with a 35% mortality rate ($p < 0.05$).

ICP 79% of patients with ICP <20 had a functional recovery ($p < 0.001$), and no patients with uncontrolled ICU (>60 mmHg) survived ($p < 0.0001$).

Initial Neurological Examination Characteristics of the group that died included 57% with bilaterally absent pupillary light reflexes ($p < 0.02$), 70% with absent or impaired oculomotor function ($p < 0.05$), and 56% with a decerebrate or flaccid motor exam ($p < 0.05$).

Multimodality-Evoked Potentials These were obtained in 40/82 patients. 25 patients had normal or mildly focal changes in potentials with 19 patients with functional recovery, 2 with severely/vegetative state, and 4 patients died of secondary issues ($p < 0.001$). 15 patients with severe abnormalities all died.

Study Limitations This was a retrospective study, and the ASDH group was pulled from the larger 366-patient group for analysis. Six patients did not have their surgery recorded.

Conclusion The key finding in this study was that comatose patients with ASDH who underwent rapid surgical decompression within 4 hours of injury demonstrated improved outcomes compared to those who were operated on after 4 hours. Postoperative elevation of ICP was also associated with a poor outcome. Preoperative neurological examination, including fixed dilated pupils, decerebrate rigidity, and impaired oculomotor function, had statistically significant increases in mortality compared to those who did not. Normal postoperative evoked potentials in the absence of other insults portended a functional recovery, whereas those with severely abnormal responses died.

Reviewer Commentary It is important to understand the historical context of this paper to fully appreciate its impact. At the time of this paper's publication, mortality rates in comatose patients with traumatic ASDH ranged from 60–90%.[1] While the overall mortality rate of 57% among the 82 patients in this series was significantly different from that of patients in the previously published series, the 30% mortality rate in patients operated on within 4 hours was the best reported rate of recovery in any published series at the time and advanced the idea that operating in a timely fashion was important.

The authors mentioned that this information was "critically important for rescue squads, emergency-room physicians and tertiary physicians who are directly involved in the transport, diagnosis, and treatment of these patients."[1] This was a prescient comment. This study spanned 1972–1980. Legislation requiring state development of EMS systems was passed in 1966, and in 1973, the Emergency Medical Services (EMS) Systems Act provided grants to support regional EMS systems, emergency medical technician training, and the development of air transport services. The American College of Surgeons released a report outlining criteria for the development of trauma centers in 1976. The need to quickly transport patients to qualified centers and physicians was driven by the recognition of improved outcomes seen with timely access to high-level medical care.[2]

The modern surgeon would look at the average time to operation in this study of 325 minutes (5½ hours) and wonder why it took so long to get there. Definitive identification and diagnosis of a subdural hematoma took longer. Early in this study, patients underwent air ventriculography to diagnose mass lesions, as it was "quicker than angiography." A head computed tomography (CT) scan was developed in England, with the first scan performed in October 1971; post-processing the images took 2 days! The first head CT in the United States took place at the Mayo Clinic in June 1973; however, early scanners only produced 2 image slices per 5-minute gantry rotation, taking an hour to get a complete study.[3] Patients in this study underwent CT scanning after mid-1975. The authors did not clarify if this improved the time to the OR in the latter group, although one could expect it might.

Ultimately, the study was published against the backdrop of a perfect storm of better diagnostic imaging and better access to trauma hospitals, which may have decreased the time to diagnosis and care. Unexplained in the study is why women, on average, got to the OR 2 hours sooner than their male counterparts, although as males represented 75% of study subjects with ASDH, the study may not have been powered to detect a difference.

The first Brain Trauma Foundation (BTF) guidelines for the medical management of severe TBI were not published until 1996, and the fourth edition was published in 2016.[4,5] The Seelig paper had a protocol for patient care (preoperative hyperventilation, steroids, IV Dilantin, IM phenobarbitol, and mannitol with postoperative monitoring of ICP with treatment thresholds at 20 mmHg). Modern neurosurgeons know from the BTF guidelines that steroids and prolonged hyperventilation to a $PaCO_2$ of 25 are not recommended and may be deleterious; information that was not available at the time of this paper's publication. Dosing of the antiepileptic drugs has changed. The protocol to monitor ICP, treat at >20 mmHg, and use of mannitol and CSF drainage echoes current guidelines, although cerebral perfusion pressure was not utilized in the study. The BTF guidelines have improved the care of patients with TBI and ASDH throughout the world.

In 2006, guidelines were published on the surgical management of acute subdural hematomas.[6] An ASDH was defined as one diagnosed within 14 days of injury, with quoted mortality rates between 40 and 60%. Three class III recommendations for surgery were derived from the available literature, which included evidence from case series and uncontrolled cohorts. First, ASDH "with a thickness greater than 10 mm or midline shift >5 mm on CT should be surgically evacuated, regardless of the patient's Glasgow Coma Scale (GCS) score." Second, all patients with ASDH and a "GCS less than 9 should undergo intracranial pressure monitoring." Third, a comatose patient with a ASDH "<10 mm thick and midline shift <5 mm should undergo surgical evacuation if the GCS score decreased between the time of injury and hospital admission by 2 or more points on the GCS and/or the patient presents with asymmetric or fixed and dilated pupils and/or the ICP is >20 mmHg." Recommendation for the timing of surgery was "as soon as possible," stating that time from injury to operative intervention was one of the few factors that could be affected by intervention. The method of surgical evacuation recommended was a craniotomy with or without removing the bone flap and duroplasty.[6]

Recommended areas for further study included craniotomy vs decompressive craniectomy, and prehospital hypotension and hypoxia on outcomes. A meta-analysis from 2017 found patients undergoing craniectomy had increased odds of poor outcome compared to craniotomy (60.1% vs 50.1%) and death ($p = 0.0004$), but lower-presenting GCS scores in the craniectomy group may have reflected greater injury at the onset.[7] Analysis of National Trauma Data Bank data 2007–2010 did not identify differences in in-hospital mortality between decompressive craniectomy vs craniotomy.[8] Hutchinson et al.[9] found no significant difference in outcomes at 6 and 12 months in patients undergoing decompressive craniectomy vs craniotomy. Patients were randomized in the operating room and patients whose brains were too swollen to allow bone flap replacement were excluded.

Surgery vs conservative therapy is also debated. A 2023 meta-analysis/review noted that mortality after surgery for comatose patients was 41% in the modern series (after 2000) and 12% in non-comatose patients.[10] Conservative treatment for the same period in comatose patients was 64% vs 2% in non-comatose patients. Weaknesses included death as the endpoint (no survivor outcome data) and possible publication bias of good outcomes constituting the available literature. Moribund patients who would not have survived regardless may have been included in the conservative group.

Summary Ultimately, this paper showed that time to surgery was a critical factor in both reducing mortality and improving good-quality survival in ASDH, a diagnosis with a dismal morbidity and mortality at that time. It highlighted the importance of ICP monitoring for both treatment and prognostication. Their use of a treatment protocol in these patients foreshadowed the BTF guidelines that followed and has improved care in survival in this vulnerable population.

REFERENCES

1. Seelig JM, Becker DP, Miller JD, Greenberg RP, Ward JD, Choi SC. Traumatic acute subdural hematoma: major mortality reduction in comatose patients treated within four hours. N Engl J Med. 1981;304(25):1511–1518.
2. American College of Surgeons. https://www.facs.org/quality-programs/trauma/systems/trauma-series/part-i/
3. McCollough CH, Rajiah PS. Milestones in CT: past, present, and future. Radiology. 2023;309(1):e230803.
4. Volovici V, Steyerberg EW, Cnossen MC, et al. Evolution of evidence and guideline recommendations for the medical management of severe traumatic brain injury. J Neurotrauma. 2019;36(22):3183–3189.
5. Carney N, Totten AM, O'Reilly C, et al. Guidelines for the Management of Severe Traumatic Brain Injury, Fourth Edition. Neurosurgery. 2017;80(1):6–15.
6. Bullock MR, Chesnut R, Ghajar J, et al. Surgical management of acute subdural hematomas. Neurosurgery. 2006;58(3 Suppl):S16–S24; discussion Si-iv.
7. Phan K, Moore JM, Griessenauer C, et al. Craniotomy versus decompressive craniectomy for acute subdural hematoma: systematic review and meta-analysis. World Neurosurg. 2017;101:677–685.e672.
8. Ahmed N, Greenberg P, Shin S. Mortality outcome of emergency decompressive craniectomy and craniotomy in the management of acute subdural hematoma: a national data analysis. Am Surg. 2021;87(3):347–353.
9. Hutchinson PJ, Adams H, Mohan M, et al. Decompressive craniectomy versus craniotomy for acute subdural hematoma. N Engl J Med. 2023;388(24):2219–2229.
10. van Essen TA, Res L, Schoones J, et al. Mortality reduction of acute surgery in traumatic acute subdural hematoma since the 19th century: systematic review and meta-analysis with dramatic effect: Is surgery the obvious parachute? J Neurotrauma. 2023;40(1–2):22–32.

CHAPTER 35

Use of Drains versus No Drains after Burr-Hole Evacuation of Chronic Subdural Haematoma: A Randomised Controlled Trial

Santarius T, Kirkpatrick PJ, Ganesan D, et al., Lancet. 2009;374(9695):1067–1073

Reviewed by Ben M Davies and Thomas Santarius

Objective/Research Question The objective of this study was to determine whether the use of a postoperative subdural drain following burr-hole evacuation of a chronic subdural haematoma (CSDH) reduces the recurrence rate of the haematoma.

Study Design This was a single-centre, block-randomised controlled trial (RCT) conducted at Addenbrooke's Hospital in Cambridge, UK. The study recruited participants from November 2004 until November 2007, when it was stopped early based on significant findings. Block randomisation with variable block sizes (ranging from 8 to 12) was used to allocate participants in a 1:1 ratio to either receive a subdural drain or not, post-surgery.

Sample Size The trial aimed to enrol 219 participants in each group to detect a reduction in the recurrence rate from 20 to 10% with 80% power and a significance level of 0.05. The trial was terminated early with a total of 108 patients in the drain group and 107 in the no-drain group due to a significant difference in recurrence rates.

Inclusion/Exclusion Criteria

- Inclusion Criteria
  - Patients aged 18 years or older.
  - Patients presenting with a symptomatic chronic subdural haematoma (CSDH) confirmed by computerised tomography (CT) scan and indicated for burr-hole drainage.

- Exclusion Criteria
  - Patients with ipsilateral haematomas treated within the last 6 months.
  - Patients with cerebrospinal fluid diversion shunts in situ.

DOI: 10.1201/9781003416197-35

- Patients requiring surgical procedures other than burr-hole evacuation.
- Patients deemed unsafe for drain insertion by the operating surgeon (determined preoperatively or at surgery after drainage of the haematoma).

Intervention or Treatment Received

Participants underwent burr-hole evacuation of CSDH. The procedure involved:

- Drilling two 14 mm burr holes approximately 7 cm apart over the haematoma.
- Opening the dura mater and washing out the haematoma with warm Ringer's lactate saline.
- For the drain group, the subdural space was filled with Ringer's lactate saline; a soft silicon drain was inserted into the subdural space and connected to a collection bag for 48 hours. The drain was tunnelled at least 5 cm from the scalp incision.
- For the no-drain group, the subdural space was filled with Ringer's lactate saline, and the scalp was closed without a drain.

Results

- *Primary outcome (recurrence rate)*: The recurrence rate was significantly lower in the drain group (9.3%) compared to the no-drain group (24%), with a p-value of 0.0031. Time-to-recurrence was longer in the drain group (median 15.5 days) than in the no-drain group (median 8 days) ($p = 0.0247$).
- *Mortality*: There was no significant difference in mortality at 30 days between the groups, but more patients with drains were alive at 6 months compared to those without drains.
- *Neurological outcomes*: More patients in the drain group had a Glasgow Coma Score of 15 at discharge compared to the no-drain group. At discharge, gross neurological deficits were significantly less frequent in the drain group, though this difference was not observed at 6 months.
- *Functional outcomes*: Favourable modified Rankin Scale (mRS) scores (0–3) at discharge and 6 months were more common in the drain group. However, after adjusting for confounding factors, the drain was not predictive of mRS at 6 months.
- *Hospital stay*: The duration of the neurosurgical hospital stay was significantly longer in cases with recurrence.
- *Complications*: Postoperative complications included subdural empyema, intracerebral haematoma, acute subdural haematoma, pneumonia, renal failure, urinary tract infection, myocardial infarction, new-onset atrial fibrillation, and gastritis, with no significant differences between groups.

Summary This comprehensive analysis suggests that the use of postoperative subdural drains in burr-hole evacuation of chronic subdural haematomas significantly reduces recurrence rates and improves short-term neurological outcomes without increasing adverse events.

Reviewer Commentary

Paper Significance and Impact The significance of this trial lies not only in its practice changing findings, but also in the enduring legacy it catalysed, stimulating subsequent randomised controlled trials and elevating research focus on chronic subdural haematomas.

Analysis of long-term follow-up data has reinforced the trial's findings, demonstrating normalised survival among patients who received an adjuvant drain.[1] This has since been externally validated by real-world evidence in multiple global settings, confirming both its effectiveness and efficacy, alongside confirming its successful knowledge translation.[2,3]

Numerous further randomised trials around surgical management have followed, including the number of burr holes, position of the drain, type of drainage, and the intraoperative irrigation fluid temperature and volume.[4] Broadly, these trials have indicated potential opportunities to rationalise the surgical technique, but none so far have replicated a superiority finding or practice change, reinforcing the landmark status of this trial. Research interest in CSDH has also expanded beyond open surgery, through adjuvant medical treatment and alternative therapies such as middle meningeal artery embolisation.[5]

Finally, the trial offers an important lesson in research opportunity and pragmatism. Randomised controlled trials have an increasing reputation for being costly and cumbersome. Pressures to rapidly achieve sample size, while ensuring generalisation and supporting implementation, favour multicentre trials. This demands huge human resources to deliver, and consequently, research investment. Despite this, only rarely do surgical trials deliver a "positive result," and only seldom are these results confirmed in subsequent clinical studies. The Cambridge drains trial was unfunded and conducted in a single centre, yet it has had a global practice-changing impact. This trial, therefore, represents an important lesson for researchers that "bigger is not always better," particularly as most surgical trials recruit predominantly from the host centre (i.e. a single centre).

Study Limitations Limitations include the trials being conducted at a single centre, alongside the use of a surrogate primary endpoint. The former always raises questions in trials around wider generalisation, the latter, meaningfulness. As outlined above, the confirmation of benefit in other key outcomes, such as survival and neurological recovery, alongside subsequent external validation, indicates these are not significant concerns in this instance.

One more notable limitation, however, was the definition of the intervention. The choice of 48-hour drainage was poorly defined or evidenced. This has committed the field to 48 hours of drainage. Follow-on RCTs (drain time 1 and drain time 2) indicate that 24 hours is likely sufficient, with benefits of earlier discharge and reduced neurosurgical centre resource usage; however, implementation is at an early stage.[6,7]

Further, there has been a suggestion that sub-galeal positioned drains (as opposed to subdural drains) offer equivalence in terms of the recurrence rate, with fewer adverse events related to insertion.[4,8]

Relevant Studies A large network meta-analysis encompassing 455 studies and 103,645 patients provided a comprehensive comparative assessment of surgical and adjunctive treatments for chronic subdural haematomas.[4] This analysis demonstrated that commonly used surgical techniques, including single vs multiple burr holes and burr-hole drainage vs craniotomy, are largely equivalent with respect to clinical outcomes. In contrast, the use of an adjuvant drain was associated with a meaningful reduction in recurrence, with no significant difference between subdural and subgaleal drain placement. The study also found that corticosteroid therapy can reduce recurrence rates; however, this benefit is offset by an increased risk of morbidity, underscoring the need to balance recurrence prevention against treatment-related complications.

Conclusion This trial provided the first level 1 evidence of superiority in placing a drain as part of the surgical treatment of chronic subdural haematomas. Its significance can be seen in the durable findings and widespread adoption, but also a legacy of further randomised controlled trials in CSDH.

REFERENCES

1. Guilfoyle MR, Hutchinson PJA, Santarius T. Improved long-term survival with subdural drains following evacuation of chronic subdural haematoma. Acta Neurochirurgica. 2017;159(5):903–905.
2. Aljabali A, Sharkawy AM, Jaradat B, Serag I, Al-Dardery NM, Abdelhady M, Abouzid M. Drainage versus no drainage after burr-hole evacuation of chronic subdural hematoma: a systematic review and meta-analysis of 1961 patients. Neurosurg Rev. 2023;46(1):251.
3. Brennan PM, Kolias AG, Joannides AJ, Shapey J, Marcus HJ, Gregson BA, Grover PJ, Hutchinson PJ, Coulter IC; British Neurosurgical Trainee Research Collaborative. The management and outcome for patients with chronic subdural hematoma: a prospective, multicenter, observational cohort study in the United Kingdom. J Neurosurg. 2017;1–8.
4. Henry J, Amoo M, Kissner M, Deane T, Zilani G, Crockett MT, Javadpour M. Management of chronic subdural hematoma: a systematic review and component network meta-analysis of 455 studies with 103 645 cases. Neurosurgery. 2022. doi:10.1227/neu.0000000000002144
5. Gillespie CS, Fung KW, Alam AM, et al. How does research activity align with research need in chronic subdural haematoma: a gap analysis of systematic reviews with end-user selected knowledge gaps. Acta Neurochir. 2023;165(7):1975–1986.
6. Grønhøj MH, Jensen TSR, Miscov R, et al. Optimal drainage time after evacuation of chronic subdural haematoma (DRAIN TIME 2): a multicentre, randomised, multiarm and multistage non-inferiority trial in Denmark. Lancet Neurol. 2024;23(8):787–796.
7. Jensen TSR, Haldrup M, Grønhøj MH, et al. National randomized clinical trial on subdural drainage time after chronic subdural hematoma evacuation. J Neurosurg. 2022;137(3):799–806.
8. Chen C, Xiong Y, Huang X, et al. Subperiosteal/subgaleal drainage vs. subdural drainage for chronic subdural hematoma: a meta-analysis of postoperative outcomes. PLoS One. 2023;18(8):e0288872.

Chapter 36

Significance of Intracranial Hypertension in Severe Head Injury

Miller JD, Becker DP, Ward JD, Sullivan HG, Adams WE, Rosner MJ, J Neurosurg. 1977 Oct;47(4):503–517

Reviewed by Allie Heineman, Kyle Mcgrath, and Laura B Ngwenya

Research Question/Objective This study determined the frequency, extent, and significance of intracranial hypertension measured with an intracranial pressure (ICP) monitor in patients with traumatic brain injury (TBI).

Study Design Prospective cohort study.

Sample Size $n = 160$ patients

Inclusion/Exclusion Criteria

- Inclusion Criteria
  - A blunt head injury resulting in a decreased level of consciousness with the inability to obey commands.
- Exclusion Criteria
  - Those who met the criteria of brain death.

Intervention or Treatment Received All patients had airways secured and deemed hemodynamically stable before a 9/64" frontal twist-drill hole was made in the emergency room. The frontal horn of the lateral ventricle was punctured with an 18-g cannula or polyethylene catheter connected to a glass manometer. Initial ICP was recorded and a ventriculogram was obtained by injecting 7–10 cc of air into the ventricles followed by obtaining a brow-up skull X-ray. All patients with a ≥5 mm midline shift were immediately treated by craniotomy for decompression. Patients with no shift but ICP >15 mmHg were referred for further study to exclude bilateral lesions. Patients with no shift and ICP <15 mmHg were directly admitted to the ICU.

With an average midline shift of 9 mm, 62 patients had mass lesions requiring surgical decompression while 24 patients had cerebral contusions and/or hematoma affecting the frontal and/or temporal lobes. Surgical decompression consisted of a large craniotomy for decompression and the removal of focal mass lesions. Bone flaps

DOI: 10.1201/9781003416197-36

were replaced except for a few extreme cases where a craniectomy was necessary to permit closure. The remaining 98 patients had little to no midline shift and were labeled as having "diffuse brain injury."

ICP was monitored in all patients by either a polyethylene cannula in the ventricle or by a subarachnoid screw. Measurement of ICP was by an external arterial range pressure transducer mounted on a disposable plastic manifold system, which was connected to a manometer, fluid reservoir, a tuberculin syringe for flushing and volume-pressure response tests, and a drainage bag, which could be raised or lowered to adjust the hydrostatic pressure.

Each morning after the initial 48 hours, the necessity of continued ICP monitoring was reassessed. Indications for treating elevated ICP were sustained >40 mmHg (threshold later adjusted to 30 mmHg), or any increase in ICP associated with neurological deterioration. After ruling out mechanical or metabolic causes of increased ICP, further treatment included hyperventilation, CSF diversion, or IV mannitol. The outcomes were classified as good recovery, moderately disabled, severely disabled, vegetative, or dead.

Results This study demonstrated that elevated ICP may indicate the presence of intracranial mass lesions or diffuse brain swelling. Elevated ICP on admission (>40 mmHg) was associated with poor outcomes (69% mortality) in patients with both mass lesions and diffuse brain injury. Conversely, normal ICP upon admission (≤10 mmHg) was associated with a relatively low mortality (14%). The relationship between ICP and outcome became clearer when patients were stratified by the presence or absence of a focal mass lesion. Patients with mass lesions exhibited greater neurological dysfunction and higher mortality (40%) compared to those with diffuse brain injury (no mass lesion) (23%). Even with elevated initial ICP (>40 mmHg), 28% of these patients had good recovery or were only moderately disabled. This suggested that other factors, such as primary brain dysfunction, brain herniation, and timing of surgical intervention, may play a significant role in determining outcomes. Furthermore, patients with diffuse brain injury appeared to have a strong correlation between ICP on presentation and overall outcome. Normal ICP (≤10 mmHg) was associated with an 85% rate of good recovery, with morbidity and mortality increased with increasing ICP. With ICP slightly elevated (11–20 mmHg), mortality rose to 25%, and severe morbidity increased to 11%, corresponding to a decrease in patients with good recovery or moderate disability (64%). In the setting of an abnormal motor response, ICP >10 mmHg was associated with 83% of patients having bad outcomes. Conversely, in patients with purposeful motor responses, ICP levels were not significantly related to outcome.

With aggressive treatment, 64 patients experienced increased ICP that could be adequately controlled, whereas 23 patients experienced refractory ICP. Persistent or recurrent intracranial hypertension was a greater problem in patients with mass lesions and brain shift on admission, affecting 52% of these patients compared to only 32% of those with diffuse injury. In cases of diffuse injury, intracranial hypertension was seen in one-third of cases, of which 25% were fatal.

Patient outcomes based on three ICP patterns were compared: uncontrollable, controllable, and normal ICP. All patients with uncontrollable ICP died. Controlled ICP led to poorer outcomes as compared to normal ICP. For patients with mass lesions, 53% with controllable ICP had poor outcomes (severe disability, vegetative state, or death), vs 23% with normal ICP. For those with diffuse injury, 46% with controllable ICP had poor outcomes, compared to 21% with normal ICP. Patients with normal ICP had only 5% with poor outcomes.

Of 160 patients, 48 (30%) died. In 22 cases, death was due to uncontrollable ICP. In the remaining 26 patients who died, death was attributed to systemic complications such as pulmonary embolism, sepsis, or renal failure. Of the 25 patients with mass lesions, 14 of those (56%) died from uncontrollable intracranial hypertension. In comparison, 8 out of 23 patients (35%) who died following diffuse brain injury experienced the same cause of death. This difference was not statistically significant. The likelihood of dying from uncontrollable ICP increased with higher ICP levels upon admission. Only 25% of patients with normal admission ICP died from high ICP, compared to 37% with ICP of 11–20 mmHg and 57% with ICP of 21–40 mmHg. Of the 48 patients who died, 79% were flexure posturing or flaccid upon admission compared to 46% of the overall cohort; 73% had impaired or absent oculocephalic responses compared to the 40% of the overall cohort; and 50% had absent bilateral pupillary light responses compared to the 17% overall. These were all statistically significant.

Reviewer Commentary

Paper Impact and Significance This landmark study by Miller and colleagues fundamentally transformed the understanding and management of severe TBI by establishing intracranial pressure (ICP) as a central pathophysiological determinant of outcome rather than a secondary or epiphenomenal observation. At a time when the management of head injury was largely reactive and based on clinical examination alone, this work provided the first rigorous, systematic evidence that sustained intracranial hypertension is common after severe head injury, is strongly associated with mortality and poor neurological outcome, and represents a modifiable target for intervention.

Crucially, the authors demonstrated a clear relationship between elevated ICP, reduced cerebral perfusion pressure, and adverse outcome, thereby reframing secondary brain injury as a dynamic and preventable process. This study moved the field beyond descriptive neuropathology and toward physiologically guided, data-driven neurocritical care. By showing that patients with persistently elevated ICP had markedly worse outcomes – and that episodes of intracranial hypertension often preceded neurological deterioration – the paper established ICP monitoring as an essential clinical tool rather than an experimental adjunct.

The impact of this work extended far beyond its immediate findings. It laid the conceptual and practical foundation for modern neurocritical care by legitimizing continuous ICP monitoring, informing the development of tiered therapeutic strategies (including hyperosmolar therapy, ventilation strategies, and surgical decompression), and catalyzing subsequent trials focused on cerebral perfusion–based management. Nearly every contemporary guideline for severe TBI management traces its intellectual lineage to the principles articulated in this study.

In retrospect, this paper represents a pivotal inflection point in the evolution of TBI care: it defined intracranial hypertension as a pathological process requiring active surveillance and treatment, introduced physiological thresholds that would shape decades of clinical decision-making, and helped establish the modern paradigm of preventing secondary brain injury. Its influence persists in daily neurocritical care practice, making it one of the most consequential contributions to the field of TBI.

Study Limitations This study reflects the methodological norms and technological constraints of neurotrauma research in the 1970s. Detailed demographic variables such as age, sex, and ethnicity were not routinely reported at the time and therefore, were not addressed, despite their recognized relevance in contemporary TBI research. The observational design limits causal inference between intracranial pressure and outcome; however, randomized or protocolized interventional trials were not yet feasible in this clinical context.

Importantly, the study's contribution was not prescriptive but conceptual. Rather than defining specific treatment algorithms, it established intracranial hypertension as a measurable, prognostically significant pathological process requiring active monitoring. While modern advances such as multimodality neuromonitoring now refine this approach, the physiological framework introduced by this work provided the foundation for subsequent interventional studies and the evolution of modern neurocritical care.

Relevant Studies ICP monitoring is now widely considered of utmost importance in TBI management. While this historical paper states abnormal ICP as >10 and ICP >30 as requiring intervention, current guidelines recommend a treatment threshold of ICP >22, and attention to personalized approaches to management.[1–3] A critical advance since the publication of this landmark paper has been the advent of multimodality neuromonitoring as an adjunct to ICP monitoring. Brain physiological parameters such as cerebral blood flow, electrocorticography (ECoG) and brain tissue oxygen ($PbtO_2$) can be monitored in real time with available technologies today. Specifically, using $PbtO_2$ in addition to ICP to guide the management of TBI has been suggested to improve outcomes and reduce mortality in TBI patients, with definitive evidence pending results of an ongoing randomized controlled trial.[4–6] The use of ECoG to measure seizures and cortical spreading depolarizations (CSDs) is also of growing clinical interest in monitoring and predicting secondary injury in TBI patients. CSDs are waves of self-propagating mass depolarization that have been shown to predict worse outcomes in TBI patients[7] and, hence, management of TBI patients using this additional electrophysiologic information is also a source of ongoing clinical investigation.[8] Given the availability of more advanced physiologic monitoring in the brain today, ICP monitoring may only be a small component of a much larger, more holistic approach to treating TBI.[9]

Although the optimal management of severe head injuries remains under some debate, the use of surgical decompression has become routine. In this historical paper, only a fraction of patients received decompressive craniectomies. Modern guidance recommends primary decompressive craniectomy (as opposed to lobectomy) in patients with significant herniation and cerebral edema associated with mass lesions. Surgical decompressive craniectomies are also a tier 3 option in episodes of refractory elevated ICP, even in patients with diffuse injury.[10]

Summary This landmark study established intracranial pressure monitoring as a foundational element of severe TBI management. By demonstrating the pathological and prognostic significance of intracranial hypertension, it laid the groundwork for continuous ICP-guided critical care strategies that remain central to modern TBI treatment and outcome optimization.

REFERENCES

1. Brain Trauma Foundation. Guidelines for Management of Severe Traumatic Brain Injury, Fourth Edition. 2016. http://www.braintrauma.org.
2. American College of Surgeons. Best practice guidelines: the management of traumatic brain injury. 2024 [cited 2024 December 14, 2024]. Available from: https://www.facs.org/media/vgfgjpfk/best-practices-guidelines-traumatic-brain-injury.pdf.
3. Stein KY, et al. Intracranial pressure monitoring and treatment thresholds in acute neural injury: a narrative review of the historical achievements, current state, and future perspectives. Neurotrauma Rep. 2023;4(1):478–494.
4. Okonkwo DO, et al. Brain oxygen optimization in severe traumatic brain injury phase-II: a phase II randomized trial. Crit Care Med. 2017;45(11):1907–1914.
5. Bernard F, et al. Brain oxygen optimization in severe traumatic brain injury (BOOST-3): a multicentre, randomised, blinded-endpoint, comparative effectiveness study of brain tissue oxygen and intracranial pressure monitoring versus intracranial pressure alone. BMJ Open. 2022;12(3):e060188.
6. Chesnut R, et al. A management algorithm for adult patients with both brain oxygen and intracranial pressure monitoring: the Seattle International Severe Traumatic Brain Injury Consensus Conference (SIBICC). Intensive Care Med. 2020;46(5):919–929.
7. Hartings JA, et al. Prognostic value of spreading depolarizations in patients with severe traumatic brain injury. JAMA Neurol. 2020;77(4):489–499.
8. Hartings JA, et al. Improving neurotrauma by depolarization inhibition with combination therapy: a phase 2 randomized feasibility trial. Neurosurgery. 2023;93(4):924–931.
9. Le Roux P, et al. The International Multidisciplinary Consensus Conference on Multimodality Monitoring in Neurocritical Care: a list of recommendations and additional conclusions: a statement for healthcare professionals from the Neurocritical Care Society and the European Society of Intensive Care Medicine. Neurocrit Care. 2014;21(Suppl 2):S282–S296.
10. Hutchinson PJ, et al. Consensus statement from the International Consensus Meeting on the role of decompressive craniectomy in the management of traumatic brain injury: consensus statement. Acta Neurochir (Wien). 2019;161(7):1261–1274.

Chapter 37

A Randomized, Double-Blind Study of Phenytoin for the Prevention of Post-Traumatic Seizures

Temkin NR, Dikmen SS, Wilensky AJ, Keihm J, Chabal S, Winn HR, N Engl J Med. 1990 Aug 23;323(8):497–502

Reviewed by Derryl Miller

Research Question/Objective Does phenytoin prevent early and late post-traumatic seizures compared to placebo?

Study Design This was a single-center, randomized double-blind controlled trial conducted from 1983 to 1987 for patients with serious head trauma. Patients were randomized to phenytoin or placebo for 1 year with the goal of maintaining high therapeutic levels throughout the treatment course before weaning. Maintaining high therapeutic phenytoin levels was significant because previous studies randomized patients to phenytoin or a combination of phenytoin and phenobarbital but did not maintain high drug levels and showed no statistical significance.[1–3] Patients continued the assigned drug for 12 months in the absence of seizures or intolerable side effects before weaning. Phenytoin was given in an unblinded fashion if seizures occurred after day 8. Consent was acquired from the patient, a relative, or by the investigators with deferred consent. Patients could withdraw participation at any time.

Outcome Measures The primary endpoints were (1) the occurrence of early seizures ≤7 days after injury or (2) late seizures ≥8 days after injury. Seizures were determined based on ictal semiology, including involuntary movements, abnormal sensations, altered mental status, or other positive symptoms consistent with aura. Families and patients received education about auras and could call a study nurse to describe their symptoms. The scalp electroencephalogram was only utilized for some patients. Events were called seizures by a blinded neurologist only if there was no doubt by semiology. Patients having early seizures were still included in the analysis of late seizures. Secondary endpoints were side effects of phenytoin and neuropsychological testing (unpublished data). Patients were studied with an intention-to-treat analysis.

Sample Size 404 patients were randomized, with 208 receiving phenytoin and 196 receiving a placebo.

DOI: 10.1201/9781003416197-37

Table 37.1 Inclusion and Exclusion Criteria of the RCT

Category	Criteria
Inclusion Criteria	• Cortical contusion on a head CT • Intracranial hemorrhage (subdural, epidural, or intracerebral hemorrhage) • Depressed skull fracture • Penetrating head injury • Seizure <24 hours from injury • Admission Glasgow Coma Scale <10 • Criteria intended to capture seizure risk >20% (variable).
Exclusion Criteria	• Age <16 years old • >24 hours between injury and study drug load • Pregnancy or breastfeeding • Lacking English proficiency • History of alcohol abuse • Previous head injury • Seizures prior to head injury or drug load • Previous neurosurgery through dura • Previous diagnosis of epilepsy.

Follow-Up 24 months.

Inclusion/Exclusion Criteria This is outlined in Table 37.1.

Intervention or Treatment Received Subjects were randomized to phenytoin or placebo with a loading dose of 20 mg/kg intravenously ≤24 hours from injury, with oral maintenance for 1 year. Serum phenytoin levels were measured three times a day in the intensive care unit, weekly in acute care units, and during clinic visits at 1, 3, 5, 9, and 12 months. Goal total phenytoin serum was 40–80 µmol/L and free phenytoin serum was 3–6 µmol/L. Phenytoin doses were adjusted by an unblinded staff member to maintain high therapeutic levels. The placebo was also dose-adjusted for blinding. Drug levels were measured 7–10 days after each dose adjustment.

Results While 586 patients were enrolled, only 404 were studied due to late loads of study drug, a complete history demonstrating an exclusion criterion, or withdrawal of consent. Eighty-five patients assigned to phenytoin and 97 patients assigned to placebo were ineligible. Eligibility was determined by a blinded study nurse and an unblinded statistician. Treatment groups showed balanced demographics and injury severity.

The phenytoin group showed 73% reduction in early seizures compared to placebo (3.6 ± 1.3% vs 14.2 ± 2.6% with $p < 0.001$). There was no reduction in seizures at 1 year between the phenytoin and placebo groups (21.5 ± 3.6% vs 15.7 ± 3.2% with $p > 0.05$) or following study drug wean at 2 years (27.5 ± 4.0% vs 21.1 ± 3.7% with $p > 0.05$). There was no difference in mortality between phenytoin and placebo groups at 8 days (14% vs 15% with $p > 0.05$), 1 month (19% vs 19% with $p > 0.05$), 1 year (22% vs 20% with $p > 0.05$), or 2 years (24% vs 21% with $p > 0.05$).

The most common side effect was rash in both phenytoin and placebo groups (25% vs 17%), with 17 patients stopping phenytoin and 4 stopping placebo ($p < 0.01$). Leukopenia and elevated transaminases occurred equally between groups.

Conclusion This study showed that phenytoin prevents early seizures in the week following a serious head injury compared to placebo. There is no significant difference between seizure rates or mortality between the phenytoin and placebo groups after 7 days for patients presenting with trauma.

Reviewer Commentary Temkin and colleagues performed the first high-quality randomized, double-blind, placebo-controlled trial to rigorously evaluate whether prophylactic antiseizure medication could reduce the risk of seizures following traumatic brain injury (TBI). This landmark study demonstrated that high-dose phenytoin administered during the first week after severe head injury significantly suppresses **early post-traumatic seizures**, while conferring no protective effect against **late seizures**. In doing so, the authors provided definitive evidence that seizure prophylaxis in TBI is temporally limited and effective only during the acute post-injury period. As a result, seizure precautions, patient education, and expert neurologic evaluation, including additional workup to estimate the risk of seizures beyond 7 days, remain necessary once the early high-risk window has passed.[4–7]

The accepted risk threshold for the diagnosis of epilepsy is a recurrence risk exceeding 60%. Seizures are broadly classified as **provoked** or **unprovoked**, with provoking factors including metabolic derangements (hyponatremia, hypocalcemia, hypoglycemia, hypomagnesemia, hyperglycemia), hypoxia, intracranial structural lesions (hemorrhage, tumors, abscesses), and substance intoxication or withdrawal.[8,9] In the absence of such provoking factors, seizures are considered unprovoked and prompt further diagnostic evaluation to estimate future seizure risk.

Importantly, no antiseizure medication (ASM) has demonstrated true antiepileptogenic properties. Rather, ASMs raise seizure threshold, reducing seizure occurrence in the setting of acute provocation or established epilepsy without altering the underlying disease process.[10,11] Temkin et al. clarified that post-traumatic seizures occur along two biologically distinct timelines, early and late, and showed that pharmacologic suppression is effective only for early seizures. This distinction remains foundational to modern seizure management in TBI.

Although phenytoin was the agent studied, the enduring contribution of this trial lies in the **clinical principle** it established rather than the specific drug employed. Subsequent retrospective and prospective studies have demonstrated that levetiracetam is equally effective as phenytoin for the prevention of early seizures in both traumatic and non-traumatic neurosurgical populations, including patients undergoing craniectomy.[12,13] Levetiracetam offers practical advantages, including the absence of serum drug-level monitoring and minimal reliance on cytochrome P450 metabolism, thereby reducing drug–drug interactions.[14] Following benzodiazepines, levetiracetam has also been shown to be non-inferior to valproic acid and fosphenytoin in the treatment of status epilepticus.[15] Accordingly, many providers now favor levetiracetam (20–60 mg/kg/day) in place of phenytoin for 7 days following severe head injury,[12] a practice that directly extrapolates from the biologic and temporal framework defined by Temkin et al.

Study Limitations This study does not show that treatment of early seizures after serious head injury results in a reduction of risk of post-traumatic epilepsy, as they incompletely assessed the risk of occurrence of unprovoked seizures with their workup. Children from 16–18 years were included, but this study was otherwise limited to adults. Patients with seizures are a heterogeneous group with a wide variety of networks and etiologies; structural, genetic, metabolic, infectious, autoimmune, and idiopathic. Generalization of the conclusions of this study to patients with seizures from an etiology other than early post-traumatic seizure is difficult.[16,17]

Despite these limitations, the study's conclusions remain highly influential. By clearly distinguishing early seizure suppression from epileptogenesis, Temkin et al. established a durable clinical paradigm that continues to guide modern TBI care. Contemporary antiseizure practices, including the widespread use of levetiracetam, are direct extensions of this landmark trial's core insight: antiseizure medications effectively prevent early post-traumatic seizures but do not prevent the development of post-traumatic epilepsy.

NOTES

1 Servit Z, Musil F. Prophylactic treatment of posttraumatic epilepsy: results of a long-term follow-up in Czechoslovakia. Epilepsia. 1981;22:315–320.
2 Wohns RN, Wyler AR. Prophylactic phenytoin in severe head injuries. J Neurosurg. 1979;51:507–509.
3 Young B, Rapp R, Brooks WH, Madauss W, Norton JA. Posttraumatic epilepsy prophylaxis. Epilepsia. 1979;20:671–681.
4 Rank WP. Seizure first aid for bystanders. Nursing. 2020;50(10):11–12.
5 Al Sawaf A, Arya K, Murr NI. Seizure Precautions. 2023 Jan 23. In: StatPearls [Internet]. Treasure Island (FL): StatPearls Publishing; 2026 Jan.
6 Bösel J. SOP: first-ever epileptic seizure in adult patients. Neurol Res Pract. 2019;1:3.
7 Gulati S, Kaushik JS. How I treat a first single seizure in a child. Ann Indian Acad Neurol. 2016;19(1):29–36.
8 Misra UK, Kalita J. Management of provoked seizure. Ann Indian Acad Neurol. 2011;14(1):2–8.
9 Miller D. Childhood Epilepsies and When to Refer for Epilepsy Surgery Evaluation. In: Common Childhood Diseases – Diagnosis, Prevention, and Management [Working Title]. IntechOpen; 2024. doi:10.5772/intechopen.1005271
10 Pitkänen A, Lukasiuk K, Dudek FE, Staley KJ. Epileptogenesis. Cold Spring Harb Perspect Med. 2015;5(10):a022822.
11 Marques FVBS, Kawamura LRdM, Quintanilha MVT, Mota IFL, Vasconcelos AS, da Silva JFF, Mortari MR. Pharmacological perspectives and mechanisms involved in epileptogenesis. Beni Suef Univ J Basic Appl Sci. 2022;11:97.
12 Milligan TA, Hurwitz S, Bromfield EB. Efficacy and tolerability of levetiracetam versus phenytoin after supratentorial neurosurgery. Neurology. 2008;71(9):665–669.
13 Rahman M, Eisenschenk S, Melnick K, Wang Y, Heaton S, Ghiaseddin A, Hodik M, McGrew N, Smith J, Murad G, Roper S, Cibula J. Duration of prophylactic levetiracetam after surgery for brain tumor: a prospective randomized trial. Neurosurgery. 2023;92(1):68–74.
14 Wright C, Downing J, Mungall D, Khan O, Williams A, Fonkem E, Garrett D, Aceves J, Kirmani B. Clinical pharmacology and pharmacokinetics of levetiracetam. Front Neurol. 2013;4:192.

15 Chamberlain JM, Kapur J, Shinnar S, Elm J, Holsti M, Babcock L, Rogers A, Barsan W, Cloyd J, Lowenstein D, Bleck TP, Conwit R, Meinzer C, Cock H, Fountain NB, Underwood E, Connor JT, Silbergleit R; Neurological Emergencies Treatment Trials; Pediatric Emergency Care Applied Research Network Investigators. Efficacy of levetiracetam, fosphenytoin, and valproate for established status epilepticus by age group (ESETT): a double-blind, responsive-adaptive, randomized controlled trial. Lancet. 2020;395(10231):1217–1224.
16 Fisher RS, Cross JH, French JA, Higurashi N, Hirsch E, Jansen FE, Lagae L, Moshé SL, Peltola J, Roulet Perez E, Scheffer IE, Zuberi SM. Operational classification of seizure types by the International League Against Epilepsy: position paper of the ILAE commission for classification and terminology. Epilepsia. 2017;58(4):522–530.
17 Wirrell EC, Nabbout R, Scheffer IE, Alsaadi T, Bogacz A, French JA, Hirsch E, Jain S, Kaneko S, Riney K, Samia P, Snead OC, Somerville E, Specchio N, Trinka E, Zuberi SM, Balestrini S, Wiebe S, Cross JH, Perucca E, Moshé SL, Tinuper P. Methodology for classification and definition of epilepsy syndromes with list of syndromes: report of the ILAE task force on nosology and definitions. Epilepsia. 2022;63(6):1333–1348.

Chapter 38

Final Results of MRC CRASH, a Randomised Placebo-Controlled Trial of Intravenous Corticosteroid in Adults with Head Injury – Outcomes at 6 Months

Edwards P, et al.; for the CRASH (Corticosteroid Randomisation After Significant Head Injury) Trial Investigators, Lancet. 2005 Jun;365(9475):1957–1959[1]

Reviewed by Mark Wilson

Research Question/Objective In adults with head injury, does the use of early corticosteroids compared to placebo reduce death and disability?

Study Design Prospective, randomized controlled trial. Clinicians and patients were blinded with concealed allocation randomization (21% centralized, 79% non-centralized). Intention-to-treat analysis. Powered to detect a 2% difference in mortality from a baseline of 15% with an accepted type 1 error of 0.01 chance of false positive if 20,000 patients are recruited.

Annual interim analysis would unmask if proof beyond reasonable doubt was found between the two groups.

Sample Size 10,008 adults in 239 hospitals from 49 countries. Europe 38%, Asia 27%, South America 16%, Africa 14%, North America 4%, and Oceania 1%.

Follow-Up 6 months.

Inclusion/Exclusion Criteria

- Inclusion Criteria
  - Adults over 16 years of age with head injuries who present in less than 8 hours of injury.
  - A GCS of 14 or less.

- Exclusion Criteria
  - Clear indication or contraindication to steroids.

DOI: 10.1201/9781003416197-38

Intervention or Treatment Received

- Methylprednisolone for 48 hours.
- Loading dose of 2 g over 1 hour in 100 mL 0.9% saline.
- Maintenance of 0.4 g/hour for 48 hours run at 20 mL/hour in 0.9% saline.
- Control: Same regime of placebo.

Results After 10,008 patients, a clear difference in mortality at 2 weeks was found between the treatment and placebo arms and unmasking therefore occurred.

The corticosteroid group had a 21% mortality vs 18% for placebo (relative risk 1.18; absolute increased risk of 3.15%).

Six-month follow-up (a secondary outcome) also favored placebo for mortality and severe disability.

Primary Outcome

Outcome	Corticosteroids	Placebo	Relative Risk	Absolute Risk Reduction	Number Needed to Harm
2-week mortality	1,052 (21.1%)	893 (17.9%)	1.18 (95% confidence interval [CI] = 1.09–1.27, $p = 0.0001$)	–3.15% (95% CI = 1.60 to 4.70%)	31

Secondary Outcomes

Outcome	Corticosteroids	Placebo	Relative Risk	Absolute Risk Reduction	Number Needed to Harm
6-month mortality	1,248 (25.7%)	1,075 (22.3%)	1.15 (95% CI = 1.07–1.24, $p = 0.0001$)	–3.40% (95% CI = 1.70 to 5.10%)	29
6-month mortality or severe disability	1,828 (38.1%)	1,728 (36.3%)	1.05 (95% CI = 0.99–1.10, $p = 0.079$)	–1.80% (95% CI = –0.12 to 3.72%)	55

Summary Corticosteroids should not be used routinely in the treatment of head injury.

Author/Reviewer Commentary The use of steroids in neurotrauma (both for spinal and brain injury) was once a popular treatment for both brain and spinal cord injury, though it lacked any evidence of benefit. The series of National Acute Spinal Cord Injury Studies, the first being in 1984, brought into question the role of methylprednisolone in spinal cord injury.[2–4]

CRASH-1 investigated steroids in traumatic brain injury (TBI). The results, as outlined above, overturned what was often considered routine treatment. The prospective randomization of many patients meant that this level 1 evidence was quickly taken up by the Brain Trauma Foundation and guidelines against the use of steroids rapidly emerged. Of note, there have been other studies stopped early where what has been assumed to be a beneficial treatment has actually been associated with harm, one of the more recent ones being the Eurotherm 3235 trial, which demonstrated that cooling caused increased mortality following TBI.[5]

CRASH 1 did not investigate why mortality was higher in those receiving steroids, but like all things in medicine, there is a balance between desired effects (e.g. a reduction in swelling/edema) and undesired effects (e.g. raised blood glucose, risk of infection). CRASH 1 convincingly demonstrated that the routine use of methylprednisolone results in more harm. It does not, however, say steroids should never be used. If clinical judgement is such that the perceived life-threatening problem is edematous brain swelling, then in the young/those less susceptible to steroid complications, there may be an overall benefit, but CRASH 1 did not investigate this. The important thing is that a clinician should document and explain the reasoning for giving a drug associated with increased mortality.

It should be noted that the authors talk about "early" use of steroids being within the first 8 hours following injury. If a study looked at the "early use of CPR" in the first 8 hours of cardiac arrest, it would not show benefit. Eight hours was chosen for pragmatic reasons to ensure adequate recruitment. It may be that steroids in the first 10 minutes are of benefit, but that was not investigated in this study, and sadly, the negative view of steroids from this study may inhibit such a future study.

It should also be noted that there have been two further CRASH studies and there is currently a fourth ongoing. Crash 2 investigated the use of tranexamic acid (TXA) in polytrauma patients. Crash 3 demonstrated that TXA use did not alter 28-day mortality in TBI patients when given within 3 hours of injury (the primary outcome), but did reduce 28-day mortality in those who were not GCS 3 or did not have fixed dilated pupils (TXA group = 12.5% vs placebo = 14%), and also reduced mortality in the mild-to-moderate TBI group (TXA group = 5.8% vs placebo = 7.5%). Crash 4 is investigating the use of intramuscular TXA.

It is interesting that the first neuroprotective drug in TBI is one that reduces bleeding (TXA) and not steroids or another drug acting on the cytotoxic cascade. Reducing further brain damage (e.g. from bleeding) still appears more effective than trying to intervene on neurons already compromised.

Study Limitations The study was terminated early. While this demonstrates a difference in the two arms, this could be extreme chance.

Hyperglycemia in the steroid group may have unwittingly unblinded clinicians.

The cause of death was not investigated, which makes it difficult to interpret why steroids cause harm.

Conclusion The routine use of methylprednisolone within 8 hours of a traumatic brain injury is associated with increased mortality.

REFERENCES

1. Edwards P, Arango M, Balica L et al. Final results of MRC CRASH, a randomised placebo-controlled trial of intravenous corticosteroid in adults with head injury: outcomes at 6 months. Lancet. 2005;365(9475):1957–1959.
2. Bracken MB. Efficacy of methylprednisolone in acute spinal cord injury. JAMA. 1984;251(1):45.
3. Bracken MB, Shepard MJ, Collins WF, et al. A randomized, controlled trial of methylprednisolone or naloxone in the treatment of acute spinal-cord injury. N Engl J Med. 1990;322(20):1405–1411.
4. Bracken MB. Administration of methylprednisolone for 24 or 48 hours or tirilazad mesylate for 48 hours in the treatment of acute spinal cord injury. JAMA. 1997;277(20):1597.
5. Andrews PJD, Sinclair HL, Rodríguez A, et al. Therapeutic hypothermia to reduce intracranial pressure after traumatic brain injury: the Eurotherm3235 RCT. Health Technol Assess (Rockv). 2018;22(45):1–133.

CHAPTER 39

Trial of Decompressive Craniectomy for Traumatic Intracranial Hypertension (RESCUEicp Trial)

Hutchinson P, et al.; RESCUEicp Trial Collaborators, N Engl J Med. 2016 Sep 22;375(12):1119–1130

Reviewed by Angelos G Kolias and Peter J Hutchinson

Research Question/Objective The RESCUEicp trial examined the effectiveness of decompressive craniectomy as a last-tier intervention for patients with severe traumatic brain injury and refractory intracranial hypertension.[1]

Study Design Multicenter randomized, controlled trial.

Sample Size A total of 408 patients were enrolled in the trial; 206 were assigned to receive a decompressive craniectomy (surgical group) and 202 were to continue with medical treatment (medical group).

Follow-Up 6, 12, and 24 months after randomization. The primary outcome was evaluated with the Extended Glasgow Outcome Scale (GOS-E) at 6 months after randomization. The secondary outcomes included GOS-E at 12 and 24 months after randomization; mortality at 6, 12, and 24 months; quality of life at 6, 12, and 24 months; and assessment of intracranial pressure (ICP) control.

Inclusion/Exclusion Criteria

- Inclusion Criteria
  - Patients with a traumatic brain injury.
  - 10–65.
  - Abnormal CT scan requiring ICP monitoring.
  - Raised ICP (>25 mmHg for >1–12 hours) refractory to stage 1 and 2 treatment measures.

- Exclusion Criteria
  - Bilateral fixed and dilated pupils.
  - Bleeding diathesis.
  - Devastating injury; not expected to survive for 24 hours.

DOI: 10.1201/9781003416197-39

- Follow-up not possible.
- It should be noted that patients who had undergone an immediate operation for evacuation of an intracranial hematoma could be included if the bone flap was replaced at the end of the procedure. In total, 14% of the patients had craniotomy for evacuation of an intracranial hematoma before randomization.

Intervention or Treatment Received All patients were managed in Intensive Care Units (ICUs) following a tiered protocol with the aim of maintaining an ICP of 25 mmHg or less. The first tier included sedation, analgesia, neuromuscular paralysis (optional), and head elevation. If the ICP was not controlled, the second tier included the following treatment options: ventriculostomy (if an external ventricular drain had not already been inserted for intracranial pressure monitoring), blood pressure augmentation, osmotherapy, moderate hypocapnia, and therapeutic hypothermia (not < 34°C).

If the ICP remained above 25 mmHg for 1 to 12 hours despite first and second tier treatments, patients were randomized to undergo a decompressive craniectomy (unilateral or bifrontal) with ongoing medical therapy (surgical group) or to continue medical therapy with the option of adding barbiturates (medical group). It should be noted that a large unilateral frontotemporoparietal craniectomy (hemicraniectomy) was recommended for patients with unilateral hemispheric swelling; a bifrontal craniectomy was recommended for patients with diffuse brain swelling that affected both hemispheres. The decision regarding the type of craniectomy was left to the discretion of the treating neurosurgeons.

Results A total of 408 patients were randomized at 52 centers in 20 countries. Due to loss to follow-up and withdrawal of consent, 389 patients were assessed for the primary outcome (201 patients in the surgical group and 188 in the medical group), 373 were evaluated at 12 months (194 in the surgical group and 179 in the medical group), and 356 at 24 months (182 in the surgical group and 174 in the medical group).[1,2] The characteristics of the two groups were similar at baseline.

In the surgical group, 92.6% of the patients underwent a decompressive craniectomy, while in the medical group, 87.2% of the patients received a barbiturate infusion. A decompressive craniectomy was performed in 37.2% of the patients in the medical group; this was allowed by the protocol and left at the discretion of the treating clinicians in order not to deny patients a potentially life-saving treatment.

The GOS-E distributions are shown in Table 39.1. At 6 months, favorable outcomes, which were prespecified as upper severe disability or better on the GOS-E, were observed in 42.8% of the patients in the surgical group and in 34.6% of those in the medical group ($p = 0.12$). At 12 months, favorable outcomes were observed in 45.4% of the patients in the surgical group, as compared with 32.4% of those in the medical group ($p = 0.01$). At 24 months, favorable outcomes were observed in 45.1% of the

Table 39.1 GOS-E at 6, 12, and 24 Months

	Surgical Group (n =202)	**Medical Group (n =196)**	**Absolute Difference (95% CI) Percentage Points**	***p*-Value**
GOS-E at 6 months, n/total (%)				**<0.001***
Death	54/201 (26.9)	92/188 (48.9)	−22.1 (−31.5 to −12.7)	
Vegetative state	17/201 (8.5)	4/188 (2.1)	6.3 (1.9 to 10.7)	
Lower severe disability	44/201 (21.9)	27/188 (14.4)	7.5 (−0.2 to 15.2)	
Upper severe disability	31/201 (15.4)	15/188 (8.0)	7.4 (1.2 to 13.6)	
Lower moderate disability	20/201 (10.0)	19/188 (10.1)	−0.2 (−6.1 to 5.7)	
Upper moderate disability	27/201 (13.4)	18/188 (9.6)	3.9 (−2.4 to 10.2)	
Lower good recovery	5/201 (2.5)	6/188 (3.2)	−0.7 (−4.0 to 2.6)	
Upper good recovery	3/201 (1.5)	7/188 (3.7)	−2.2 (−5.4 to 1.0)	
GOS-E at 12 months, n/total (%)				**<0.001***
Death	59/194 (30.4)	93/179 (52.0)	−21.5 (−31.4 to 11.6)	
Vegetative state	12/194 (6.2)	3/179 (1.7)	4.5 (0.4 to 8.6)	
Lower severe disability	35/194 (18.0)	25/179 (14.0)	4.1 (−3.4 to 11.6)	
Upper severe disability	26/194 (13.4)	7/179 (3.9)	9.5 (3.8 to 15.2)	
Lower moderate disability	20/194 (10.3)	14/179 (7.8)	2.5 (−3.1 to 8.1)	
Upper moderate disability	23/194 (11.9)	22/179 (12.3)	−0.4 (−7.2 to 6.4)	
Lower good recovery	14/194 (7.2)	7/179 (3.9)	3.3 (−1.3 to 7.9)	
Upper good recovery	5/194 (2.6)	8/179 (4.5)	−1.9 (−5.7 to 1.9)	
GOS-E at 24 months, n/total (%)				**0.001***
Death	61/182 (33.5)	94/174 (54.0)	−20.5 (−30.8 to −10.2)	
Vegetative state	12/182 (6.6)	4/174 (2.3)	4.3 (0.0 to 8.6)	
Lower severe disability	27/182 (14.8)	22/174 (12.6)	2.2 (−5.4 to 9.8)	
Upper severe disability	16/182 (8.8)	4/174 (2.3)	6.5 (1.8 to 11.2)	
Lower moderate disability	19/182 (10.4)	10/174 (5.7)	4.7 (−0.9 to 10.3)	
Upper moderate disability	27/182 (14.8)	21/174 (12.1)	2.8 (−4.2 to 9.8)	
Lower good recovery	14/182 (7.7)	9/174 (5.2)	2.5 (−2.8 to 7.8)	
Upper good recovery	6/182 (3.3)	10/174 (5.7)	−2.5 (−6.9 to 1.9)	

Abbreviations: GOS-E = Glasgow Outcomes Score Extended; CI = Confidence interval.* p values were calculated by the unordered X^2-test for differences between the two randomized groups.
Source: From References 1 and 2.

patients in the surgical group, as compared with 31.0% of those in the medical group ($p = 0.006$). Control of ICP was significantly better in the surgical group than in the medical group but there was no between-group difference in the median values of time to discharge from the ICU.

Conclusion Decompressive craniectomy for severe and refractory intracranial hypertension after traumatic brain injury (TBI) resulted in a substantial reduction in mortality compared to medical management. Surgery was also associated with higher rates of vegetative state, lower severe disability, upper severe disability, and moderate disability compared to medical management.

Author/Reviewer Commentary The RESCUEicp trial was a well-conducted trial that enrolled patients worldwide.[3] The results showed that decompressive craniectomy, as a rescue intervention for severe and refractory intracranial hypertension, reduces mortality by about 20%. For every 100 patients treated surgically rather than medically, there were 21 additional survivors. At 24 months, about 70% of the additional survivors were at least independent at home or better.[2] The rest were dependent on others.

These results led the Brain Trauma Foundation to update its guidelines in 2020, stating that:

> Secondary decompressive craniectomy (DC) performed for *late* refractory ICP elevation is recommended to improve mortality and favorable outcomes.[3]

Nevertheless, the operation is not a panacea. 30% of the additional survivors were dependent on others or in a persistent vegetative state. After severe TBI, patients who survive have varying levels of disability, ranging from vegetative state to moderate disability on the GOS-E. Vegetative state and lower severe disability (dependent on others for care) are considered unfavorable outcomes in most Western societies.[4] However, patients with upper severe disability are independent at home but require assistance outside (e.g. for shopping or traveling), and patients with moderate disability are usually employed in a paid or a voluntary capacity but have not returned to their pre-TBI employment.[5] Bearing in mind these descriptions is useful, as it is evident that lower severe disability is very different from upper severe disability. In fact, when discussing with families in the acute setting, we advocate against using terms such as "favorable" or "unfavorable," which inevitably reflect our own value judgments.[4,6] It is preferable to simply state that the best available evidence suggests that:

1. Decompressive craniectomy, as a rescue intervention when most other interventions have failed, reduces mortality by about 20% in severe and refractory intracranial hypertension.
2. At 24 months, about 70% of these additional survivors will be at least independent at home. The rest will be dependent at home or will remain in a vegetative state.

Our experience is that, when presented with this information, some families favor surgery, and some do not. This is because the degree of acceptable disability varies from person to person and is dependent on many factors, such as culture, social environment, and religion.[7] Moreover, one should also bear in mind that patients can adapt to a level of significant disability that they may have previously regarded as unacceptable.[8] For these reasons, we do not think that clinicians should be unilaterally deciding whether a given degree of disability is "acceptable" or "unacceptable"; the person who needs to accept an outcome is the patient.[6] Therefore, the indirect input of patients through their families is critical when determining the degree of acceptable disability, and consequently, whether a secondary decompressive craniectomy should be undertaken.

Study Limitations More than one-third of the medical group received a decompressive craniectomy as a result of medical treatment failure, which could have diluted the observed treatment effect.[1] Furthermore, we analyzed GOS-E scores in this trial to explore global functional outcomes after TBI; the granularity of the GOS-E outcome categories may not have allowed us to adequately capture outcome differences between the two treatment groups in the context of severe TBI.[9] Because of the trial's pragmatic nature, long-term data on cranioplasty and rehabilitation was not collected systematically.

Relevant Studies The DECRA (decompressive craniectomy) trial aimed to address the role of early, neuroprotective bifrontal DC for patients with severe TBI and mild/moderate intracranial hypertension not controlled by first-tier therapies.[10,11] At 12 months, the mortality was similar in both groups (21% surgical group vs 19% medical group), but more surgical patients had an unfavorable GOS-E, defined as upper severe disability or worse (59% surgical group vs 48% medical group; $p = 0.16$). It is important to understand that the DECRA and RESCUEicp trials had different hypotheses, inclusion criteria, and ultimately addressed different research questions.[4] The DECRA trial, compared to RESCUEicp, enrolled patients with a lower ICP threshold (20 mmHg vs 25 mmHg) for shorter intervals (15 min vs 1–12 hours), after lower intensity therapies (tier 1 interventions vs tier 1 and 2 interventions), and within a shorter interval after injury (all patients enrolled within 72 h after injury vs 44% of patients enrolled >72 h after injury).[4] Moreover, patients with mass lesions were enrolled in the RESCUEicp trial, but not in the DECRA trial. At enrollment, the populations also differed with respect to expected outcome, as the requirement for tier 2 interventions increases the relative risk of death by 60%.[12] Although DECRA has been widely criticized mostly for its hypothesis and enrollment criteria, we view it as a valuable trial that addressed a very specific question.[13,14] On the basis of its findings, we can conclude that bifrontal DC should not be used as a neuroprotective measure for moderate intracranial hypertension after TBI in well-resourced ICUs that have the means to manage elevated ICP with medical measures and external ventricular drainage.[4]

Finally, the RESCUE-ASDH trial was a multicenter, randomized, controlled trial that compared the outcomes of craniotomy vs decompressive craniectomy in adult patients with a traumatic acute subdural hematoma.[15] The results showed no significant difference across GOS-E categories between the craniotomy group (bone flap replaced) and the decompressive craniectomy group (bone flap left out) at 12 months. Most secondary outcomes were similar between the two groups but additional cranial operations within 2 weeks after randomization were performed more frequently in the craniotomy group and most of them were decompressive craniectomies for brain swelling. However, patients in the decompressive craniectomy group had more wound-related complications and surgical-site infections. Based on the results of the RESCUE-ASDH trial, we recommend that if the bone flap can be replaced without compression of the brain, surgeons may consider doing so, as opposed to performing a preemptive decompressive craniectomy.[15]

Summary RESCUEicp trial is a landmark study in neurotrauma that definitively established **secondary decompressive craniectomy as an effective rescue therapy** for refractory intracranial hypertension after severe traumatic brain injury. It demonstrated a meaningful reduction in mortality while clearly defining the long-term functional outcomes of survivors, shifting clinical decision-making from survival alone to informed discussions about disability and quality of life.

REFERENCES

1. Hutchinson PJ, Kolias AG, Timofeev IS, et al. Trial of decompressive craniectomy for traumatic intracranial hypertension. N Engl J Med. 2016;375(12):1119–1130. doi:10.1056/NEJMoa1605215
2. Kolias AG, Adams H, Timofeev IS, et al. Evaluation of outcomes among patients with traumatic intracranial hypertension treated with decompressive craniectomy vs standard medical care at 24 months: a secondary analysis of the RESCUEicp randomized clinical trial. JAMA Neurol. 2022;79(7):664–671. doi:10.1001/JAMANEUROL.2022.1070
3. Hawryluk GWJ, Rubiano AM, Totten AM, et al. Guidelines for the management of severe traumatic brain injury: 2020 update of the decompressive craniectomy recommendations. Neurosurgery. 2020;87(3):427–434. doi:10.1093/neuros/nyaa278
4. Kolias AG, Paschalis A, Fountas KN, Hutchinson PJ. The Value of Decompressive Craniectomy in Traumatic Brain Injury. In: Evidence for Neurosurgery. Cham: Springer International Publishing; 2019:5–18. doi:10.1007/978-3-030-16323-5_2
5. Wilson JT, Pettigrew LE, Teasdale GM. Structured interviews for the Glasgow Outcome Scale and the extended Glasgow Outcome Scale: guidelines for their use. J Neurotrauma. 1998;15(8):573–585.
6. Menon DK, Kolias AG, Servadei F, Hutchinson PJ. Survival with disability. Whose life is it, anyway? Br J Anaesth. 2017;119(5):1062–1063. doi:10.1093/bja/aex374
7. Kolias AG, Viaroli E, Rubiano AM, et al. The current status of decompressive craniectomy in traumatic brain injury. Curr Trauma Rep. 2018;4(4):1–7. doi:10.1007/s40719-018-0147-x
8. Honeybul S, Janzen C, Kruger K, Ho KM. Decompressive craniectomy for severe traumatic brain injury: Is life worth living? J Neurosurg. 2013;119(6):1566–1575. doi:10.3171/2013.8.JNS13857
9. Kolias A, Adams H, Timofeev I, et al. Outcomes of decompressive craniectomy compared to medical treatment for traumatic intracranial hypertension at 2 years: a secondary analysis of the RESCUEicp randomized trial. JAMA Neurol. 2022;1;79(7):664–671. doi: 10.1001/jamaneurol.2022.1070.
10. Cooper DJ, Rosenfeld JV, Murray L, et al. Decompressive craniectomy in diffuse traumatic brain injury. N Engl J Med. 2011;364(16):1493–1502. doi:10.1056/NEJMoa1102077.
11. Cooper DJ, Rosenfeld JV, Murray L, et al. Patient outcomes at twelve months after early decompressive craniectomy for diffuse traumatic brain injury in the randomized DECRA clinical trial. J Neurotrauma. 2020;37(5):810–816. doi:10.1089/neu.2019.6869

12. Stocchetti N, Zanaboni C, Colombo A, et al. Refractory intracranial hypertension and "second-tier" therapies in traumatic brain injury. Intensive Care Med. 2008;34(3): 461–467. doi:10.1007/s00134-007-0948-9
13. Timmons SD, Ullman JS, Eisenberg HM. Craniectomy in diffuse traumatic brain injury. N Engl J Med. 2011;365(4):373–376. doi:10.1056/NEJMc1106421
14. Appelboom G, Piazza M, Zoller SD, Connolly ES. Clinical trials in decompressive craniectomy after severe diffuse traumatic brain injury. World Neurosurg. 2013; 80(5):e153–e155. doi:10.1016/j.wneu.2011.05.013
15. Hutchinson PJ, Adams H, Mohan M, et al. Decompressive craniectomy versus craniotomy for acute subdural hematoma. N Engl J Med. 2023;388(24):2219–2229. doi:10.1056/ NEJMOA2214172

Chapter 40

Surgical Management of Acute Epidural Hematomas

Bullock MR, et al., Neurosurgery. 2006;58:S2-7–S2-15

Reviewed by Shelly D Timmons

Recommendations

- Indications for surgery
  - An epidural hematoma (EDH) greater than 30 cm^3 should be surgically evacuated regardless of the patient's Glasgow Coma Scale (GCS) score.
  - An EDH less than 30 cm^3 and with less than a 15 mm thickness and with less than a 5 mm midline shift in patients with a GCS score greater than 8 without focal deficit can be managed nonoperatively with serial computed tomographic (CT) scanning and close neurological observation in a neurosurgical center.

- Timing
  - It is strongly recommended that patients with an acute EDH in coma (GCS score < 9) with anisocoria undergo surgical evacuation as soon as possible.

- Methods
  - There is insufficient data to support one surgical treatment method. However, craniotomy provides a more complete evacuation of the hematoma.

Research Question/Objective The aim of this analysis was to provide evidence-guided recommendations for the surgical evacuation of traumatic intracranial epidural hemorrhage or hematoma (EDH). Topics addressed included timing to surgery, risk factors predicting the need for surgery, predictors of outcome, and factors that favor lower risk of nonoperative management.

Study Design Evidence-based guidelines.

DOI: 10.1201/9781003416197-40

Sample Size N/A. However, the review included 190 articles published between 1975 and 2001, with 41 final references, and details of 18 of these articles were included in the evidentiary tables.

Follow-Up N/A

Inclusion/Exclusion Criteria

- Inclusion Criteria
  - Search terms included "traumatic brain injury" or "head injury" and "epidural" or "extradural" and "hematoma," or "hematoma," or "hemorrhage."
  - The search was narrowed by the addition of the keywords "surgical treatment," or "surgery" or "operation" or "craniotomy" or "craniectomy" or "craniostomy" or "burr holes."

- Exclusion Criteria
  - The search excluded "spinal."

Intervention or Treatment Received N/A. However, the evidentiary review included all forms of cranial surgery for the evacuation of epidural hematomas in the setting of traumatic brain injury (TBI).

Results The background literature review revealed that common mechanisms of injury resulting in EDH include: traffic-related accidents (53%, range 30–73%), falls (30%, range 7–52%), and assaults (8%, range 1–19%). EDH is more commonly seen in younger patients, peaking in the second decade, and is rarely seen in patients older than 50–60 years old. The data indicated that EDH occurred in 2.7–4% of TBI patients, and that, among those presenting in coma, up to 9% suffered from an evacuable EDH.

EDH can emanate from a lacerated middle meningeal artery (MMA), middle meningeal vein, diploic veins, venous sinuses, or (as not reported in these guidelines but commonly seen) bone fracture lines, particularly in the frontal fossa/anterior skull base and posterior fossa. While the "classic" etiology of EDH has been described as a squamous temporal bone fracture with an MMA injury, one report cited in this manuscript described that mechanism in only 36% of adults and 18% of children ($n = 387$, all ages). A bleeding source could not be identified in about a third of pediatric patients and venous sources accounted for about a third of EDH in both pediatric and adult subpopulations. Temporal and temporoparietal locations were cited as the most common, and a small proportion (5%) presented with bilateral EDH.

Studies reviewed included both those case series and cohorts in which all patients were treated operatively initially and those in which some were initially observed and underwent delayed surgery.

Immediate Surgery Two studies examined findings associated with immediate surgery. Servadei et al. prospectively analyzed 158 consecutive patients admitted to three hospitals with a GCS of 14–15, although no treatment protocol was in place. The report merely described the characteristics of those undergoing immediate surgery (n = 116/158). The majority of those operated on had MLS > 5 mm (93%), hematoma thickness >15 mm (91%), and MLS and thickness were shown by linear regression analysis as factors associated with surgery. Location and the existence of other lesions did not rise to significance. Outcomes were similar, as they also were in a separate study of pediatric patients who had similar findings (20/33 undergoing surgery) (Bejjani). While children showed no difference in outcomes based upon GCS or age, the variables of MLS (4 mm vs 0.5 mm) and volume (41 cm^3 vs 8 cm^3), as well as temporal location, were related to early operation vs observation. Finally, a review comparing 30 operative patients to 18 nonoperative patients demonstrated that those with surgery had overall lower GCS scores, more frequent pupillary abnormalities, hemiparesis, higher-volume hematomas, and greater MLS, whereas in this series, location and presence of fracture were not associated with the decision (Hamilton).

Successful Observational Management Was associated with presenting neurological status, size, midline shift, and location. Initial observation was seen more often in patients in a conscious state, i.e. not in coma. GCS scores ranged from 12–15 in one study (Bullock 1985) in which 12/123 patients were treated nonoperatively. GCS ranged from 10 to 15 for observed patients in another retrospective cohort (Cucciniello). Observation was also associated with smaller hematoma volumes (12–38 cm^3; mean 26.8 cm^3), and less MLS [MLS <10 mm on first computed tomography (CT) scan (Bullock) or <12 mm (Cuccianiello)]. In the Bullock study, none of the observed lesions were in the temporal fossa and in the Cucciniello study, only 5 out of 57 were temporal.

Conversion to Surgical Management Was associated with similar findings to those that prompted immediate/early surgery in three studies cited (Bezircioglu, Chen, and Knuckey). The first was a prospective study in which 80 patients with GCS 9–15 were observed initially if they also had EDH volume less than 30 cm^3, thickness <2 cm, and no neurological deficit. Of these 80 patients, five progressed to need surgery because of deterioration, one of whom died. The factor associated with deterioration and progression to surgery was temporal location (100% of these 5 patients but present in only 24% of the 75 who did not progress). The second study of 74 patients with initially asymptomatic EDH indicated that 14 progressed to require surgery due to deterioration or increased hematoma size. EDH thickness >15 mm, MLS >5 mm, or volume >30 cm^3 were associated with a higher likelihood of eventual surgery. This group also assessed the effects of fractures, time to CT scan, and location of hematoma; these findings were not associated with outcomes. Finally, a very small study of 22 patients, seven of whom converted to later surgery, concluded that a time interval of less than 6 hours from injury to the first CT scan and a fracture that crossed a major vessel were significantly related to surgery.

Timing of Surgery Was studied vis-a-vis impact on outcome in four studies. The key factor impacting outcome was the duration of brain compression (as evidenced by anisocoria or alteration in consciousness), not the time from injury or admission to surgery (Lee, Cohen, Haselsberger, and Sakas). Another topic related to timing that was addressed included the question of surgery by non-neurosurgeons prior to transfer. All patients in one study of 83 patients (Wester) showed that all 11 of the 28 who underwent surgery by non-neurosurgeons before transfer had worse outcomes compared to those directly admitted, due mostly to the technical inadequacy of the primary operation. Two other studies showed that patients directly admitted to the index institution had more rapid surgery and better outcomes than those who required a transfer.

Conclusion Higher-volume epidural hematomas, those with significant mass effect, and those causing neurological deficit should be surgically evacuated as soon as possible via craniotomy. Other factors that may prompt evacuation in clinically better-appearing patients include the temporal location of the hematoma. If patients are to be observed, the authors recommended that they should be observed in a neurosurgical center with close neurological evaluation and with serial CT scanning, with the first follow-up scan done within 6 to 8 hours of injury, since those who get to the operating room shortly after they deteriorate do better and this is the most common window for enlargement. The authors concluded that surgical evacuation should be performed as soon as feasible after the onset of neurological deficits "because every hour delay in surgery is associated with progressively worse outcome."

Study Limitations Evidentiary review of primarily retrospective or observational studies. Prospective, randomized trials comparing surgical treatment with nonoperative management were not available and would be unethical to conduct. No studies of strictly nonoperative EDH management in TBI patients in coma were found.

Relevant Studies Other chapters in this evidence-based guidelines set included: Introduction, Methodology, Surgical Management of Subdural Hematomas, Surgical Management of Traumatic Parenchymal Lesions, Surgical Management of Posterior Fossa Mass Lesions, Surgical Management of Depressed Cranial Fractures, Appendix I: Post-Traumatic Mass Volume Measurement in Traumatic Brain Injury Patients, and Appendix II: Evaluation of Relevant Computed Tomographic Scan Findings.

In the years since this analysis was performed, the use of antiplatelet and anticoagulant medications (antithrombotic medications [ATMs]) has dramatically risen and patients admitted with ATMs on board have become much more prevalent. As a result, the use of ultra-early and early follow-up CT scans has become common for all types of structural lesions, not just EDH.

Moskopp et al. performed a retrospective review using an administrative database and ICD10 codes to assess whether early CT scanning was a significant predictor of outcome or influenced surgical decision-making in TBI patients with EDH, subdural hematoma, traumatic contusion, traumatic subarachnoid hemorrhage, and mixed lesions. Of 213 patients included, only nine had isolated EDH, and of these, none had ATMs or laboratory-confirmed clotting derangements. They concluded that, unlike all other forms of intracranial hemorrhage, those with EDH alone had outcomes more closely related to the mechanism of injury than coagulopathy. While their other findings suggested that early CT at 6 hours did not impact surgical timing or decision-making, but rather clinical deterioration did, the subset of isolated EDH patients was too small to make an exception to the prior recommendations from Bullock et al. (2006).

Paper Significance and Impact While this evidentiary review is now two decades past its publication date, the data reviewed support similar conclusions for surgical recommendations in a clinical entity that does not lend itself well to other forms of study due to the life-threatening nature of the lesions, and precious few publications have addressed the surgical management of EDH since. Epidural hematomas should be completely and rapidly evacuated through open surgery as early as possible if they are associated with signs of significant mass effect, as described in the abstract.

BIBLIOGRAPHY

1. Bezircioglu H, Ersahin Y, Demircivi F, Yurt I, Donertas K, Tektas S: Nonoperative treatment of acute extradural hematomas: Analysis of 80 cases. **J Trauma** 41:696–698, 1996.
2. Bejjani G, Donahue D, Rusin J, Broemeling L: Radiological and clinical criteria for the management of epidural hematomas in children. **Pediatr Neurosurg** 25:302–308, 1996.
3. Bullock R, Smith R, van Dellen JR: Nonoperative management of extradural hematoma. **Neurosurgery** 16:602–606, 1985.
4. Chen T, Wong C, Chang C, Lui T, Cheng W, Tsai M, Lin T: The expectant treatment of asymptomatic supratentorial epidural hematomas. **Neurosurgery** 32:176–179, 1993.
5. Cohen J, Montero A, Israel Z: Prognosis and clinical relevance of anisocoria-craniotomy latency for epidural hematoma in comatose patients. **J Trauma** 41:120–122, 1996.
6. Cucciniello B, Martellotta N, Nigro D, Citro E: Conservative management of extradural haematomas. **Acta Neurochir (Wien)** 120:47–52, 1993.
7. Haselsberger K, Pucher R, Auer L: Prognosis after acute subdural or epidural haemorrhage. **Acta Neurochir (Wien)** 90:111–116, 1988.
8. Knuckey N, Gelbard S, Epstein M: The management of asymptomatic epidural hematomas. A prospective study. **J Neurosurg** 70:392–396, 1989.
9. Lee E, Hung Y, Wang L, Chung K, Chen H: Factors influencing the functional outcome of patients with acute epidural hematomas: Analysis of 200 patients undergoing surgery. **J Trauma** 45:946–952, 1998.
10. Sakas D, Bullock M, Teasdale G: One-year outcome following craniotomy for traumatic hematoma in patients with fixed dilated pupils. **J Neurosurg** 82:961–965, 1995.
11. Servadei F, Faccani G, Roccella P, Seracchioli A, Godano U, Ghadirpour R, Naddeo M, Piazza G, Carrieri P, Taggi F, Pagni CA: Asymptomatic extradural haematomas. Results of a multicenter study of 158 cases in minor head injury. **Acta Neurochir (Wien)** 96:39–45, 1989.
12. Wester K: Decompressive surgery for pure epidural hematomas: Does neurosurgical expertise improve the outcome? **Neurosurgery** 44:495–500, 1999.

CHAPTER 41

Validity of a Set of Clinical Criteria to Rule Out Injury to the Cervical Spine in Patients with Blunt Trauma

Hoffman JR, Mower WR, Wolfson AB, Todd KH, Zucker MI; National Emergency X-Radiography Utilization Study Group, N Engl J Med. 2000 Jul 13;343(2):94–99

Reviewed by Jamie Bradbury and Jae Hyun Kwon

Research Question/Objective This prospective study aimed to validate the five clinical criteria for identifying patients who are at extremely low risk of clinically significant cervical spine injuries after blunt trauma, eliminating the need for imaging studies.

Study Design Prospective observational study.

Sample Size 34,069 patients from 21 centers across the United States of varying backgrounds.

Inclusion/Exclusion Criteria

- Inclusion Criteria
  - Patients with blunt trauma who underwent radiography of the cervical spine in the emergency department.

- Exclusion Criteria
  - Patients with penetrating trauma.
  - Patients who underwent cervical spine imaging unrelated to the blunt trauma.

Intervention or Treatment Received As an observational and prospective study, the protocol neither required nor directed any element of the care for enrolled patients.

Results A total of 34,069 patients underwent cervical spine imaging and data regarding the following criteria were collected: no tenderness at the posterior midline of the cervical spine, no focal neurologic deficit, normal level of alertness, no evidence of intoxication, and no clinically apparent, painful injury that might distract them from the pain of a cervical spine injury.

DOI: 10.1201/9781003416197-41

Of these patients, 818 (2.4%) had radiographically documented cervical spine injuries. The decision instrument yielded a false-negative result for 8 of the 818 patients (those who met the criteria yet had positive radiographic findings). The remaining 810 patients with injury were all correctly identified by the decision instrument and met at least one of the five criteria. 4,309 patients were deemed to have a low probability of cervical spine injury, and the instrument yielded a true negative in 4,301 patients (those who met the criteria and had negative radiographic findings).

The sensitivity of the instrument was an impressive 99.0% (95% confidence interval [CI], 98.0 to 99.6%), and the negative predictive value reached 99.8% (95% CI, 99.6 to 100%). Achieving such high sensitivity required careful assessment of all five criteria, as many patients met only one.

Of the 8 patients with false negatives, 2 met the predefined criteria of a "clinically significant injury." The first was a 54-year-old male with an endplate avulsion injury that, in one report, was described as a teardrop fracture; he opted for no treatment beyond a soft collar, which he subsequently removed after discharge. Notably, he remained asymptomatic at a 6-week follow-up. The second was a 57-year-old male who sustained a fracture of the sixth cervical lamina and later developed paresthesia in his right arm. He underwent a laminectomy and fusion, resulting in clinical improvement.

Based on the decision instrument, 4,309 (12.6%) of the patients could have avoided radiographic evaluation.

Conclusion This prospective study validated an easily replicable decision instrument that clinicians can readily use for evaluating cervical spine injuries in blunt trauma patients and the need for radiographs with a high degree of confidence. This instrument offers healthcare providers a reliable method to minimize unnecessary imaging, reducing healthcare costs and patient exposure to ionizing radiation, ultimately enhancing patient safety and care efficiency.

Reviewer Commentary Missing an occult cervical spine injury in a trauma patient can lead to catastrophic neurological injury and structural instability. This fear leads to unnecessary radiographic studies to evaluate the cervical spine, frequently going beyond plain radiographs. While it can ease the mind of the clinician, it results in significant healthcare costs and unnecessary ionizing radiation to the patient. One study suggested a high cost-effectiveness ratio of computed tomography to prevent paralysis in low-risk patients was >$80,000 per quality-adjusted life year in 1999.[1] Adjusted for inflation, this figure would be approximately $155,000 in 2026.

The National Emergency X-Radiography Utilization Study (NEXUS) criteria offer a straightforward clinical framework to identify blunt trauma patients who are at low risk of cervical spine injury. The 5-criteria decision instrument is a simple and easy modality to apply, as evidenced by the heterogeneous nature of the centers involved in the study. Before this study, the NEXUS criteria suffered from having a lower confidence interval of 89% sensitivity.[2] This multicenter prospective study validated the high 95% confidence interval sensitivity (98.0 to 99.6%) of the criteria in identifying patients who are at a low risk for clinically significant cervical spine injury. Around 12.6% of the patients enrolled in the study could have avoided unnecessary imaging based on the decision instrument.

With its validity confirmed, this study provides clinicians with a replicable tool for assessing blunt trauma patients, effectively minimizing the need for unnecessary imaging. This not only spares patients from exposure to ionizing radiation, but also conserves valuable resources for both the patient and the healthcare system.

Study Limitations A main limitation was the low specificity of 12.9% and positive predictive value of 2.7%, meaning that a positive finding from the NEXUS criteria rarely led to a clinically significant image finding. However, most clinicians will likely appreciate a decision instrument that errs on the side of over-testing to obtain such a high negative predictive value to avoid a possibly devastating injury. Additionally, the criterion "no painful, distracting injury" is a subjective criterion that could be interpreted differently by the evaluating clinician. Some have raised questions about the reproducibility of this criterion.[3]

Its application for pediatric patients raises caution due to differences in developmental and anatomic differences compared to the adult population. When applied specifically to patients under the age of 18, the NEXUS criteria still had a high sensitivity of 100%, but more significantly had a lower 95% confidence interval of 87.8% compared to the 98% in the original study.[4]

Relevant Studies The Canadian C-spine Rule (CCR) is often discussed as an alternative decision instrument for evaluating a cervical spine injury in blunt trauma patients. It demonstrated a high sensitivity of 100% (95% confidence interval, 98–100%).[5] The instrument was applied to alert and stable patients, assessing the lack of high-risk factors, the presence of low-risk factors that allowed safe assessment of the range of motion, and the ability to rotate the neck in sequential order. Cervical spine imaging was indicated for any patients who could not meet these criteria.

Authors of the CCR study published a prospective cohort study comparing CCR and NEXUS. It showed that CCR was more sensitive than the NEXUS (99.4% vs 90.7%, $p < 0.001$) and more specific (45.1% vs 36.8%, $p < 0.001$), leading to lower radiography rates (55.9% vs 66.6%, $p < 0.001$).[3] However, some have questioned the validity of this comparison study due to different patient eligibility criteria, location of the study sites (institutions from which the CCR was derived), and an altered definition of the NEXUS criteria.[6,7]

Summary This study is a landmark in trauma care because it validated the NEXUS criteria as a safe, simple, and widely applicable clinical decision instrument for ruling out clinically significant cervical spine injury after blunt trauma. By demonstrating near-perfect sensitivity in a large, prospective, multicenter cohort, it provided clinicians with confidence to safely forgo unnecessary cervical spine imaging in low-risk patients, reducing radiation exposure, costs, and resource utilization without compromising patient safety. The NEXUS criteria is an essential tool that is embedded in emergency and trauma care worldwide.

REFERENCES

1. Blackmore CC, Ramsey SD, Mann FA, Deyo RA. Cervical spine screening with CT in trauma patients: a cost-effectiveness analysis. Radiology. 1999;212(1):117–125. doi:10.1148/radiology.212.1.r99jl08117
2. Hoffman, JR, Schriger, DL, Mower, WR, Luo, JS, Zucker, M. Low-risk criteria for cervical-spine radiography in blunt trauma: a prospective study. Ann Emerg Med. 1992;12:1454–1460.
3. Stiell IG, Clement CM, McKnight RD, Brison R, Schull MJ, Rowe BH, Worthington JR, Eisenhauer MA, Cass D, Greenberg G, MacPhail I, Dreyer J, Lee JS, Bandiera G, Reardon M, Holroyd B, Lesiuk H, Wells GA. The Canadian C-spine rule versus the NEXUS low-risk criteria in patients with trauma. N Engl J Med. 2003;349(26): 2510–2518. doi:10.1056/NEJMoa031375
4. Viccellio P, Simon H, Pressman BD, Shah MN, Mower WR, Hoffman JR; NEXUS Group. A prospective multicenter study of cervical spine injury in children. Pediatrics. 2001;108(2):E20. doi:10.1542/peds.108.2.e20
5. Stiell IG, Wells GA, Vandemheen KL, et al. The Canadian C-spine Rule for radiography in alert and stable trauma patients. JAMA. 2001;286(15):1841–1848. doi:10.1001/jama.286.15.1841
6. Mower WR, Wolfson AB, Hoffman JR, Todd KH. The Canadian C-spine Rule. N Engl J Med. 2004;350(14):1467–1469. doi:10.1056/NEJM200404013501420
7. Yealy DM, Auble TE. Choosing between clinical prediction rules. N Engl J Med. 2003;349(26):2553–2555. doi:10.1056/NEJMe038184

CHAPTER 42

The Subaxial Cervical Spine Injury Classification System: A Novel Approach to Recognize the Importance of Morphology, Neurology, and Integrity of the Disco-Ligamentous Complex

Vaccaro AR, Hulbert RJ, Patel AA, Fisher C, Dvorak M, Lehman RA Jr, Anderson P, Harrop J, Oner FC, Arnold P, Fehlings M, Hedlund R, Madrazo I, Rechtine G, Aarabi B, Shainline M; Spine Trauma Study Group,
Spine. 2007 Oct 1;32(21):2365–2374

Reviewed by Alexander Vaccaro

Research Question/Objective To define a novel classification system for subaxial cervical spine trauma that conveys information about injury pattern, severity, treatment considerations, and prognosis. To evaluate the reliability and validity of this system.

Study Design The classification system was derived through a literature review and expert opinion of experienced spine surgeons. In addition, a multicenter reliability and validity study of the system was conducted on a collection of trauma cases.

Summary of Background Data The classification of subaxial cervical spine injuries remains largely descriptive, lacking standardization and prognostic information.

Methods Clinical and radiographic variables encountered in subaxial cervical trauma were identified by a working section of the Spine Trauma Study Group. Significant limitations of existing systems were defined and addressed within the new system. This system, as well as the Harris, and Ferguson and Allen systems, was applied by 20 spine surgeons to 11 cervical trauma cases. Six weeks later, the cases were randomly reordered and again scored. Interrater reliability, intrarater reliability, and validity were assessed.

Results Each of the three main categories (injury morphology, disco-ligamentous complex [DLC], and neurologic status) identified as integrally important to injury classification was assigned a weighted score; the injury

DOI: 10.1201/9781003416197-42

severity score was obtained by summing the scores from each category. Treatment options were assigned based on threshold values of the severity score. Interrater agreement, as assessed by the intraclass correlation coefficient of the DLC, morphology, and neurologic status scores, was 0.49, 0.57, and 0.87, respectively. The intrarater agreement, as assessed by the intraclass correlation coefficient of the DLC, morphology, and neurologic status scores, was 0.66, 0.75, and 0.90, respectively. Raters agreed with the treatment recommendations of the algorithm in 93.3% of cases, suggesting high construct validity. The reliability compared favorably to the Harris, and Ferguson and Allen systems.

Conclusion The Subaxial Injury Classification and Severity Scale provides a comprehensive classification system for subaxial cervical trauma. Early validity and reliability data is encouraging.

Author/Reviewer Commentary Cervical spine injuries are common and demand a precise understanding of the injury and detailed treatment plans. Accordingly, a classification system categorizing these injuries to guide treatment is of great interest. In 1970, Sir Frank Holdsworth pioneered a classification system that grouped patterns of spine injuries into the categories of flexion, flexion rotation, extension, vertebral compression, and shearing.[1] Holdsworth emphasized the anatomic stability provided by the posterior ligamentous complex and described patterns of injury in terms of their disruption of this stabilizing structure.[2] Holdsworth created a simple foundation for classification systems with his observations; however, it did not provide a robust enough guide for treatment, nor has it been clinically validated.

This was followed by Allen and Ferguson's classification in 1982 and the Harris classification in 1986. Both used mechanism of injury to categorize subaxial cervical spine injuries. Allen and Ferguson created groupings or "phylogenies" of compression and distraction, flexion, and extension, as well as vertical or lateral-based loading. Harris would add rotational forces as well. These groups were determined by radiographic findings and stratified according to severity.[3] Both systems aimed to correlate the mechanism of cervical injury to the extent of neurological deficit. In doing so, this created numerous permutations of injury mechanisms, but ultimately lacked a bridge to guiding treatment decisions.

In 2007, we developed and validated the Subaxial Cervical Spine Classification System (SLICS) with the goal of creating a classification system for cervical spine injuries that was both comprehensive in its descriptions of trauma and straightforward in clinical practice. The major elements involved in the SLICS are (1) injury morphology (compression, distraction, or translation/rotation), (2) the integrity of the DLC, and (3) the neurologic status of the patient.[5] Each category is then scored and this score helps the provider determine surgical (scores > 4) or nonsurgical (scores < 4) recommendations.[5] This format was modeled off the thoracolumbar classification (TLIC)[6] in combination with the clinical expertise of the Spine Trauma Study Group (STSG).

As Holdsworth recognized the importance of the posterior ligamentous structures, we too felt that the DLC provided significant cervical spine stability in various planes of movement.[5] The SLICS, therefore, accounts for obvious injury or abnormalities within the components of the DLC. Doing so, however, did introduce limitations to the classification, as we observed low inter- and intrarater scores in the assessment of DLC integrity in our internal validation.

Finally, we believed that neurologic status was key to providing clinical applicability that was missing in prior systems.[5] Neurologic status allows the surgeon to account for the integrity of the spinal cord, the preservation of which is arguably the goal of all spine surgery. No neurologic deficit is scored as 0, an injury to the nerve root is scored as 1, a complete cord injury is scored as 2, and an incomplete cord injury is scored as a 3. We felt it crucial to provide a greater severity score for the incomplete cord injury patient, as there may be a greater opportunity for recovery with surgical intervention.[5]

To assess reliability, we applied the SLICS, Allen and Ferguson,[3] and Harris[4] systems to 11 subaxial trauma cases. 20 surgeons from the STSG assessed these 11 cases with respect to each classification system at 2 time points, 6 weeks apart.[5] We found neurologic status had the highest inter- and intrarater agreement, followed by injury morphology and finally, the DLC category.[5] In terms of clinical validation, we found that raters agreed with the classification score and the correlating management plan. We also found a 71.5% agreement between the injury morphology category of the SLICS and the Allen and Ferguson classification.[5]

While the SLICS only provided guidance on surgical vs nonsurgical management, Dvorak et al. developed an algorithm to recommend surgical approaches based on a comprehensive literature review and expert recommendations.[7] Their study proposed that a single anterior approach is often favored in compression or distraction extension injury morphologies, while translation/rotational injuries generally call for a posterior or a combination anterior and posterior approach.[7]

Studies analyzing the SLICS have demonstrated excellent reliability, validity, and accessibility, as agreement has been observed in treatment plans based on independent surgeon preferences.[8–14] Some studies, however, have indicated that the injury morphology section of the SLICS demonstrated lower interrater agreement.[15–17] Since the development of the SLIC, other classification systems have been developed. Moore et al.[18] devised a classification system called the Cervical Spine Injury Severity Score (CSISS), which focuses on the stability of the spine.[19] Despite strong inter- and intraobserver reliability, the CSISS lacked a neurologic component, thus making its clinical application less robust.[20-21] Similarly, in 2019, Hitti et al.[22] created a modified SLICS score, which included a “time to evaluation/treatment” section, as they found this correlated to better nonoperative outcomes.[22]

As previously mentioned, some studies have still postulated that the morphological categories in the SLICS have not been as widely accepted, as many surgeons have found it challenging to fit into the limited specifications.[15–17, 23] Due to this lack of consensus, in 2016, the Arbeitsgemeinschaft für Osteosynthesefragen (AO) Spine Classification group created the AO Spine Subaxial Cervical Spine Injury Classification System.[24] This classification system describes morphological injuries as compression injuries, tension band injuries, and translational injuries with various subtypes dependent on the degree of injury. This system also utilizes criteria specific to facet injury, case-specific modifiers, and a neurologic component, making it a comprehensive model for classification. The literature on this system has shown it to be highly reliable, suggesting it will have a strong impact on future studies and clinical applications.[24]

REFERENCES

1. Holdsworth F. Fractures, dislocations, and fracture-dislocations of the spine. J Bone Joint Surg Am. 1970;52(8):1534–1551.
2. Aarabi B, Walters BC, Dhall SS, Gelb DE, Hurlbert RJ, Rozzelle CJ, Ryken TC, Theodore N, Hadley MN. Subaxial cervical spine injury classification systems. Neurosurgery. 2013;72(Suppl 2):170–186. doi:10.1227/NEU.0b013e31828341c5
3. Allen BL Jr, Ferguson RL, Lehmann TR, O'Brien RP. A mechanistic classification of closed, indirect fractures and dislocations of the lower cervical spine. Spine. 1982;7(1): 1–27. doi:10.1097/00007632-198200710-00001
4. Harris JH Jr, Edeiken-Monroe B, Kopaniky DR. A practical classification of acute cervical spine injuries. Orthop Clin North Am. 1986;17(1):15–30.
5. Vaccaro AR, Hulbert RJ, Patel AA, Fisher C, Dvorak M, Lehman RA Jr, Anderson P, Harrop J, Oner FC, Arnold P, Fehlings M, Hedlund R, Madrazo I, Rechtine G, Aarabi B, Shainline M; Spine Trauma Study Group. The subaxial cervical spine injury classification system: a novel approach to recognize the importance of morphology, neurology, and integrity of the disco-ligamentous complex. Spine. 2007;32(21):2365–2374. doi:10.1097/BRS.0b013e3181557b92
6. Vaccaro AR, Lehman RA Jr, Hurlbert RJ, Anderson PA, Harris M, Hedlund R, Harrop J, Dvorak M, Wood K, Fehlings MG, Fisher C, Zeiller SC, Anderson DG, Bono CM, Stock GH, Brown AK, Kuklo T, Oner FC. A new classification of thoracolumbar injuries: the importance of injury morphology, the integrity of the posterior ligamentous complex, and neurologic status. Spine. 2005;30(20):2325–2333. doi:10.1097/01.brs.0000182986.43345.cb
7. Dvorak MF, Fisher CG, Fehlings MG, Rampersaud YR, Oner FC, Aarabi B, Vaccaro AR. The surgical approach to subaxial cervical spine injuries: an evidence-based algorithm based on the SLIC classification system. Spine. 2007;32(23):2620–2629. doi:10.1097/BRS.0b013e318158ce16
8. Lee WJ, Yoon SH, Kim YJ, Kim JY, Park HC, Park CO. Interobserver and intraobserver reliability of sub-axial injury classification and severity scale between radiologist, resident and spine surgeon. J Korean Neurosurg Soc. 2012;52(3):200–203. doi:10.3340/jkns.2012.52.3.200
9. Stone AT, Bransford RJ, Lee MJ, Vilela MD, Bellabarba C, Anderson PA, Agel J. Reliability of classification systems for subaxial cervical injuries. Evid Based Spine Care J. 2010;1(3):19–26. doi:10.1055/s-0030-1267064
10. Whang PG, Patel AA, Vaccaro AR. The development and evaluation of the subaxial injury classification scoring system for cervical spine trauma. Clinical Orthopaedics and Related Research. 2011;469(3):723–731. doi:10.1007/s11999-010-1576-1

11. Cruz HY, Joaquim AF, Tedeschi H, Patel AA. Evaluation of the SLICS use in the treatment of subaxial cervical spine injuries. Arquivos de neuro-psiquiatria. 2015;73(5): 445–449. doi:10.1590/0004-282X20150022
12. Joaquim AF, Lawrence B, Daubs M, Brodke D, Patel AA. Evaluation of the subaxial injury classification system. J Craniovertebr Junction Spine. 2011;2(2):67–72. doi:10.4103/0974-8237.100057
13. Joaquim AF, Ghizoni E, Tedeschi H, da Cruz HY, Patel AA. Clinical results of patients with subaxial cervical spine trauma treated according to the SLIC score. J Spinal Cord Med. 2014;37(4):420–424. doi:10.1179/2045772313Y.0000000143
14. Samuel S, Lin JL, Smith MM, Hartin NL, Vasili C, Ruff SJ, Cree AK, Ball JR, Sergides IG, Gray R. Subaxial injury classification scoring system treatment recommendations: external agreement study based on retrospective review of 185 patients. Spine. 2015; 40(3):137–142. doi:10.1097/BRS.0000000000000666
15. van Middendorp JJ, Audigé L, Bartels RH, Bolger C, Deverall H, Dhoke P, Diekerhof CH, Govaert GA, Guimerá V, Koller H, Morris SA, Setiobudi T, Hosman AJ. The subaxial cervical spine injury classification system: an external agreement validation study. Spine J. 2013;13(9):1055–1063. doi:10.1016/j.spinee.2013.02.040
16. Sharif S, Ali MYJ, Sih IMY, Parthiban J, Alves ÓL. Subaxial cervical spine injuries: WFNS spine committee recommendations. Neurospine. 2020;17(4):737–758. doi:10.14245/ns.2040368.184
17. Schroeder GD, Canseco JA, Patel PD, Divi SN, Karamian BA, Kandziora F, Vialle EN, Oner FC, Schnake KJ, Dvorak MF, Chapman JR, Benneker LM, Rajasekaran S, Kepler CK, Vaccaro AR; AO Spine Cervical Classification Validation Group. Establishing the injury severity of subaxial cervical spine trauma: validating the hierarchical nature of the AO spine subaxial cervical spine injury classification system. Spine. 2021;46(10): 649–657. doi:10.1097/BRS.0000000000003873
18. Moore TA, Vaccaro AR, Anderson PA. Classification of lower cervical spine injuries. Spine. 2006;31(11 Suppl):S37–S61. doi:10.1097/01.brs.0000217942.93428.f7
19. Nicoll EA. Fractures of the dorsolumbar spine. J Bone Joint Surg Br. 1949;31:376–394.
20. White AA, Panjabi MM. Clinical Biomechanics of the Spine. Philadelphia: Lippincott, 1970.
21. Anderson PA, Moore TA, Davis KW, Molinari RW, Resnick DK, Vaccaro AR, Bono CM, Dimar JR, 2nd, Aarabi B, Leverson G; Spinal Trauma Study Group. Cervical spine injury severity score. Assessment of reliability. J Bone Joint Surg Am. 2007;89(5):1057–1065. doi:10.2106/JBJS.F.00684
22. Hitti FL, McShane BJ, Yang AI, Rinehart C, Albayar A, Branche M, Malhotra NR, Janjua MB, Ali ZS, Schuster JM, Ozturk AK. Predictors of failure of nonoperative management following subaxial spine trauma and creation of modified subaxial injury classification system. World Neurosurg. 2019;122:e1359–e1364. doi:10.1016/j.wneu.2018.11.048
23. Vaccaro AR, Koerner JD, Radcliff KE, Oner FC, Reinhold M, Schnake KJ, Kandziora F, Fehlings MG, Dvorak MF, Aarabi B, Rajasekaran S, Schroeder GD, Kepler CK, Vialle LR. AOSpine subaxial cervical spine injury classification system. Eur Spine J. 2016;25(7):2173–2184. doi:10.1007/s00586-015-3831-3
24. Halliday AL, Henderson BR, Hart BL, et al. The management of unilateral lateral mass/ facet fractures of the sub-axial cervical spine: the use of magnetic resonance imaging to predict stability. Spine. 1997;22:2614–2621.

CHAPTER 43

A New Classification of Thoracolumbar Injuries: The Importance of Injury Morphology, the Integrity of the Posterior Ligamentous Complex, and Neurologic Status

Vaccaro AR, Lehman RA Jr, Hurlbert RJ, Anderson PA, Harris M, Hedlund R, Harrop J, Dvorak M, Wood K, Fehlings MG, Fisher C, Zeiller SC, Anderson DG, Bono CM, Stock GH, Brown AK, Kuklo T, Oner FC, Spine (Phila Pa 1966). 2005 Oct 15;30(20):2325–2333

Reviewed by Alexander Vaccaro

Research Question/Objective To devise a practical, yet comprehensive, classification system for TL injuries that assists in clinical decision-making in terms of the need for operative versus nonoperative care and surgical treatment approach in unstable injury patterns.

Study Design A new proposed classification system for thoracolumbar (TL) spine injuries, including injury severity assessment, designed to assist in clinical management.

Methods Clinical spine trauma specialists from a variety of institutions around the world were canvassed with respect to information they deemed pivotal in the communication of TL spine trauma and the clinical decision-making process. Traditional injury patterns were reviewed and reconsidered in light of these essential characteristics. An initial validation process to determine the reliability and validity of an earlier version of this system was also undertaken.

Results A new classification system called the Thoracolumbar Injury Classification and Severity Score (TLICS) was devised based on three injury characteristics: (1) morphology of injury determined by radiographic appearance, (2) integrity of the posterior ligamentous complex, and (3) neurologic status of the patient. A composite injury severity score was calculated from these characteristics, stratifying

DOI: 10.1201/9781003416197-43

patients into surgical and nonsurgical treatment groups. Finally, a methodology was developed to determine the optimum operative approach for surgical injury patterns.

Conclusion Although there will always be limitations to any cataloging system, the TLICS reflects accepted features cited in the literature important in predicting spinal stability, future deformity, and progressive neurologic compromise. This classification system is intended to be easy to apply and to facilitate clinical decision-making as a practical alternative to the cumbersome classification systems already in use. The TLICS may improve communication between spine trauma physicians and the education of residents and fellows. Further studies are underway to determine its reliability and validity.

Author/Reviewer Commentary Significant controversy exists regarding the optimal methods for categorizing and managing thoracolumbar spinal fractures. Prior classification systems for these injuries were often too complex to be utilized in clinical practice or failed to consider significant factors in determining whether a patient should undergo operative or nonoperative treatment. For instance, the Denis classification system was the first to establish the three-column model of the spine. This system focused on the biomechanical stability of thoracolumbar fractures but neglected to consider neurologic deficits in the classification and treatment of these injuries.[1,2] The Magerl classification system, established in 1994, divided thoracolumbar injuries into three different groups, including compression injuries (Type A), distraction injuries (Type B), and rotational and translational injuries (Type C). While this system provided more precise categorization, it was very complex and exhibited only moderate inter- and intraobserver reliability, which restricted its widespread use in clinical practice.[1,3]

My colleagues and I within the Spine Trauma Study Group (STSG) developed the Thoracolumbar Injury Classification and Severity Score (TLICS) to provide a universal classification system for thoracolumbar injuries and guide clinical decision-making. At the time, STSG comprised 40 spine experts. Collectively, we believed one of the major drawbacks of prior thoracolumbar trauma classifications was their systematic difficulty in predicting spinal instability. In response to the challenge, we developed a framework aimed at categorizing groups of instability with consideration for immediate mechanical stability, long-term stability, and neurologic stability. This methodological approach allows for a more clinically pertinent assessment of injury severity than previous classification systems. Furthermore, incorporating the categorization allowed us to create a composite injury severity score, using a point system to determine whether patients would benefit more from operative versus non-operative treatment.

Since the advent of the TLICS system, its widespread adoption among both orthopedic spine surgeons and neurosurgeons underscores its significant unifying framework for assessing thoracolumbar injuries. A significant contribution to this validation was the multicenter reliability study performed by Rampersaud et al. to evaluate agreement in injury classification and clinical management between these distinct specialties utilizing the TLICS algorithm. Notably, this study demonstrated consistent recommendations between orthopedic surgeons and neurosurgeons, indicating the potential of the TLICS classification system to mitigate variability in the management of thoracolumbar injuries across diverse disciplines.[4,5]

Subsequent studies have underscored the modest learning curve with high reliability of the TLICS system. Patel et al. pioneered the first prospective clinical assessment of the TLICS system, using two consecutive patient cohorts with thoracolumbar injuries to gauge the interobserver reliability of the algorithm over time. Their findings revealed improvement in interobserver reliability on the second assessment, suggesting the TLICS system could be readily implemented into clinical practice.[4,6] Furthermore, in a complementary study, TLICS was applied to a series of spinal trauma cases to assess the validity of the classification system. The results indicated concordance between TLICS recommendations and clinical treatment in 96% of cases, affirming its excellent validity in informing clinical decision-making.[1,7]

While the TLICS system offers many advantages, it is not exempt from limitations. For instance, all burst fractures are given two points, without distinguishing an incomplete burst fracture (single endplate involvement) from a complete burst fracture (both endplate involvement), which could vary significantly in severity and therefore their natural history of healing. Moreover, TLICS employs MRI assessment of the posterior ligamentous complex integrity to allocate scores, yet the accuracy of the imaging modality for evaluating the complex remains uncertain. Although TLICS equips clinicians with a numerical score to direct their clinical management, it presents a "gray zone" at a score of 4 points where neither operative nor non-operative treatment is recommended. This leaves the treating surgeon in a situation where they must make treatment decisions for thoracolumbar injuries based on clinical judgment, rather than objective measures.[1]

In 2015, the TLICS evolved into the AO Spine Thoracolumbar Injury Classification System and Treatment Algorithm to address some of these limitations. The TL AOSIS not only retained elements of TLICS but also incorporated aspects of the Magerl classification system. This updated system considered the integrity of the posterior ligamentous complex and neurologic status in the injury severity score, and also categorized thoracolumbar injuries into three groups (Type A, Type B, and Type C). In 2020, further updates were made to the TL AOSIS, specifically assigning a score of 3 points to A3 burst fractures and 5 points to A4 burst fractures in neurologically intact patients. This adjustment aimed to clarify the treatment approach for these types of fractures, establishing specific management recommendations based on severity.[8] Despite its increased complexity, the TL AOSIS has demonstrated higher interrater and intrarater reliability.[1,9] Additional studies showed a stronger correlation between treatment recommendations and actual surgical management when using the TL AOSIS compared to the TLICS framework.[10–12]

The TLICS system has generated algorithms that integrate critical factors, resulting in meaningful classifications of thoracolumbar injuries. The update of the TL AOSIS has significantly improved the clinical management of the original algorithm, addressing the need for a validated, evidence-based surgical algorithm in treating thoracolumbar spinal trauma.[13]

REFERENCES:

1. Kweh, B. T. S., Tee, J. W., Dandurand, C., Vaccaro, A. R., Lorin, B. M., Schnake, K., Vialle, E., Rajasekaran, S., El-Skarkawi, M., Bransford, R. J., Kanna, R. M., Aly, M. M., Holas, M., Canseco, J. A., Muijs, S., Popescu, E. C., Camino-Willhuber, G., Joaquim, A. F., Chhabra, H. S., Bigdon, S. F., … Schroeder, G. (2024). The AO Spine Thoracolumbar Injury Classification System and Treatment Algorithm in Decision Making for Thoracolumbar Burst Fractures Without Neurologic Deficit. Global spine journal, 14(1_suppl), 32S–40S. https://doi.org/10.1177/21925682231195764
2. Denis F. (1983). The three column spine and its significance in the classification of acute thoracolumbar spinal injuries. Spine, 8(8), 817–831. https://doi.org/10.1097/00007632-198311000-00003
3. Sethi, M. K., Schoenfeld, A. J., Bono, C. M., & Harris, M. B. (2009). The evolution of thoracolumbar injury classification systems. The spine journal: official journal of the North American Spine Society, 9(9), 780–788. https://doi.org/10.1016/j.spinee.2009.04.003
4. Rihn, J. A., Anderson, D. T., Harris, E., Lawrence, J., Jonsson, H., Wilsey, J., Hurlbert, R. J., & Vaccaro, A. R. (2008). A review of the TLICS system: a novel, user-friendly thoracolumbar trauma classification system. Acta orthopaedica, 79(4), 461–466. https://doi.org/10.1080/17453670710015436
5. Raja Rampersaud, Y., Fisher, C., Wilsey, J., Arnold, P., Anand, N., Bono, C. M., Dailey, A. T., Dvorak, M., Fehlings, M. G., Harrop, J. S., Oner, F. C., & Vaccaro, A. R. (2006). Agreement between orthopedic surgeons and neurosurgeons regarding a new algorithm for the treatment of thoracolumbar injuries: a multicenter reliability study. Journal of spinal disorders & techniques, 19(7), 477–482. https://doi.org/10.1097/01.bsd.0000211237.14211.21
6. Patel, A. A., Vaccaro, A. R., Albert, T. J., Hilibrand, A. S., Harrop, J. S., Anderson, D. G., Sharan, A., Whang, P. G., Poelstra, K. A., Arnold, P., Dimar, J., Madrazo, I., & Hegde, S. (2007). The adoption of a new classification system: time-dependent variation in interobserver reliability of the thoracolumbar injury severity score classification system. Spine, 32(3), E105–E110. https://doi.org/10.1097/01.brs.0000254107.57551.8a
7. Patel, A. A., Dailey, A., Brodke, D. S., Daubs, M., Harrop, J., Whang, P. G., Vaccaro, A. R., & Spine Trauma Study Group (2009). Thoracolumbar spine trauma classification: the Thoracolumbar Injury Classification and Severity Score system and case examples. Journal of neurosurgery. Spine, 10(3), 201–206. https://doi.org/10.3171/2008.12.SPINE08388
8. Vaccaro, A. R., Lehman, R. A., Jr, Hurlbert, R. J., Anderson, P. A., Harris, M., Hedlund, R., Harrop, J., Dvorak, M., Wood, K., Fehlings, M. G., Fisher, C., Zeiller, S. C., Anderson, D. G., Bono, C. M., Stock, G. H., Brown, A. K., Kuklo, T., & Oner, F. C. (2005). A new classification of thoracolumbar injuries: the importance of injury morphology, the integrity of the posterior ligamentous complex, and neurologic status. Spine, 30(20), 2325–2333. https://doi.org/10.1097/01.brs.0000182986.43345.cb
9. Kaul, R., Chhabra, H. S., Vaccaro, A. R., Abel, R., Tuli, S., Shetty, A. P., Das, K. D., Mohapatra, B., Nanda, A., Sangondimath, G. M., Bansal, M. L., & Patel, N. (2017). Reliability assessment of AOSpine thoracolumbar spine injury classification system

and Thoracolumbar Injury Classification and Severity Score (TLICS) for thoracolumbar spine injuries: results of a multicentre study. European spine journal: official publication of the European Spine Society, the European Spinal Deformity Society, and the European Section of the Cervical Spine Research Society, 26(5), 1470–1476. https://doi.org/10.1007/s00586-016-4663-5

10. An, Z., Zhu, Y., Wang, G., Wei, H., & Dong, L. (2020). Is the Thoracolumbar AOSpine Injury Score Superior to the Thoracolumbar Injury Classification and Severity Score for Guiding the Treatment Strategy of Thoracolumbar Spine Injuries?. World neurosurgery, 137, e493–e498. https://doi.org/10.1016/j.wneu.2020.02.013
11. Lambrechts MJ, Schroeder GD, Tran K, Li S, Huang A, Chu J, Karamian BA, Canseco JA, Hilibrand AS, Oner C, Dvorak M, Schnake K, Kepler CK, Vaccaro AR. Validation of the AO Spine Thoracolumbar Injury Classification System Treatment Algorithm: Should it be used to Guide Fracture Management? Spine (Phila Pa 1976). 2023 Jul 15;48(14):994–1002. doi: 10.1097/BRS.0000000000004693. Epub 2023 Apr 27. PMID: 37141491.
12. Morrissey PB, Shafi KA, Wagner SC, Butler JS, Kaye ID, Sebastian AS, Schroeder GD, Kepler CK, Aarabi B, Oner FC, Vaccaro AR. Surgical Management of Thoracolumbar Burst Fractures: Surgical Decision-making Using the AOSpine Thoracolumbar Injury Classification Score and Thoracolumbar Injury Classification and Severity Score. Clin Spine Surg. 2021 Feb 1;34(1):4–13. doi: 10.1097/BSD.0000000000001038. PMID: 32657842.
13. Vaccaro, A. R., Schroeder, G. D., Kepler, C. K., Cumhur Oner, F., Vialle, L. R., Kandziora, F., Koerner, J. D., Kurd, M. F., Reinhold, M., Schnake, K. J., Chapman, J., Aarabi, B., Fehlings, M. G., & Dvorak, M. F. (2016). The surgical algorithm for the AOSpine thoracolumbar spine injury classification system. European spine journal: official publication of the European Spine Society, the European Spinal Deformity Society, and the European Section of the Cervical Spine Research Society, 25(4), 1087–1094. https://doi.org/10.1007/s00586-015-3982-2

CHAPTER 44

A Clinical Practice Guideline for the Management of Patients with Acute Spinal Cord Injury: Recommendations on the Use of Methylprednisolone Sodium Succinate

Fehlings MG, Wilson JR, Tetreault LA, Aarabi B, Anderson P, Arnold PM, Brodke DS, Burns AS, Chiba K, Dettori JR, Furlan JC, Hawryluk G, Holly LT, Howley S, Jeji T, Kalsi-Ryan S, Kotter M, Kurpad S, Kwon BK, Marino RJ, Martin AR, Massicotte E, Merli G, Middleton JW, Nakashima H, Nagoshi N, Palmieri K, Skelly AC, Singh A, Tsai EC, Vaccaro A, Yee A, Harrop JS, Global Spine J. 2017 Sep;7(3 Suppl):203S–211S

Reviewed by Karlo M Pedro and Michael G Fehlings

Research Question/Objective This guideline aims to clarify the appropriate use of methylprednisolone sodium succinate (MPSS) in acute spinal cord injury (SCI) by reviewing existing evidence and providing updated clinical recommendations.

Study Design This guideline is based on a systematic review and meta-analysis of existing randomized controlled trials (RCTs) and observational studies that were controlled for baseline neurological status. The GRADE (Grading of Recommendations, Assessment, Development, and Evaluation) guideline development tool was used to weigh the benefits and harms of treatment options and evaluate the strength of recommendations.[1]

Sample Size This review included three RCTs (four publications) and one prospective cohort study assessing MPSS efficacy and safety.

Follow-Up Outcomes were analyzed at 6-month and 12-month follow-up periods to assess neurological recovery and the incidence of complications.

DOI: 10.1201/9781003416197-44

Inclusion/Exclusion Criteria

- Inclusion Criteria
  - Adult patients with acute traumatic SCI
  - Studies evaluating MPSS compared to no steroids
  - RCTs and observational studies controlling for baseline severity

- Exclusion Criteria
  - Non-randomized studies without controlled baseline characteristics
  - Studies without relevant neurological outcome data

Intervention or Treatment Received Patients receiving MPSS infusions in different durations and dosages:

1. 24-hour infusion initiated within 8 hours of injury
2. 24-hour infusion initiated after 8 hours of injury
3. 48-hour infusion of MPSS

Results Key findings from the systematic review:

- No significant differences in motor score recovery at any time point between patients receiving MPSS and those who did not.
- MPSS administered within 8 hours was associated with a modest improvement in motor score at 6 and 12 months, but the clinical significance continues to be debated.
- No statistical differences in complication rates between MPSS and control groups; however, a longer 48-hour infusion increased the risk of severe pneumonia and sepsis.

Conclusion The guideline provides weak recommendations regarding MPSS use:

- Do not offer a 24-hour infusion of high-dose MPSS if initiated after 8 hours of injury.
- Consider offering a 24-hour infusion within 8 hours as a treatment option.
- Do not offer a 48-hour infusion, as it lacks supporting evidence and increases the risk of infections.

Study Limitations This guideline is informed by a robust synthesis of high-quality studies, yet several limitations must be acknowledged. First, there is significant heterogeneity among the included trials with respect to injury severity, timing of intervention, and outcome measures. Second, the foundational evidence base, specifically the National Acute Spinal Cord Injury (NASCIS) trials, has been widely criticized for its methodological limitations, including the reliance on post-hoc subgroup analysis and the disputed clinical relevance of the observed effect sizes.[2] Third, while RCTs offer the highest level of evidence, many of the more recent studies assessing MPSS in SCI have been observational in nature, introducing potential confounding factors such as selection bias, particularly the tendency to administer steroids to more severely injured patients.

Another limitation is the lack of stratified long-term outcomes data. Most studies measure efficacy at 6 to 12 months, with few extending follow-up to evaluate lasting functional outcomes or quality of life. Additionally, there is insufficient evidence on cost-effectiveness, despite MPSS being a low-cost, off-patent drug. Moreover, the guideline development group acknowledged a paucity of high-quality studies comparing 24- vs 48-hour infusion or directly assessing outcomes based on timing post-injury. These gaps in evidence were accounted for in the GRADE methodology by downgrading the quality of evidence for imprecision or indirectness. Lastly, the rapid decline in the MPSS use across institutions may be driven more by risk aversion or medicolegal concerns than by new clinical trial data, which complicates the interpretation of real-world trends.[3]

Author/Reviewer Commentary The discussion around steroid use in SCI has evolved through distinct eras. In the 1980s and 1990s, the NASCIS I, II, and III trials formed the backbone of support for MPSS administration. These trials found statistically significant, albeit modest, improvement in motor scores when steroids were administered within 8 hours post-injury. Based on these findings, the use of MPSS became widely accepted, despite criticisms surrounding the trials' methodology.

By the early 2000s, skepticism began to grow. The 2002 CNS/AANS guidelines acknowledged that while MPSS could be offered for 24 or 48 hours, the evidence of potential harm was more consistent than the evidence of benefit. Around the same time, multiple non-randomized studies reported no meaningful improvement in outcomes with steroid use. This culminated in the 2013 CNS/AANS guideline update, which issued a level 1 recommendation against MPSS use in acute SCI.

In response to the polarized landscape, the 2017 AO Spine guideline provided a more nuanced recommendation, differentiating between 24- and 48-hour regimens and between administration within and after 8 hours of injury. The meta-analysis found a small but statistically significant improvement in motor scores when MPSS was administered within 8 hours, leading to a recommendation of this approach as a treatment option.

However, widespread clinical acceptance of these recommendations has been slow, likely due to lingering concerns about safety, perceived lack of efficacy, and medicolegal implications.[4] Moving forward, it will be critical to personalize treatment strategies based on individual patient characteristics and preferences. Enhanced shared decision-making, especially in cases where patients can participate in discussions or where surrogate decision-makers are present, may allow for more tailored approaches that align with the values of those most affected.

Ultimately, while MPSS may no longer be a universally endorsed intervention, it continues to be a reasonable option in specific SCI contexts, such as in the young, non-polytrauma cases. As research methodologies advance to address the persistent challenges of patient heterogeneity, and our basic scientific understanding of SCI biology deepens, paving the way for novel neuroprotective strategies, MPSS stands as a case study in the evolving nature of evidence-based medicine, where certainty is elusive and clinical nuance remains essential.[5]

Relevant Studies (Annotated)

1. **Bracken et al. (1990): A Randomized, Controlled Trial of Methylprednisolone or Naloxone in the Treatment of Acute Spinal Cord Injury (NASCIS II)**[2]
   This landmark multicenter RCT found that MPSS, when administered within 8 hours of injury, significantly improved motor and sensory outcomes at 6 months compared to placebo. No benefit was observed in patients treated after 8 hours, and naloxone showed no effect. Mortality and morbidity were similar across all treatment arms.

   Key Limitations: Critics argue that the benefit was based on post-hoc subgroup analyses involving only a fraction (about 27%) of the original cohort, making the results vulnerable to chance findings. Concerns were also raised about selective reporting (e.g. only right-sided motor scores were presented) and the use of arbitrary time windows without a priori justification, which weakens the robustness and reproducibility of the findings.
2. **Bracken et al. (1997): NASCIS III – Administration of Methylprednisolone for 24 or 48 Hours or Tirilazad for 48 Hours in the Treatment of Acute SCI**[6]
   NASCIS III compared 24-hour and 48-hour MPSS regimens and found that extending MPSS to 48 hours provided modest motor benefits in patients treated between 3 and 8 hours post-injury. However, this extended regimen was also associated with higher rates of severe sepsis and pneumonia. Tirilazad did not demonstrate superiority over 24-hour MPSS.

   Key Limitations: As with NASCIS II, primary outcomes showed no significant differences, and positive findings were based on post-hoc subgroup analyses of patients treated in a narrow 3- to 8-hour window. The study lacked a true placebo group, used compliance-based analyses, and omitted key motor and sensory data (e.g. left-sided scores), raising concerns of data instability and bias.
3. **Bracken (2012): Cochrane Systematic Review of Steroids for Acute Spinal Cord Injury**[7]
   This review concluded that high-dose MPSS improves motor outcomes if given within 8 hours of injury, with the additional benefit when treatment is extended to 48 hours in patients treated between 3 and 8 hours post-injury. The review

highlighted the consistency of findings in NASCIS and Japanese trials and found no significant increase in complications or mortality with MPSS.

Key Limitations: Critics argue that the Cochrane review heavily relied on the NASCIS studies, which themselves have methodological issues. The positive conclusions may be overstated due to the inclusion of low-quality and unblinded studies, and limited generalizability due to variation in patient populations and outcome measures.

4. **Evaniew et al. (2016): Systematic Review and Meta-Analysis of MPSS in Acute SCI**[8]
   This comprehensive meta-analysis found no significant long-term motor benefit of MPSS when considering all RCTs and observational studies. Short-term improvements were observed only in patients treated within 8 hours, but confidence in the evidence was low due to risk of bias and imprecision. There was a significantly increased risk of gastrointestinal bleeding associated with MPSS in observational studies.

   Key Limitations: The study's confidence in its pooled effect estimates was limited by heterogeneity among included trials, the predominance of low-quality observational studies, and the lack of blinding. Additionally, the meta-analysis confirmed that much of the supporting evidence for MPSS stems from a narrow subgroup of patients, which limits the ability to make strong or generalized clinical recommendations.

5. **Geisler et al. (2023): Reanalysis of NASCIS II and Sygen Trials**[9]
   Using modern statistical methods, this case-matched study reanalyzed pooled patient-level data from NASCIS II and the Sygen trial. The results confirmed that the previously reported positive effects of MPSS were confined to a sub-subgroup (right-sided motor scores within 8 hours), a finding that current standards consider clinically insignificant due to lack of pre-specification and correction for multiple comparisons. No benefit of MPSS was found on American Spinal Injury Association motor score recovery or sensory level improvement at 26 weeks.

   Key Limitations: While robust in its methodology, this retrospective reanalysis may still be limited by inherent differences between historical cohorts and the evolving SCI standards of care.

REFERENCES

1. Guyatt G, Oxman AD, Akl EA, et al. GRADE guidelines: 1. Introduction-GRADE evidence profiles and summary of findings tables. J Clin Epidemiol. 2011;64(4):383–394. doi:10.1016/j.jclinepi.2010.04.026
2. Bracken MB, Shepard MJ, Collins WF, et al. A randomized, controlled trial of methylprednisolone or naloxone in the treatment of acute spinal-cord injury. Results of the Second National Acute Spinal Cord Injury Study. N Engl J Med. 1990;322(20): 1405–1411. doi:10.1056/NEJM199005173222001

3. Rispoli R, Cappelletto B. Unraveling the controversy: high-dose steroids in spinal cord injury. Forty years of inquiry. J Neurosurg Sci. 2024;68(3):251–253. doi:10.23736/S0390-5616.24.06238-6
4. Hejrati N, Moghaddamjou A, Pedro K, et al. Current practice of acute spinal cord injury management: a global survey of members from the AO spine. Global Spine J. 2022;14(2):546–560. doi:10.1177/21925682221116888
5. Pedro KM, Fehlings MG. Progress and future directions in spinal cord injury trials. Lancet Neurol. 2025;24(1):3–5. doi:10.1016/S1474-4422(24)00482-4
6 Bracken MB, Shepard MJ, Holford TR, et al. Administration of methylprednisolone for 24 or 48 hours or tirilazad mesylate for 48 hours in the treatment of acute spinal cord injury. Results of the Third National Acute Spinal Cord Injury Randomized Controlled Trial. National Acute Spinal Cord Injury Study. JAMA. 1997;277(20):1597–1604. PMID: 9168289.
7. Bracken MB. Steroids for acute spinal cord injury. Cochrane Database Syst Rev. 2012;1(1):CD001046. doi:10.1002/14651858.CD001046.pub2
8. Evaniew N, Belley-Côté EP, Fallah N, Noonan VK, Rivers CS, Dvorak MF. Methylprednisolone for the treatment of patients with acute spinal cord injuries: a systematic review and meta-analysis. J Neurotrauma. 2016;33(5):468–481. doi:10.1089/neu.2015.4192
9. Geisler FH, Moghaddamjou A, Wilson JRF, Fehlings MG. Methylprednisolone in acute traumatic spinal cord injury: case-matched outcomes from the NASCIS2 and Sygen historical spinal cord injury studies with contemporary statistical analysis. J Neurosurg Spine. 2023;38(5):595–606. doi:10.3171/2022.12.SPINE22713

Chapter 45

Effect of High-Dose Dexamethasone in Carcinomatous Metastatic Spinal Cord Compression Treated with Radiotherapy: A Randomised Trial

Sørensen S, Helweg-Larsen S, Mouridsen H, Hansen HH, Eur J Cancer. 1994;30A(1):22–27

Reviewed by Gordan Mao

Research Question/Objective To evaluate the effectiveness of high-dose dexamethasone as an adjunct treatment for patients with solid-tumor metastatic spinal cord compression treated with radiotherapy.

Study Design Single-blind, randomized controlled trial. Patients were allocated randomly to treatment with either high-dose dexamethasone or no steroidal treatment.

Sample Size 57 patients (18 male and 39 female) with a median age of 62 years (range 25–82) were randomized.

Follow-Up Ambulatory status at the end of radiotherapy, 3 weeks, 3 months, and then at intervals of 3 months for 2 years.

Inclusion/Exclusion Criteria

- Inclusion Criteria
  - A confirmed diagnosis of metastatic spinal cord compression via myelography or MRI
- Exclusion Criteria
  - Lymphoma
  - Previously treated epidural metastasis
  - Meningeal carcinomatosis
  - Infectious diseases

DOI: 10.1201/9781003416197-45

- Patients with diagnosed peptic ulcers (due to increased risk with steroid therapy)
- Patients who had undergone spinal surgical intervention for a tumor

Intervention or Treatment Received

- Patients in the high-dose dexamethasone arm received an intravenous (IV) bolus of 96 mg after MRI or myelography confirmed metastatic spinal cord compression, followed by 96 mg IV or oral dexamethasone for 3 days, divided into 4 doses per day, then tapered over 10 days in adjunct to radiotherapy.
- Patients in the no-steroid treatment arm received radiotherapy alone.
- The radiotherapy protocol included 6 MV photon beams in two parallel opposing anterior and posterior fields to cover one normal vertebra that was cranial and caudal to the block/cord compression on myelography/MRI. This was administered at a dose of 20 Gy in fractions of 4 Gy for 7 consecutive days, with the first dose within 1–20 hours after imaging.

Primary Endpoint Regaining ambulation in non-ambulatory patients or preservation of ambulation in ambulatory patients within 3 months.

Secondary Endpoint Survival after treatment.

Results A total of 57 patients were randomized, with 27 assigned to high-dose dexamethasone plus radiotherapy and 30 to radiotherapy alone. The interval between cancer diagnosis and the onset of spinal cord compression symptoms ranged widely from 0 to 17 years. Baseline characteristics, including age, sex, level of spinal cord compression, pretreatment gait function, and myelographic findings of complete vs partial block, were well balanced between the 2 groups.

At 3 months post-treatment, both gait preservation and restoration were more frequent in the high-dose dexamethasone group (81%) compared with the radiotherapy-alone group (63%). Notably, all patients who were ambulatory at baseline remained ambulatory in the dexamethasone arm, whereas 2 initially ambulatory patients in the no-dexamethasone arm lost gait function. Although ambulation declined in both groups by 6 months, a significantly greater proportion of patients remained ambulatory in the dexamethasone group (59% vs 33%). By 1 year, there was no difference between groups in ambulation or survival, with 30% of patients in the dexamethasone group and 20% in the radiotherapy-alone group remaining ambulatory.

Overall survival was poor and similar between groups, with a median survival of 6 months; only 3 patients were alive beyond 2 years after radiographic diagnosis. Subgroup analyses demonstrated that breast cancer was associated with a more favorable prognosis, with a significantly higher rate of ambulation success (82%) compared with other primary tumors (57%). Although ambulatory outcomes among breast cancer patients were higher in the dexamethasone group (94%) than in the no-dexamethasone group (69%), this difference did not reach statistical significance.

The thoracic spine was the most common site of epidural metastasis (21 patients), followed by the lumbar (11 patients) and cervical spine (1 patient). Gait function was present before treatment and preserved in all patients with lumbar involvement. Among patients with thoracic epidural metastases, gait preservation was substantially higher in the high-dose dexamethasone group (92%) compared with the radiotherapy-alone group (50%). Reported dexamethasone-related adverse effects included hyponatremia in one patient, psychosis in one patient, and a perforated gastric ulcer requiring surgery in one patient. Dexamethasone therapy was discontinued in patients who developed psychosis, a perforated ulcer, and in an additional patient with a systemic infection.

Conclusion High-dose glucocorticoid therapy, in conjunction with radiotherapy, may preserve or restore gait function and ambulation status in patients with metastatic epidural spinal cord compression but does not affect survival.

Reviewer Commentary The randomized trial by Sørensen and colleagues represents one of the earliest prospective studies to rigorously evaluate the role of high-dose corticosteroids in the acute management of metastatic spinal cord compression (MSCC). At a time when treatment strategies were largely empiric, this study provided critical evidence demonstrating that early administration of high-dose dexamethasone, in conjunction with prompt radiotherapy, significantly improved short-term gait preservation and restoration compared with radiotherapy alone. By selecting ambulation as the primary endpoint, the authors emphasized functional independence and quality of life as central outcomes in a patient population with limited life expectancy.

This work had substantial practice-changing implications. It helped establish corticosteroids as a standard early intervention in patients with suspected or radiographically confirmed MSCC, reinforcing the concept that MSCC constitutes a neurological emergency requiring immediate medical treatment. The study's findings directly influenced clinical algorithms in neurosurgery, oncology, and radiation oncology, where high-dose dexamethasone became widely adopted as part of first-line management.

Biological Rationale and Interpretation The early preservation or restoration of gait observed in the dexamethasone-treated cohort is most plausibly attributed to steroid-mediated reduction of spinal cord edema at the site of compression, thereby alleviating secondary ischemic injury and transiently improving spinal cord function. The transient nature of this benefit, diminishing beyond 6 months, provides important mechanistic insight, suggesting that corticosteroids do not meaningfully reduce tumor burden in solid epidural metastases. Lymphoma patients were excluded from the study, in whom corticosteroids are known to induce tumor cytoreduction.

Radiotherapy, delivered within hours of diagnosis using a total dose of 28 Gy in 4-Gy fractions over 7 consecutive days, likely contributed to delayed neurological improvement in both treatment arms by reducing tumor burden. This likely explains why some patients in the no-steroid group experienced partial gait recovery, albeit to a lesser degree than those receiving dexamethasone. The findings therefore highlight the complementary roles of immediate edema control with steroids and longer-term tumor control with radiotherapy.

Study Limitations Several limitations warrant consideration. The study's modest sample size limits statistical power, particularly for subgroup analyses. Gait function, the primary endpoint, was assessed by a single neurologist blinded to treatment allocation, but the authors did not specify the objective criteria or standardized testing used to evaluate ambulation. Additionally, the role of adjunctive therapies, such as physical or occupational therapy, was not reported, introducing potential confounding in functional outcomes.

The authors also did not provide data on the interval between symptom onset and diagnosis. Given the uniformly poor median survival of 6 months in both groups, delayed presentation with advanced systemic disease may have limited the potential impact of treatment on long-term neurological and survival outcomes. Furthermore, patients undergoing surgical decompression were excluded, precluding comparison with operative management and limiting conclusions regarding the relative benefits of medical vs surgical approaches. Criteria guiding surgical decision-making, including radiographic instability, were not discussed.

Steroid-related adverse effects, although infrequent, were clinically significant. Reported complications included hypomania, psychosis, gastrointestinal perforation requiring surgical intervention, and clinical deterioration due to systemic infection. These events underscore the narrow therapeutic window of high-dose dexamethasone and highlight the importance of balancing neurological benefit against systemic toxicity.

Relevant Studies

The findings of this trial were consistent with anecdotal reports and experimental observations cited by the authors suggesting a beneficial effect of steroids in MSCC.[1] However, uncertainty regarding optimal dosing remained. Subsequent studies, including those comparing different dexamethasone dosing regimens, failed to demonstrate clear differences in pain or ambulation outcomes, reinforcing concerns about escalating doses without proportional benefit.[2,3]

Since the publication of this study, treatment paradigms for MSCC have evolved substantially. Advances in surgical decision-making, including the development of the Spinal Instability Neoplastic Score, now provide structured guidance for identifying patients who may benefit from decompression and stabilization.[4]

In parallel, modern radiotherapy techniques such as stereotactic body radiotherapy (SBRT) have emerged as promising alternatives or adjuncts to conventional external beam radiotherapy, offering improved local control in selected patients.[4,5] These developments have prompted renewed interest in defining the role of dexamethasone within a contemporary multimodal treatment framework.[2,3,6]

Summary In summary, although high-dose dexamethasone did not confer a survival advantage, this landmark study demonstrated that early neurological function could be preserved or restored in patients with MSCC. Its lasting contribution lies in establishing corticosteroids as a foundational component of acute management and in framing MSCC as a neurological emergency requiring rapid, coordinated intervention.

REFERENCES

1. Versteeg AL, Elkaim LM, Sahgal A, et al. Steroids in the management of preoperative neurological deficits in metastatic spine disease: results from the EPOSO study. Neurospine. 2022;19(1):43–50.
2. Graham PH, Capp A, Delaney G, et al. A pilot randomised comparison of dexamethasone 96 mg vs 16 mg per day for malignant spinal-cord compression treated by radiotherapy: TROG 01.05 Superdex study. Clin Oncol (R Coll Radiol). 2006;18(1):70–76.
3. Jawad MS, Fahim DK, Gerszten PC, et al. Vertebral compression fractures after stereotactic body radiation therapy: a large, multi-institutional, multinational evaluation. J Neurosurg Spine. 2016;24(6):928–936.
4. Fisher CG, DiPaola CP, Ryken TC, et al. A novel classification system for spinal instability in neoplastic disease: an evidence-based approach and expert consensus from the Spine Oncology Study Group. Spine (Phila Pa 1976). 2010;35(22):E1221–E1229. doi:10.1097/BRS.0b013e3181e16ae2
5. Ito K, Ogawa H, Shimizuguchi T, et al. Stereotactic body radiotherapy for spinal metastases: clinical experience in 134 cases from a single Japanese Institution. Technol Cancer Res Treat. 2018;17:1533033818806472.
6. Skeoch GD, Tobin MK, Khan S, Linninger AA, Mehta AI. Corticosteroid treatment for metastatic spinal cord compression: a review. Global Spine J. 2017;7(3):272–279.

CHAPTER 46

Direct Decompressive Surgical Resection in the Treatment of Spinal Cord Compression Caused by Metastatic Cancer: A Randomised Trial

Patchell RA, Tibbs PA, Regine WF, Payne R, Saris S, Kryscio RJ, Mohiuddin M, Young B, Lancet. 2005 Aug;366(9486):643–648

Reviewed by Obeng-Gyasi, Barnabas, Miracle Anokwute, and Gordan Mao

Research Question/Objective To assess the efficacy of direct decompressive surgery followed by radiotherapy compared to radiotherapy alone in patients with metastatic epidural spinal cord compression (MESCC).

Study Design This was a randomized, multi-institutional, non-blinded trial that included two treatment groups: one receiving direct decompressive surgery followed by radiotherapy, and the other receiving radiotherapy alone.

All patients underwent magnetic resonance imaging (MRI) of the entire spinal cord, including whole spine sagittal T1 (thoracic vertebra) and T2 imaging and axial T1 imaging. The imaging was centrally reviewed to confirm MESCC. Upon diagnosis, all patients received an initial dose of 100 mg dexamethasone followed by 24 mg every 6 hours until the start of radiotherapy or surgery. For patients with severe diabetes or other contraindications, reduced corticosteroid doses were administered as appropriate.

Patients were stratified by treating institution, tumor type, ambulatory status, and spinal stability, which was assessed according to Cybulski's guidelines. Randomization within strata was performed using permuted blocks at each institution with a computerized technique to ensure immediate allocation at study entry.

Sample Size 101 patients were randomized (50 to surgery + radiotherapy, 51 to radiotherapy alone).

DOI: 10.1201/9781003416197-46

Inclusion/Exclusion Criteria

- Inclusion Criteria
  - Patients aged 18 or older with a tissue-proven diagnosis of cancer (excluding central nervous systems CNS or spinal column origin) and MRI evidence of MESCC
  - One neurological sign or symptom (e.g. pain), with the symptomatic MESCC restricted to a single area (including contiguous spinal or vertebral segments)
  - An expected survival of at least 3 months and be in sufficient health to be considered surgical candidates

- Exclusion Criteria – Patients with:
  - Highly radiosensitive tumors (e.g. lymphoma, leukemia, multiple myeloma, and germ-cell tumors)
  - Multiple discrete compressive lesions
  - Multiple non-compressive lesions
  - Total paraplegia for over 48 hours
  - Previous MESCC
  - Prior spinal radiation
  - Pre-existing or concomitant neurological dysfunction not directly related to their MESCC

Intervention or Treatment Received

- *Radiotherapy group*: Patients began radiotherapy within 24 hours of randomization, receiving a total dose of 30 Gy in ten fractions (3 Gy per fraction). Treatment ports encompassed one vertebral body above and below the visible lesion. Radiotherapy treatment plans were centrally reviewed to ensure protocol compliance.
- *Surgery group*: Surgery was performed within 24 hours of randomization, aiming for immediate direct circumferential decompression of the spinal cord. The surgical approach was tailored to the tumor's location, with anterior, lateral, or posterior approaches as needed. Spinal stabilization was performed if instability was present, using cement, metallic rods, bone grafting, or other fixation devices. Post-surgery, patients received radiotherapy within 14 days, following the same schedule as the radiotherapy group. Steroid administration was consistent across both groups.

Outcome Measures

- *Primary endpoint*: The ability to walk post-treatment. Ambulatory status was assessed by the patient's ability to take at least two steps with each foot unassisted, even if using a cane or walker.

- *Secondary endpoints*: Included urinary continence, changes in Frankel functional scale scores, American Spinal Injury Association (ASIA) motor scores, use of corticosteroids and opioid analgesics, and survival time. Neurological assessments were conducted before treatment, weekly during radiotherapy, and at regular intervals post-treatment for up to 2 years.

Statistical Analysis The study used an intention-to-treat analysis throughout. Multivariate analyses were based on a Cox regression model, incorporating covariates such as treatment group, age, sex, primary tumor type, spinal level involved, position of metastasis, spinal stability, Frankel and ASIA scores at entry, duration of motor symptoms, and time between primary tumor diagnosis and cord compression development. Sample size calculations assumed a 20% difference in post-treatment ambulatory rates between groups, with an interim analysis planned at the halfway point of the trial.

Monitoring and Compliance Operative reports and post-surgery radiotherapy plans were reviewed within 1 month to monitor compliance. Regular follow-up assessments were conducted every 4 weeks until the end of the trial or the patient's death.

Results In this randomized trial, 101 patients with metastatic spinal cord compression were assigned to receive either surgical decompression followed by radiotherapy ($n = 50$) or radiotherapy alone ($n = 51$). Functional outcomes strongly favored the combined treatment approach. Post-treatment ambulation was achieved in 84% of patients undergoing surgery plus radiotherapy, compared with 57% of those treated with radiotherapy alone. Moreover, the durability of ambulation differed markedly between groups, with a median duration of 122 days in the surgical cohort versus only 13 days in the radiotherapy-only group.

Importantly, surgical intervention demonstrated substantial benefit even among patients who were non-ambulatory at presentation. In this subgroup, 62% of patients treated with surgery plus radiotherapy regained the ability to walk, compared with just 19% in the radiotherapy group. Secondary endpoints further underscored the functional advantages of surgery, with significant improvements in urinary continence, muscle strength, and overall functional status, as well as reduced reliance on corticosteroids and opioid analgesics. Median survival was modestly but significantly longer in the surgical group (126 days) compared with the radiotherapy group (100 days), supporting the role of surgical decompression as a means of improving both quality of life and clinical outcomes in appropriately selected patients.

Conclusion Direct decompressive surgery followed by radiotherapy is superior to radiotherapy alone for treating MESCC, leading to better ambulation outcomes, functional status, and longer survival times.

Reviewer Commentary The study by Patchell et al. is pivotal in shifting the treatment paradigm for MESCC, traditionally managed with corticosteroids and radiotherapy. The clear superiority of direct decompressive surgery combined with radiotherapy in improving ambulation, functional status, and survival highlights the need for a more aggressive surgical approach in appropriately selected candidates.

The significant difference in post-treatment ambulation rates (84% in the surgery group versus 57% in the radiotherapy group) underscores the efficacy of direct decompressive surgery in providing immediate relief from spinal cord compression. This immediate decompression is crucial in preventing irreversible spinal cord injury, which radiotherapy alone cannot achieve promptly.[1] Subsequent studies, such as the meta-analysis by Lee et al.[2] and the elderly patient cohort studied by Itshayek et al.,[3] have corroborated these findings, emphasizing the role of surgery in preserving neurological function.

Careful patient selection is essential to optimize outcomes, considering factors such as the extent of spinal cord compression, overall health status, and expected survival. The decision framework developed by Fisher et al.[4] based on tumor type, neurological status, spinal stability, and predicted survival, provides a useful tool for identifying surgical candidates. This framework shares similarities with the widely used NOMS (Neurologic, Oncologic, Mechanical stability, Systemic disease) framework developed at Memorial Sloan-Kettering Cancer Center for decision-making in spinal metastasis treatment. The NOMS framework integrates these four fundamental assessments to determine the optimal use of radiation, surgery, and/or systemic therapy.[5] However, further refinement of these criteria based on emerging prognostic factors, such as those identified by Ju et al. [6] and Chaichana et al.,[7] could help tailor treatment decisions more precisely. Specifically, Ju et al. found that for patients with castration-resistant prostate cancer, a Karnofsky Performance Status (KPS) ≥80% was independently associated with better survival outcomes after surgery. Chaichana et al. identified that preoperative ability to walk, pathological vertebral compression fracture, symptoms present for less than 48 hours, and postoperative radiotherapy were significant factors associated with postoperative ambulatory status.

The reduction in corticosteroid and opioid use with surgery is particularly noteworthy, as it may mitigate the significant side effects and long-term complications associated with these medications. However, the optimal dose and duration of steroid therapy in MESCC remain controversial. While some studies suggest a benefit of high-dose steroids,[8] others have found no advantage over moderate doses.[9] Judicious use of steroids, guided by patient-specific factors and treatment goals, is warranted until more definitive evidence emerges.

The Patchell study's multi-institutional design enhances the generalizability of its findings, but the potential for bias in this non-blinded trial must be acknowledged. Future studies with blinded assessments and larger sample sizes could provide more robust evidence. Additionally, long-term follow-up data would be valuable to assess the durability of the functional and survival benefits observed.

This study set the stage for further research into optimizing surgical techniques, radiation dose/fractionation, and the integration of novel systemic therapies. The advent of stereotactic body radiation therapy and minimally invasive surgical approaches holds promise for improving local control and reducing morbidity.[10,11] Cost-effectiveness analyses, such as that by Furlan et al.,[12] can help inform resource allocation and treatment guidelines. Ongoing multidisciplinary collaboration and prospective trials[13,14] are crucial to refine patient selection, treatment paradigms, and survivorship care for this complex patient population.

REFERENCES

1. Itshayek E, Candanedo C, Fraifeld S, Hasharoni A, Kaplan L, Schroeder JE, Cohen JE. Ambulation and survival following surgery in elderly patients with metastatic epidural spinal cord compression. Spine J. 2018;18(7):1211–1221.
2. Gok B, McGirt M, Sciubba DM, Ayhan S, Bydon A, Witham TF, Wolinsky JP, Gokaslan ZL. Surgical resection plus adjuvant radiotherapy is superior to surgery or radiotherapy alone in the prevention of neurological decline in a rat metastatic spinal tumor model. Neurosurgery. 2008;63(2):346–351.
3. Lee CH, Kwon JW, Lee J, Hyun SJ, Kim KJ, Jahng TA, Kim HJ. Direct decompressive surgery followed by radiotherapy versus radiotherapy alone for metastatic epidural spinal cord compression: a meta-analysis. Spine. 2014;39(9):E587–E592.
4. Fisher CG, DiPaola CP, Ryken TC, et al. A novel classification system for spinal instability in neoplastic disease: an evidence-based approach and expert consensus from the Spine Oncology Study Group. Spine. 2010;35(22):E1221–E1229.
5. Laufer I, Rubin DG, Lis E, Cox BW, Stubblefield MD, Yamada Y, Bilsky MH. The NOMS framework: approach to the treatment of spinal metastatic tumors. Oncologist. 2013;18(6):744–751.
6. Ju DG, Zadnik PL, Groves ML, Hwang L, Kaloostian PE, Wolinksy JP, Witham TF, Bydon A, Gokaslan ZL, Sciubba, DM. Factors associated with improved outcomes following decompressive surgery for prostate cancer metastatic to the spine. Neurosurgery. 2013;73(4):657–666.
7. Chaichana KL, Woodworth GF, Sciubba DM, McGirt MJ, Witham TJ, Bydon A, Wolinsky JP, Gokaslan Z. Predictors of ambulatory function after decompressive surgery for metastatic epidural spinal cord compression. Neurosurgery. 2008;62(3):683–692.
8. Furlan JC, Chan KK, Sandoval GA, Lam KC, Klinger CA, Patchell RA, Laporte A, Fehlings MG. The combined use of surgery and radiotherapy to treat patients with epidural cord compression due to metastatic disease: a cost-utility analysis. Neuro Oncol. 2012;14(5):631–640.
9. Sørensen S, Helweg-Larsen S, Mouridsen H, Hansen HH. Effect of high-dose dexamethasone in carcinomatous metastatic spinal cord compression treated with radiotherapy: a randomised trial. Eur J Cancer. 1994;30(1):22–27.
10. Vecht CJ, Haaxma-Reiche H, van Putten WL, de Visser M, Vries EP, Twijnstra A. Initial bolus of conventional versus high-dose dexamethasone in metastatic spinal cord compression. Neurology. 1989;39(9):1255–1257.
11. Jawad MS, Fahim DK, Gerszten PC, Flickinger JC, Sahgal A, Grills IS, Sheehan, J, Kersh R, Shin J, Oh K, Mantel F, Guckenberger M. Vertebral compression fractures after stereotactic body radiation therapy: a large, multi-institutional, multinational evaluation. J Neurosurg Spine. 2016;24(6):928–936.

12. Ito K, Ogawa H, Shimizuguchi T, Nihei K, Furuya T, Tanaka H, Karasawa K. Stereotactic body radiotherapy for spinal metastases: clinical experience in 134 cases from a single Japanese institution. Technol Cancer Res Treat. 2018;17:1533033818806472.
13. Spratt DE, Beeler WH, de Moraes FY, Rhines LD, Gemmete JJ, Chaudhary N, Shultz DB, Smith SR, Berlin A, Dahele M, Slotman BJ, Younge KC, Bilsky M, Park P, Szerlip NJ. An integrated multidisciplinary algorithm for the management of spinal metastases: an International Spine Oncology Consortium report. Lancet Oncol. 2017;18(12):e720–e730.
14. Lawton AJ, Lee KA, Cheville AL, Ferrone ML, Rades D, Balboni TA, Abrahm JL. Assessment and management of patients with metastatic spinal cord compression: a multidisciplinary review. J Clin Oncol. 2019;37(1):61–71.

CHAPTER 47

Surgical vs Nonoperative Treatment for Lumbar Disc Herniation: The Spine Patient Outcomes Research Trial (SPORT): A Randomized Trial

Weinstein JN, Tosteson TD, Lurie JD, Tosteson AN, Hanscom B, Skinner JS, Abdu WA, Hilibrand AS, Boden SD, Deyo RA. 2006 Nov 22;296(20):2441–2450

Reviewed by Thomas Noh, Dilon Putzler, and Meng Huang

Research Question/Objective This study reports the results of a prospective, multicenter trial with both randomized and observational cohorts designed to compare outcomes between the surgical and nonsurgical management of lumbar intervertebral disk herniation, spinal stenosis, or degenerative spondylolisthesis.

Study Design Prospective, multicenter, randomized controlled study.

Sample Size 1,244 patients were enrolled in the trial, with 743 in the observational cohort and 501 in the randomized cohort. In the randomized cohort, 245 were placed in the surgical arm with a standard discectomy and nerve root examination as the selected intervention. 256 were placed in the nonoperative arm.

Follow-Up 6 weeks, 3 and 6 months, 1 and 2 years.

Inclusion/Exclusion Criteria

- Inclusion Criteria
  - Age 18–65 years old
  - Diagnosis: Lumbar disc herniation confirmed by magnetic resonance imaging or computed tomography
  - Symptoms: Radicular pain (leg pain) consistent with the imaging findings
  - Symptoms duration: At least 6 weeks of persistent symptoms
  - Neurological signs: Presence of objective neurological deficits consistent with the affected nerve root

DOI: 10.1201/9781003416197-47

- Exclusion Criteria
  - Cauda equina syndrome or progressive neurological deficits
  - Prior lumbar surgery at the affected level
  - Spondylolisthesis/instability or significant deformity
  - Severe medical conditions conferring increased surgical risk
  - Active infection or malignancy
  - Pregnancy
  - Work-related compensation claims

Methods Beginning in March 2000, 2,720 patients aged 18+ with a diagnosis of intervertebral disk herniation were screened for enrolment at 13 spine practices in 11 states (California, Georgia, Illinois, Maine, Michigan, Missouri, Nebraska, New York, New Hampshire, Ohio, and Pennsylvania). 1,244 patients met the criteria for enrollment as stated above. Data was analyzed utilizing both intent-to-treat and as-treated analysis. The Medical Outcomes Study 36-Item Short Form Health Survey (SF-36) bodily pain and physical function scales and the American Academy of Orthopaedic Surgeons Musculoskeletal Outcomes Data Evaluation and Management System version of the Oswestry Disability Index (ODI), measured at 6 weeks, 3 and 6 months, and 1 and 2 years, were used as primary outcome measures. The Sciatica Bothersomeness Index was a secondary measure used to assess pain and disease impact on functional status.

Results In the randomized arm, 471 patients with a mean age of 42 years completed at least one follow-up and were included in the data analysis. The majority of patients were employed, white males. L5-S1 posterior-lateral herniations were the most common (61%). All patients had radicular leg pain, with 97% in classic dermatomal distributions. Treatments were not standardized in the nonoperative arm. They consisted of education (93%), anti-inflammatory medication (61%), epidural injections (50%), opioid medications (46%), physical therapy (44%), and/or activity restriction (29%). The average operative time in the surgical arm was 75 minutes, with no perioperative mortalities. 95% of patients had no complications; Dural tear was the most common complication (4%). The surgical and nonsurgical arms showed significant improvement in the SF-36 score, Oswestry Disability Index, and sciatica indices at each follow-up.

Using the intent-to-treat analysis, the surgical arm improved to a greater degree than the nonoperative arm, but this improvement was not statistically significant. The surgical arm showed a statistically significant improvement in the Sciatica Bothersomeness Index, a measure of secondary outcome, at 3 months, 1 year, and 2 years. Recontextualizing the data using the as-treated analysis showed statistically significant improvement in primary measures with surgical treatment at all follow-ups.

In the observational cohort, most patients in the surgical group (91%) had the procedure completed, with 22% of the nonsurgical arm crossing over to surgical treatment by 2 years. Patients in the surgical cohort rated their symptoms as progressively worsening. In the observational cohort, much like the randomized cohort, both the surgical and nonoperative groups showed improvement in primary measures. The surgical arm showed statistically significant improvement over the nonoperative arm. However, the difference in improvement between the two groups narrowed by a 2-year follow-up while remaining statistically significant.

Analysis of the patient population that crossed over to surgical treatment demonstrated that these patients were more likely to be of lower income, worse baseline status, more disability as measured by the ODI, and were more likely to self-report their symptoms as worsening. Conversely, those most likely to switch over to the nonoperative group were found to be older on average, with higher incomes, less baseline pain and ODI disability, as well as self-perceived improvement in pain. Additionally, these patients more commonly had an upper lumbar disc herniation and a negative straight-raise examination.

Conclusion Patients in both the surgery and the nonoperative treatment groups improved substantially over a 2-year period. Because of the large numbers of patients who crossed over in both directions, conclusions about the superiority or equivalence of the treatments are not warranted based on the intent-to-treat analysis.

Author/Reviewer Commentary The SPORT trial by Weinstein and colleagues was a landmark study because it rigorously addressed one of the most common and controversial questions in spine care: whether surgery provides superior outcomes to nonoperative management for lumbar disk herniation. As the largest multicenter, randomized and observational trial in this domain, SPORT demonstrated that patients undergoing discectomy experienced rapid and, over time, improvements in pain relief and functional outcomes that are comparable with those treated nonoperatively.

Relevant Studies The SPORT trial significantly improved on previous works, such as the Maine Lumbar Spine Study and other works conducted by Malmivaara et al. and Weber, by increasing sample size and geographic distribution and using validated disability tools. Although subject to debate, this prospective study's randomized cohort demonstrated significant improvement in the surgical and nonoperative arms over 2 years.[1] The improvement in the surgical group was greater at all points of follow-up, but this finding was not statistically significant, suggesting equal effectiveness between the two groups. For secondary measures (Sciatica Bothersome Index, satisfaction with symptoms, and self-rated progress), surgery showed a statistically significant improvement over the nonoperative treatment in the Sciatica Bothersome Index and self-measured progress. The as-treated analysis demonstrated significant improvements over nonoperative treatments at all follow-up points.

The difference in result between the intent-to-treat and as-treated analyses is the most striking finding of the trial. In any intent-to-treat trial, participants are randomized, and statistical analysis is conducted based on the originally assigned groups, regardless of whether participants adhered to treatment. The large, bidirectional crossover in the SPORT trial (i.e. operative arm to nonoperative and vice versa) complicates data analysis, likely obscuring the differences in outcomes between treatment arms. The main advantage of the intent-to-treat analysis is eliminating systematic bias when implemented correctly, a protective effect that is not preserved when data is analyzed via the as-treated protocol. The key takeaway from the data analysis in the SPORT trial and other trials with a large crossover between treatment arms is to interpret results with a healthy dose of skepticism, as the true efficacy (or inferiority) of treatments may be misrepresented.

Surgical intervention was shown to be a safe intervention with low mortality and complication rates. Dural tear was the common complication, occurring in 4% of cases. With the evolution of surgical procedures following the SPORT trial, comparisons of post-operative outcomes are inevitable. However, the literature has continually shown similar complication rates between open discectomy and comparatively newer techniques, such as microdiscectomy.[2–4] Studies evaluating open vs endoscopic discectomy have been mixed, with most studies suggesting minimal or no difference in outcomes.[5,6] More research is needed to more accurately assess the differences between surgical approaches.

Timing is a consideration that could use future study. A randomized control trial from the Hague Spine Intervention Prognostic Study Group gave some insight into this by selecting patients with symptoms ranging from 6 to 12 weeks and treating patients in the surgical arm early, resulting in high adherence to the surgical arm.[7] The outcomes between surgical and nonoperative arms did equalize near the 1-year mark by multiple disability indices (Roland Disability Questionnaire, Likert scale, and the visual-analog scale for leg pain). However, the relief of leg pain was faster for patients assigned to early surgery and patients assigned to early surgery reported a faster rate of perceived recovery. This should be an important variable, particularly in regard to quality of life and the potential impact on time off from work for future studies.

Study Limitations The primary limitation of this study relates to the significant crossover between surgical and nonoperative treatment groups in the randomized cohort. By 3 months, 30% of the nonoperative group had crossed over to surgical treatment. This number increased to 45% at 2-year follow-up. Only 40% of the surgical group had undergone the procedure by 2 years. The high crossover between treatment groups increases the risks of bias toward the null and potentially confounds data analysis by underestimating the true efficacy of surgical treatment. Additionally, to be included in this study, patients must have already failed 6 weeks of nonoperative treatment, potentially skewing the results to favor the operative arm.

The lack of standardization in the nonoperative arm also limited the interpretation of the results. While all nonoperative treatments followed published guidelines, standardization was limited by variance in patient preference and individual responses to treatment. For example, medications used in the nonoperative group ranged from

NSAIDs, COX-2 inhibitors, oral steroids, narcotics, or muscle relaxants based solely on patient and provider preference, with adjunct treatment modalities ranging from braces to injections to acupuncturists in some cases. This complicated the head-to-head comparison between groups, as "operative vs nonoperative treatment" is a significantly more complicated question than "operative vs nonoperative treatment with physical therapy and NSAIDs" per a specific protocol. This limitation results in the inability to compare surgical treatment to any specific form of nonoperative treatment.

Summary The SPORT trial was a landmark study that established discectomy as providing fast and durable improvement in pain and function for lumbar disk herniation, while also confirming that many patients improve with nonoperative care alone. By revealing the significant impact of treatment crossover and patient preference, the trial reshaped the interpretation of surgical randomized studies. Its lasting contribution is the reinforcement of individualized, evidence-based shared decision-making in the management of lumbar disk herniation.

REFERENCES

1. Weinstein JN, Tosteson TD, Lurie JD, et al. Surgical vs nonoperative treatment for lumbar disk herniation. JAMA. 2006;296(20):2441–2450. doi:10.1001/jama.296.20.2441
2. Tullberg T, Isacson J, Weidenhielm L. Does microscopic removal of lumbar disc herniation lead to better results than the standard procedure? Results of a one-year randomized study. Spine (Phila Pa 1976). 1993;18(1):24–27. doi:10.1097/00007632-199301000-00005
3. Katayama Y, Matsuyama Y, Yoshihara H, et al. Comparison of surgical outcomes between macro discectomy and micro discectomy for lumbar disc herniation: a prospective randomized study with surgery performed by the same spine surgeon. J Spinal Disord Tech. 2006;19(5):344–347. doi:10.1097/01.bsd.0000211201.93125.1c
4. Henriksen L, Schmidt K, Eskesen V, Jantzen E. A controlled study of microsurgical versus standard lumbar discectomy. Br J Neurosurg. 1996;10(3):289–293. doi:10.1080/02688699650040160
5. Barber SM, Nakhla J, Konakondla S, et al. Outcomes of endoscopic discectomy compared with open microdiscectomy and tubular microdiscectomy for lumbar disc herniations: a meta-analysis. J Neurosurg. 2019;31:802–815. doi:10.3171/2019.6.SPINE19532
6. Page PS, Ammanuel SG, Josiah DT. Evaluation of endoscopic versus open lumbar discectomy: a multi-center retrospective review utilizing the American College of Surgeons' National Surgical Quality Improvement Program (ACS-NSQIP) Database. Cureus. 2022;14(5):e25202. doi:10.7759/cureus.25202
7. Peul WC, van Houwelingen HC, van den Hout WB, et al. Surgery versus prolonged conservative treatment for sciatica. N Engl J Med. 2007;356(22):2245–2256. doi:10.1056/NEJMoa064039

Chapter 48

Cauda Equina Syndrome Secondary to Lumbar Disc Herniation: A Meta-Analysis of Surgical Outcomes

Ahn UM, Ahn NU, Buchowski JM, Garrett ES, Sieber AN, Kostuik JP, Spine (Phila Pa 1976). 2000 Jun 15;25(12):1515–1522

Reviewed by Brandon Lane

Research Question/Objective To determine the relationship between time to decompression after onset of cauda equina syndrome (CES) and clinical outcome, and to identify preoperative variables that were associated with clinical outcomes.

Study Design Meta-analysis.

Sample Size 104 citations were reviewed, with 42 that met the inclusion criteria. Outcomes were then analyzed in 322 patients from these citations.

Follow-Up Range from months to years.

Inclusion/Exclusion Criteria

- Inclusion Criteria
  - A MEDLINE search was performed for CES caused by a herniated lumbar disc from January 1966 through May 1999.
  - Studies were eligible for inclusion if they involved a clinical study of human patients with CES caused by a herniated lumbar disc.
  - Each patient from each study had to provide at least one pre- and one postoperative variable to be included in this study.
  - All patients included were treated with surgical decompression. Preoperative and postoperative variables were defined by the authors.

- Excusion Criteria
  - Articles evaluating CES by other causes were excluded. Patients in this study were drawn from the eligible articles.

Intervention or Treatment Received Surgical decompression for CES caused by a herniated lumbar disc.

DOI: 10.1201/9781003416197-48

Table 48.1 Preoperative Variables

- Age
- Gender
- Laborer occupation
- History of previous spine surgery
- History of chronic low back pain
- Duration of chronic low back pain prior to CES
- History of trauma with onset of CES
- Sudden onset of CES
- Presence of sciatica with CES
- Preoperative weakness in lower extremities
- Preoperative sensory deficit
- Preoperative loss of reflexes
- Preoperative rectal dysfunction
- Length of time to surgery from onset of CES

Abbreviation: CES, cauda equina syndrome.

Results This meta-analysis analyzes 322 patients, who were pulled from 42 articles meeting the inclusion/exclusion criteria above. Tables 48.1 and 48.2 from the article summarize the pre- and postoperative variables assessed.

The analysis was done in two parts. The first consisted of regressing postoperative outcomes on the preoperative variables with time to surgery excluded. A multivariate logistics regression was attempted to control for confounding but was unsuccessful as the majority of patients had only a few of the pre- and postoperative variables reported. Univariate logistic regression analyses were utilized and odds ratios, *p*-values, 95% confidence intervals, and the number of patients included in regression were reported for each of the six postoperative outcomes regressed on the 13 preoperative variables.

Significant associations included a worsened prognosis for urinary continence in patients who had a history of preoperative chronic low back pain or in patients with preoperative rectal dysfunction. The prognosis for rectal function after surgery worsened with a history of chronic low back pain. In addition, older patients had a worsened prognosis for the resolution of sexual dysfunction. The prognosis for the return of sensory deficit after surgery worsened with a history of preoperative rectal dysfunction.

The second analysis compared the time to decompression with each of the six postoperative outcomes. Time to decompression was initially divided into five

Table 48.2 Postoperative Variables

- Resolution of pain
- Resolution of sensory deficit
- Resolution of motor deficit
- Resolution of urinary incontinence
- Resolution of sexual dysfunction
- Resolution of rectal dysfunction

categories: <24 hours, 24–48 hours, 2–10 days, 11 days to 1 month, and more than a month. There was no significant difference in outcome among the three groups greater than 48 hours. There was no significant difference between the <24-hour group and the 24–28-hour group. There were significant differences between the <24-hour group and the >48-hour group, and the 24–28-hour group and the >48-hour group. Therefore, a univariate regression was performed for each postoperative outcome comparing <48 hours and >48 hours to surgery. There was a significant improvement in resolution of sensory deficit, resolution of motor deficit, resolution of urinary incontinence, and resolution of rectal dysfunction when decompression was performed within 48 hours compared with after 48 hours. Specifically, those patients who had surgery >48 hours after symptom onset were at 2.5 × risk of continued urinary deficit, 9.1 × risk of continued motor deficit, 9.1 × risk of continued rectal dysfunction, and 3.5 × risk of continued sensory deficit.

Conclusion There was a significant advantage to treating patients within 48 hours vs more than 48 hours after the onset of cauda equina syndrome. A significant improvement in sensory and motor deficits, as well as urinary and rectal function, occurred in patients who underwent decompression within 48 hours vs after 48 hours.

Reviewer Commentary Cauda equina syndrome (CES) is a complex of low back pain, bilateral sciatica, saddle anesthesia, lower extremity motor weakness, and rectal and urinary incontinence. However, like most clinical disease states, CES manifests as a spectrum of disorders which can include all or some of the elements above. While it occurs in only 2% of cases of herniated lumbar discs, large studies have been limited. Previous reports suggested a benefit to early decompression but largely lacked power to demonstrate significance. This study attempted to confirm or refute the conclusion by previous investigators that decompression performed within 48 hours of the onset of CES resulted in improved postoperative functional outcomes. This meta-analysis was performed to improve the statistical power of the available data in the literature, and it demonstrates a significant improvement in sensory and motor deficits as well as urinary and rectal function in patients who underwent decompression within 48 hours vs after 48 hours. This landmark paper provided the strongest evidence for earlier surgical intervention in CES.

Study Limitations (1) Wide range in reported follow-ups, spanning months to years, which may not account for patients with improvements after the last recorded follow-up. (2) Variability in types of surgical decompression performed, including hemilaminectomy, wide laminectomy, and intradural surgery, which could all contribute to different outcomes. (3) Information from the available studies was insufficient to control coexisting diseases such as spondylosis and spinal stenosis. (4) In meta-analysis, different studies report data in different ways, which leads to incomplete data and a lack of standardization across variables.

Relevant Studies Cauda equina syndrome (CES) was first described by Mixter and Barr[1] in the *New England Journal of Medicine* in 1934. Subsequent reports noted that the onset of CES is heralded by disturbances in urinary or rectal function.[2] As such, the development of urinary dysfunction is the measure defining the onset of CES in this meta-analysis. Notably, though, urinary symptoms in CES can be varied and include altered urethral sensation, poor stream, and urinary retention, as reported by Nielsen et al.[3] Several authors, including Shapiro, reported on the resolution of urinary disturbances in CES cases treated surgically within 48 hours.[4] Specifically, in his first series, of the 10 patients who had no incontinence after surgery, 7 underwent surgery within 48 hours of onset. Of the 4 patients with persistent incontinence, all underwent surgery after 48 hours. Based on these results, Shapiro subsequently published a retrospective chi 2 analysis of 44 patients surgically treated for CES due to lumbar disc herniation.[5] The statistically significant results of this study demonstrated a greater chance of persistent bladder/sphincter problem ($p = 0.008$), persistent severe motor deficit ($p = 0.006$), persistent pain ($p = 0.025$), and sexual dysfunction ($p = 0.006$) in those patients surgically treated >48 hours after CES onset.

This set the stage for the development of this meta-analysis to further investigate the postoperative functional outcomes in CES patients in an effort to improve the statistical power of the available data. As summarized above, this analysis supported significant outcome advantages to treating patients within 48 hours.

Subsequent studies have highlighted the heterogeneity in definitions and clinical presentations of CES. In a comprehensive literature review by Fraser, 17 different definitions for CES were identified.[6] No single aspect of CES within the literature achieved unanimity or consensus, but a majority view indicated that there would be bladder and sensory disturbance (74% and 66% of all articles, respectively). Fraser then proposed the following as a single definition of CES. One or more of the following must be present: (1) bladder and/or bowel dysfunction, (2) reduced sensation in the saddle area, and (3) sexual dysfunction, with possible neurologic deficit in the lower limb (motor/sensory loss, reflex change). Despite Fraser's efforts to provide a singular definition of CES, substantial controversy still exists in reporting CES definitions and a start point for the time to surgery. A systematic review in 2023 noted that only 14.5% of the 110 studies reviewed utilized previously established definitions of CES, such as the Fraser criteria (or British Association of Spine, or Gleave and MacFarlane).[7]

While there is no uniform definition for CES, it is recognized as a condition that results from the compression of nerves in the lumbosacral spinal canal, whose most commonly cited etiology is lumbar disk herniation.[8] It is also clear that this clinical phenomenon exists on a spectrum with a wide variance in radiographic and clinical presentation from one individual to another. Recognizing this broad variance has led to difficulties in standardized reporting. Although there is discordance in the literature on the definition of CES and optimal timing of surgery, there is a growing consensus that biologic systems deteriorate in a continuous rather than stepwise manner.[9] Earlier surgical intervention will therefore provide more beneficial effects for compressed nerves, especially with acute neurologic compromise.

REFERENCES

1. Mixter WJ, Barr JS. Rupture of the intervertebral disc with involvement of the spinal canal. N Engl J Med. 1934;211:210–214.
2. Love JG, Emmet JL. “Asymptomatic” protruded lumbar disk as a cause of urinary retention: Preliminary report. Mayo Clin Proc. 1967;42:249–257.
3. Nielsen B, de Nully M, Schmidt K, et al. A urodynamic study of cauda equina syndrome due to lumbar disc herniation. Urol Int. 1980;35:167–170.
4. Shapiro S. Cauda equina syndrome secondary to lumbar disc herniation. Neurosurg. 1993;32:743–747.
5. Shapiro S. Medical realities of cauda equina syndrome secondary to lumbar disc herniation. Spine. 2000;25:348–352.
6. Fraser S, Roberts L, Murphy E. Cauda equina syndrome: a literature review of its definition and clinical presentation. Arch Phys Med Rehabil. 2009;90(11):1964–1968. doi:10.1016/j.apmr.2009.03.021
7. Mustafa MA, Richardson GE, Gillespie CS, Islim AI, Wilby M, Clark S, Srikandarajah N. Definition and surgical timing in cauda equina syndrome-An updated systematic review. PLoS One. 2023;18(5):e0285006. doi:10.1371/journal.pone.0285006
8. Kuris EO, McDonald CL, Palumbo MA, Daniels AH. Evaluation and management of cauda equina syndrome. Am J Med. 2021;134(12):1483–1489. doi:10.1016/j.amjmed.2021.07.021
9. Chau AM, Xu LL, Pelzer NR, Gragnaniello C. Timing of surgical intervention in cauda equina syndrome: a systematic critical review. World Neurosurg. 2014;81(3–4):640–650. doi:10.1016/j.wneu.2013.11.007

CHAPTER 49

Surgical vs Nonsurgical Therapy for Lumbar Spinal Stenosis

Weinstein JN, Tosteson TD, Lurie JD, Tosteson AN, Blood E, Hanscom B, Herkowitz H, Cammisa F, Albert T, Boden SD, Hilibrand A, Goldberg H, Berven S, An H; SPORT Investigators, N Engl J Med. 2008 Feb 21;358(8):794–810

Reviewed by Thomas Noh and Meng Huang

Research Question/Objective To determine the comparative effectiveness of surgical decompression vs nonsurgical management for patients with lumbar spinal stenosis in terms of pain relief, functional outcomes, and overall patient satisfaction.

Study Design The Spine Patient Outcomes Research Trial (SPORT) was a prospective, multicenter study utilizing both randomized and observational cohorts to evaluate outcomes of surgical and nonsurgical treatments for lumbar stenosis. The randomized cohort was randomly assigned to surgery or nonsurgical treatment. The observational cohort selected their own treatment. Data was collected from 13 participating centers across the United States.

Sample Size The study included a total of 654 patients: 289 in the randomized cohort (138 surgery, 151 nonsurgical) and 365 in the observational cohort (219 surgery, 146 nonsurgical).

Follow-Up Outcomes were assessed at multiple time points, including 6 weeks, 3 months, 6 months, 1 year and 2 years.

Inclusion/Exclusion Criteria

- Inclusion Criteria
  - Adults with imaging-confirmed lumbar spinal stenosis and persistent symptoms (neurogenic claudication or radicular leg pain) for at least 12 weeks despite conservative management and deemed surgical candidates by their treating physician.
- Exclusion Criteria
  - Prior spine surgery
  - Significant scoliosis (>15°)

DOI: 10.1201/9781003416197-49

- Spondylolisthesis >50%
- Cauda equina syndrome
- Malignancy
- Infection
- Contraindications to surgery

Results Utilizing an intent-to-treat analysis, patients in the randomized cohort were first analyzed. At 2 years, 67% of patients assigned to surgery had undergone surgery, while 43% of those assigned to nonsurgical treatment had also undergone surgery. Surgery seemed to significantly improve pain scores on the SF-36 scale by 7.8 points (95% confidence interval [CI], 1.5 to 14.1, $p < 0.05$). There were no significant differences in the physical function of the Oswestry Disability Index (ODI) in the intent-to-treat (ITT) analysis.

When utilizing an as-treated analysis where both cohorts were combined, surgical patients had significantly better outcomes in all measures by 3 months, with sustained improvements at 2 years. SF-36 bodily pain scores improved by 15.3 points (95% CI, 10.4 to 20.2), ODI improved by 13.1 (95% CI, –16.9 to 19.2), and surgical patients were overall more satisfied with their treatment (67% vs 29%).

Conclusion Based on the combined as-treated analysis, the authors conclude that patients who underwent surgery showed significantly more improvement in all primary outcomes than did patients who were treated nonsurgically.

Reviewer Commentary Following their initial study on lumbar disc herniations,[1] the SPORT group turned their attention to lumbar stenosis, where they found differences in both their ITT and the as-treated cohorts. The results favoured surgical intervention with low and comparable complication and mortality rates. This study is important because it is one of the most rigorously conducted trials in spine surgery. It provides strong evidence supporting surgical decompression while also demonstrating that some patients also improved with conservative care.

Study Limitations As with the previous SPORT study, this trial also carried a high crossover rate (43%). While crossover is expected in surgical trials, the extent seen in SPORT introduces a rather strong bias toward the null, which really underestimates the true benefit of surgery. Given this, the fact that the ITT analysis was significant, is perhaps even more telling.

Another limitation was the heterogeneity in the nonsurgical treatment, which was not standardized. Some patients received only NSAIDs, while others underwent intensive physical therapy (PT) and epidural injections. This variability complicates the comparisons. Perhaps a more structured nonoperative protocol might strengthen a path toward the small nonsurgical group that improved without surgery.

Lastly, the generalizability is somewhat limited given the exclusion of instability and deformity. While this ensures homogeneity, patients often present with combinations thereof. Although the SPORT investigators did a separate analysis on spondylolisthesis,[2] future studies could include a broader patient base, including patients who are not mobile.

Relevant Studies It is worth noting that there was a small subset of patients who improved with conservative care. One study[3] randomized patients with surgical lumbar stenosis to PT and surgery. Despite 75% of patients refusing to consent to receiving randomization (possibly receiving PT instead of surgery) and the 57% crossover from PT to surgery, there was a subgroup of 43% of patients (35/82) assigned to PT that had avoided surgery at the 2-year mark.

Similar to our previous analysis on discectomies, this study did not address the role of minimally invasive techniques, some of which have changed since the publication of this paper. Endoscopic techniques, for example, have been shown to have statistically lower visual analog scale, lower back pain scores, fewer postoperative laboratory markers, and less decrease in multifidus muscle cross-sectional areas.[4]

Another consideration, as payer and societal costs become more relevant, is the cost-effectiveness of treatment strategies for lumbar stenosis. In a recent study looking at the cost-effectiveness of PT as compared to a single-level lumbar laminectomy for lumbar stenosis, the authors found that a laminectomy produced higher QALYs (12.11 vs 11.87) at a lower total cost ($15,735 vs $16,877). The authors concluded that virtually all iterations of their probabilistic model showed laminectomy to be the preferred treatment strategy from the outset for symptomatic lumbar stenosis.[5]

Summary In summary, this SPORT trial was a landmark study that established decompressive surgery as providing greater and more durable improvement in pain and function than nonsurgical care for lumbar spinal stenosis. It also demonstrated that selected patients can improve without surgery, underscoring the importance of individualized treatment selection. By highlighting the effects of crossover and patient preference, the study reshaped the interpretation of surgical trials and strengthened evidence-based, shared decision-making in degenerative spine care.

REFERENCES

1. Weinstein JN, Tosteson TD, Lurie JD, et al. Surgical vs nonoperative treatment for lumbar disk herniation. JAMA. 2006;296(20):2441–2450. doi:10.1001/jama.296.20.2441
2. Weinstein JN, Lurie JD, Tosteson TD, et al. Surgical compared with nonoperative treatment for lumbar degenerative spondylolisthesis. Four-year results in the Spine Patient Outcomes Research Trial (SPORT) randomized and observational cohorts. J Bone Joint Surg Am. 2009;91(6):1295–1304. doi:10.2106/JBJS.H.00913
3. Delitto A, Piva SR, Moore CG, et al. Surgery versus nonsurgical treatment for lumbar spinal stenosis: a comparative effectiveness randomized trial with 2-year follow-up. Ann Intern Med. 2015;162(7):465–473. doi:10.7326/M14-1420

4. Hwang YH, Kim JS, Chough CK, et al. Prospective comparative analysis of three types of decompressive surgery for lumbar central stenosis: conventional, full-endoscopic, and biportal endoscopic laminectomy. Sci Rep. 2024;14(1):19853. doi:10.1038/s41598-024-65923-3
5. Rajan PV, Eisenberg J, Selverian S, Wawrose R, Yoon ST. The cost-effectiveness of physical therapy versus laminectomy for lumbar spinal stenosis: a Markov decision analysis. Spine J. 2025;25(8). doi:10.1016/j.spinee.2025.02.008

Chapter 50

The Anterior Approach for the Removal of Ruptured Cervical Discs

Cloward RB, J Neurosurg. 1958 Nov;15(6):602–617

Reviewed by David Stockwell and Abdulbaki Kozan

Historical Background At the time of this publication (1958), cervical intervertebral disc pathology was primarily managed by posterior approach surgeries, which involved significant operative morbidity. With the standard posterior approach in the cervical spine, surgeons had limited safe access to ventral structural pathology. Paracentral ventral pathology required either a transdural approach with retraction on the spinal cord and nerve roots or blindly working extradurally beneath the cord.[1] Both approaches could result in significant morbidity. An anterior approach to decompression of the cervical spine was suggested during the development of discography techniques.[2,3] Modification of the lumbar interbody fusion technique for an anterior approach to cervical spine pathology offered a less invasive intervention.[4]

Research Question/Objective Technical description of an anterior surgical approach for cervical disc pathology and review of the results of this surgical intervention on patients.

Study Design A retrospective review of patients who underwent an anterior cervical approach for the removal of ruptured cervical intervertebral discs, followed by fusion.

Sample Size The study included 47 patients aged 33 to 74, with a mean age of 46.3. Of these, 29 were male and 18 were female.

Inclusion/Exclusion Criteria

- Inclusion Criteria
  - There were no specific inclusion criteria for this study
  - All patients had tried conservative treatments for neck and upper extremity pain without significant relief.
  - Patients were divided into two groups based on their symptoms: (a) patients who had only neck, shoulder, and arm pain; and (b) those who also had radiating hand and finger pain.

DOI: 10.1201/9781003416197-50

Intervention or Treatment The original technique involved general anesthesia but evolved to use only a local anesthetic in combination with anxiolytics and analgesics. The patient was positioned supine with head turned to the left and neck extended over a sandbag under the neck. Before making a skin incision, the pathologic level would be localized by lateral roentgenography and discography. The latter was added due to a wrong-level surgery. To complete the discography, digital pressure was applied to the right side of the neck to identify the anterior spine in the space between the carotid sheath and trachea. A 20-gauge needle was placed through the skin into an intervertebral disc and a lateral roentgenogram was obtained. Once confirmed to be the correct level, methylene blue was injected into the disc.

A transverse skin incision was then made from the midline to the medial border of the sternocleidomastoid. Platysma was divided longitudinally for superior cosmesis and the plane between the carotid sheath and the esophagus and trachea was developed to the prevertebral space. The pathologic disc, with methylene blue, was identified and the longus colli was dissected back and the retractor blades were engaged into the longus. The adjustable depth drill was then engaged about the pathologic disc level, with positioning determined by where the pathology was suspected: midline for the midline lesions and eccentric to the side for lateral lesions (see Figure 50.1). The drill was advanced until the smooth cortical bone that forms the ventral aspect of the spinal canal was encountered, advancing a millimeter at a time to decrease the chance of going too deep and injuring the spinal cord. Between drill attempts, the interspace was clear of tissue with small, sharp curettes. Bone dust was pushed into the sidewalls to minimize bleeding without affecting fusion. Ruptured disc fragments and posterior osteophytes were then removed with small, sharp mastoid curettes. Gel foam and thrombin were used for hemostasis from small areas of bleeding, and electrocautery was reserved for larger vessels and used at a low setting. The posterior longitudinal ligament was left intact, and the dura and nerve roots were not visualized unless there was a traumatic rent from a disc herniation.

For fusion, A bone dowel 1 mm larger than the drill hole and slightly shorter than the hole depth was then tapped into place. One patient had autologous bone from the anterior superior iliac spine; the remainder utilized fresh frozen ilium dowels from cadavers that were harvested and stored in sterile conditions. A small rubber drain was left in the operative field and the incision was closed in layers. Patients were initially braced in a cervical orthosis but this was discontinued early in the series. Patients were generally discharged home 3 to 4 days postoperatively. Patients were followed for 6 to 18 months.

Results Over a year, 47 patients (29 males and 18 females) underwent surgical treatment using this technique. The mean age was 46.3 years. All patients experienced preoperative neck and shoulder pain, and 27 of them also presented with radiculopathy. Morbidity was minimal. The primary symptom reported was difficulty swallowing, attributed to esophageal retraction and edema, which typically resolved within 2 days after the surgery. One patient had an epidural hemorrhage

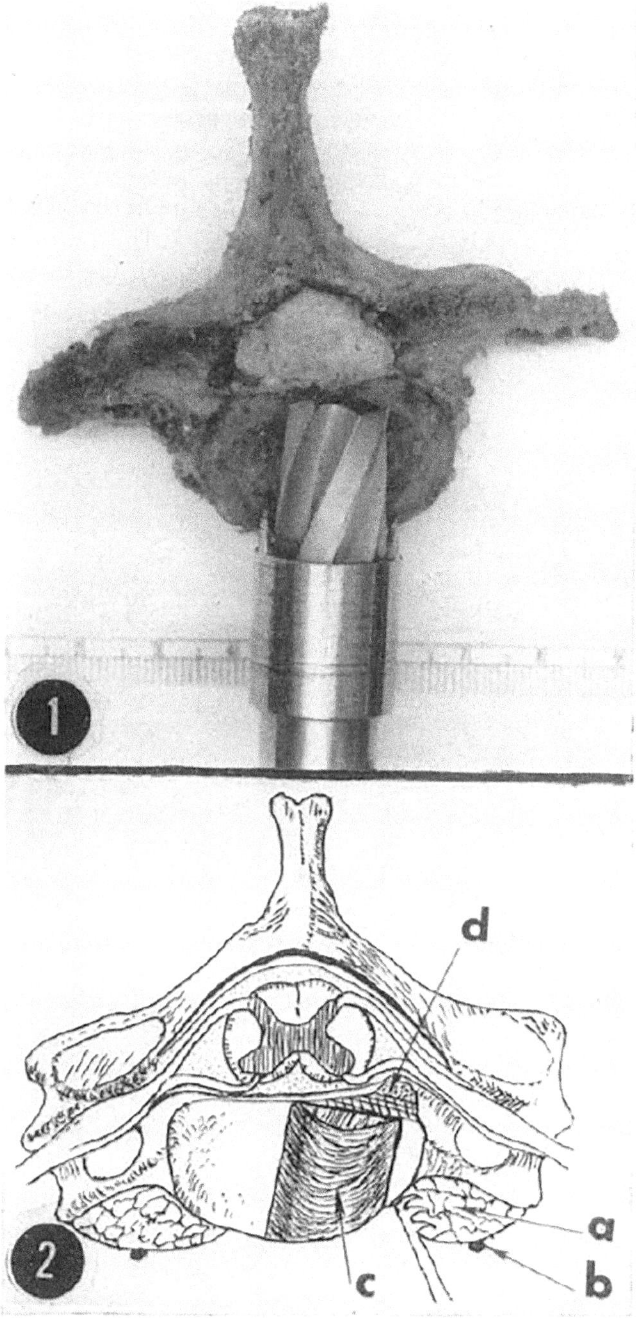

Figure 50.1 (1) Photograph of the sixth cervical vertebra with drill and guard superimposed on vertebral body. Note the width of the drill hole compared to the spinal canal (actual size). (2) Drawing to show: (a) longus coil muscle retracted from the vertical body, (b) sympathetic chain, (c) drill hole directed diagonally toward (d) unilateral disc protrusion or osteophyte.

and spinal cord injury. The patient woke with severe neurological deficits, which gradually improved with minimal residual right-hand paresis and right leg spasticity.

Significant reduction in pain was achieved with 42 patients reporting complete relief and 5 experiencing some degree of improvement. Eight patients required reoperation due to persistent or escalating pain, 2 undergoing surgeries for an additional disc pathology, 4 having their bone grafts replaced for proper fitting, and 2 underwent wound hematoma evacuation. One wrong-level surgery occurred before the methylene blue discogram to mark the operative level. Remarkably, the patients did not experience any wound infections. Fusion was successful in 43 patients within 3 to 4 months based on roentgenograms. Bone graft resorption was seen in 3 patients, one of whom remained asymptomatic, while the others experienced manageable neck and shoulder discomfort.

Conclusion This article documented technical details for the operative technique for anterior cervical discectomy and fusion, which provided a safe and reliable method to address symptomatic cervical spondylosis.

Reviewer Commentary This paper was published in 1958, the same year that Smith and Robinson published their first case series on their anterior approach to the cervical spine. Cloward's publication shared a slightly different technique to anterior decompression and fusion with a high fusion rate, reliable symptom improvement, and minimal morbidity. The technique from localization to exposure and surgical decompression was efficient and effective.

Study Limitations This study is limited by its retrospective design, small sample size, and short follow-up period. Typically, 90–95% of cervical fusion takes place within 1 to 2 years after an anterior cervical discectomy and fusion (ACDF) procedure.[5] An extended follow-up period would provide more support to the fusion evaluation. Pain assessment is subjective. Objective function and quality of life evaluations would have been ideal but not expected at that time.

Relevant Studies Robinson and Smith initially wrote the article on anterolateral cervical disc removal and interbody fusion for cervical disc syndrome in 1955.[6] Before that, they performed this method on 8 dogs in 1954. They subsequently published their seminal paper in 1958, the same year as this article was printed. Their paper included a smaller retrospective review of 14 patients who underwent ACDF.[3] They discussed comparable surgical methods, preoperative disc-level localization, and postoperative protocols. The patients were relatively young, ranging from 25 to 50 years old. The average follow-up was 2 years (15 to 36 months). No related wound infections were reported. Radiological fusion was characterized as a bony bridge between the vertebral bodies with a lack of motion on dynamic images. Eighteen-disc levels were evaluated as radiologically fused, three levels of fibrous non-union, and a pseudoarthrosis was assessed in one level. They used a "horseshoe-shaped graft" as a surgical technique, which involved harvesting the patient's own iliac crest and tapping it into the disc space following a discectomy. Bailey and Bagley described anterior cervical fusion as a "trough onlay fusion technique" without decompression for traumatic and postsurgical instabilities in 1960.[7] In 1962, Robinson published an expanded article on ACDFs with the outcomes of 56 patients with multiple degenerative levels.[8] Thanks to the pioneering work of Cloward, Smith, and Robinson, the ACDF is one of the most commonly used spinal procedures for treating cervical disc herniations today, with a high success rate of over 85–90%.[9] Interestingly, the reliability we see with ACDF procedures today, with high rates of fusion and symptom relief, is similar to what Cloward demonstrated almost 70 years ago.

Conclusion Anterior cervical discectomy and fusion (ACDF) surgery has been utilized since the 1950s with similar techniques as described here. The results were highly reliable from the start, and Cloward's technique was an eloquent approach to anterior cervical spine surgery. The impact of this work was profound and enduring. It helped to shift the surgical paradigm from indirect posterior decompression to targeted anterior pathology-based surgery, laid the technical foundation for ACDF, and influenced generations of spinal surgeons across neurosurgery and orthopedics. Nearly seven decades later, the core concepts Cloward introduced of direct anterior decompression, disc excision, and fusion are central to modern cervical spine surgery.

REFERENCES

1. Mayfield FH. Cervical spine trauma: neurosurgical aspects. Clin Neurosurg. 1954;2:83–100.
2. Cloward RB. Cervical diskography; technique, indications and use in diagnosis of ruptured cervical disks. Am J Roentgenol Radium Ther Nucl Med. 1958;79:563–574.
3. Smith GW, Robinson RA. The treatment of certain cervical-spine disorders by anterior removal of the intervertebral disc and interbody fusion. J Bone Joint Surg Am. 1958;40-A:607–624.
4. Cloward RB. The treatment of ruptured lumbar intervertebral discs; criteria for spinal fusion. Am J Surg. 1953;86:145–151. doi:10.1016/0002-9610(53)90421-8
5. Oshina M, Oshima Y, Tanaka S, Riew KD. Radiological fusion criteria of postoperative anterior cervical discectomy and fusion: a systematic review. Global Spine J. 2018;8: 739–750. doi:10.1177/2192568218755141
6. Ra R. Anterolateral cervical disc removal and interbody fusion for cervical disc syndrome. Bull Johns Hopkins Hosp. 1955;96:223–224.
7. Bailey RW, Badgley, CE. Stabilization of the cervical spine by anterior fusion. J Bone Joint Surg Am. 1960;42-a:565–594.
8. Robinson, RA, Walker AE, Ferlic DC, Wiecking DK. The results of anterior interbody fusion of the cervical spine. JBJS. 1962;44:1569–1587.
9. Buttermann, GR. anterior cervical discectomy and fusion outcomes over 10 years: a prospective study. Spine (Phila Pa 1976). 2018;43:207–214. doi:10.1097/ BRS.0000000000002273

Index

Note: Page numbers followed by "f" and "t" refer to figures and tables, respectively.